Pathogenesis and Therapy of Oral Carcinogenesis

Pathogenesis and Therapy of Oral Carcinogenesis

Editors

Marko Tarle
Ivica Lukšić

MDPI • Basel • Beijing • Wuhan • Barcelona • Belgrade • Manchester • Tokyo • Cluj • Tianjin

Editors

Marko Tarle
Department of Maxillofacial Surgery
Dubrava University Hospital
Zagreb
Croatia

Ivica Lukšić
Department of Maxillofacial Surgery
Dubrava University Hospital
Zagreb
Croatia

Editorial Office

MDPI
St. Alban-Anlage 66
4052 Basel, Switzerland

This is a reprint of articles from the Special Issue published online in the open access journal *International Journal of Molecular Sciences* (ISSN 1422-0067) (available at: www.mdpi.com/journal/ijms/special_issues/5197914FC2).

For citation purposes, cite each article independently as indicated on the article page online and as indicated below:

LastName, A.A.; LastName, B.B.; LastName, C.C. Article Title. *Journal Name* **Year**, *Volume Number*, Page Range.

ISBN 978-3-0365-8431-7 (Hbk)
ISBN 978-3-0365-8430-0 (PDF)

Contents

About the Editors

Marko Tarle

Dr. Marko Tarle is an assistant at the Department of Maxillofacial Surgery at the School of Dental Medicine, University of Zagreb, and works as a maxillofacial surgeon at Dubrava University Hospital in Zagreb, Croatia. He graduated summa cum laude from the School of Medicine in Zagreb in 2015 and was awarded two Dean's Awards: for the best student and for his contribution to the reputation of the Faculty. In October 2022, he received the title of University Master of Maxillofacial Surgery after completing his postgraduate specialist studies. In 2023, he defended his doctoral thesis at the School of Medicine, University of Zagreb. Since 2023, he has been participating in the Postgraduate Program in Head and Neck Surgery: Oncology 2023 of the European Association of Cranio-Maxillofacial Surgery (EACMFS). He won the "Primarijus Mikolji" award for the best resident in 2019 and was awarded for the best presentation at the 8th International Congress of the Croatian Society of Dental Implantology and the 14th Congress of the European Scull Base Society. He is a collaborator on the project "Toll-like receptor 3 in the development and treatment of human head and neck cancer: the role of endogenous ligands" of the Croatian Science Foundation. He has a special interest in head and neck oncology. He is the author and co-author of more than 30 scientific papers published in prestigious international journals.

Ivica Lukšić

Prof. Lukšić graduated from the School of Medicine, University of Zagreb, in 1995 and has since worked at the Department of Maxillofacial Surgery of Dubrava University Hospital. His narrow area of work has been head and neck cancer surgery. He is the Head of the Reference Center of the Ministry of Health for Surgery of Tumors of the Face, Jaws, and Mouth and Head of the Postgraduate Specialist Study of Maxillofacial Surgery at the School of Medicine, University of Zagreb. He is the author of several teaching texts, books, and monographs and the mentor of several graduate and doctoral theses. Furthermore, he is a member of the Board of Directors of the Croatian Society for Maxillofacial, Plastic, and Reconstructive Surgery of the Head and Neck, Secretary of the Croatian Society of Head and Neck Tumors, a full member of international professional societies in the field of head and neck surgery, and a reviewer of several international scientific journals.

Preface to "Pathogenesis and Therapy of Oral Carcinogenesis"

We are proud to present our reprint on oral squamous cell carcinoma (OSCC) research. This compilation contains important findings from various studies covering different aspects of OSCC.

Despite advances in diagnosis and treatment, OSCC remains a challenge for scientists and clinicians worldwide. According to recent epidemiological data, the incidence of OSCC continues to rise, with a significant increase in younger patients. Therefore, it is critical to explore new approaches to the prevention, diagnosis, and treatment of this disease.

The articles in this reprint address novel biomarkers and therapeutic targets for the prevention and treatment of OSCC. Research focuses on the combined use of signaling pathway inhibitors in cancer control and the role of specific genes and microRNAs in disease development. These studies shed light on the complex molecular pathways involved in OSCC development and provide insights into potential diagnostic biomarkers and therapeutic interventions.

In addition, epidemiological factors that influence the development of OSCC, such as smoking and HPV infection, have been investigated. These factors were found to be associated with oxidative stress and DNA damage in oral cells. The interaction between tobacco smoking and high-risk HPV infection was investigated, showing effects on superoxide dismutase 2 (SOD2) levels and DNA damage.

In addition, the importance of cholesterol in the progression of OSCC and the role of mast cells in tumor proliferation and invasion were highlighted. The results demonstrate the influence of cholesterol on cell polarity, migration, and caveolin-1 (CAV1) expression in OSCC cells. The potential for interactions between mast cells and oral cavity cancer cells and the identification of soluble factors that mediate these interactions were explored.

This reprint provides valuable insights into recent research and encourages further innovation in the field of OSCC. The researchers' comprehensive approach contributes to our understanding of the complex molecular mechanisms underlying the development and progression of OSCC.

We hope that these publications will provide you with useful information, stimulate further discussion, and point to new avenues of research. We thank the authors for their significant contributions to OSCC research.

Marko Tarle and Ivica Lukšić
Editors

International Journal of *Molecular Sciences*

MDPI

Article

Nuclear Epidermal Growth Factor Receptor Overexpression as a Survival Predictor in Oral Squamous Cell Carcinoma

Marko Tarle [1,2], Marina Raguž [3,4], Danko Muller [5,6] and Ivica Lukšić [1,6,*]

1 Department of Maxillofacial Surgery, Dubrava University Hospital, 10000 Zagreb, Croatia; tarlemarko1@gmail.com
2 School of Dental Medicine, University of Zagreb, Gundulićeva 5, 10000 Zagreb, Croatia
3 Department of Neurosurgery, Dubrava University Hospital, 10000 Zagreb, Croatia
4 School of Medicine, Catholic University of Croatia, 10000 Zagreb, Croatia
5 Department of Pathology and Cytology, Dubrava University Hospital, 10000 Zagreb, Croatia
6 School of Medicine, University of Zagreb, 10000 Zagreb, Croatia
* Correspondence: luksic@kbd.hr

Abstract: The aim of this study was to determine, by immunohistochemical methods, the expression of nEGFR and markers of cell proliferation (Ki-67), cell cycle (mEGFR, p53, cyclin D1), and tumor stem cells (ABCG2) in 59 pathohistological samples of healthy oral mucosa, 50 oral premalignant changes (leukoplakia and erythroplakia), and 52 oral squamous cell carcinomas (OSCC). An increase in the expression of mEGFR and nEGFR was found with the development of the disease ($p < 0.0001$). In the group of patients with leukoplakia and erythroplakia, we found a positive correlation between nEGFR and Ki67, p53, cyclin D1, and mEGFR, whereas in the group of patients with OSCC, we found a positive correlation between nEGFR and Ki67, mEGFR ($p < 0.05$). Tumors without perineural (PNI) invasion had a higher expression of p53 protein than tumors with PNI ($p = 0.02$). Patients with OSCC and overexpression of nEGFR had shorter overall survival ($p = 0.004$). The results of this study suggest a potentially important independent role of nEGFR in oral carcinogenesis.

Keywords: squamous cell carcinoma; oral cavity; biomarkers; nEGFR; immunocytochemistry

Citation: Tarle, M.; Raguž, M.; Muller, D.; Lukšić, I. Nuclear Epidermal Growth Factor Receptor Overexpression as a Survival Predictor in Oral Squamous Cell Carcinoma. *Int. J. Mol. Sci.* **2023**, *24*, 5816. https://doi.org/10.3390/ijms24065816

Academic Editor: Cheng-Chia Yu

Received: 26 February 2023
Revised: 14 March 2023
Accepted: 17 March 2023
Published: 18 March 2023

1. Introduction

Oral Squamous Cell Carcinoma (OSCC) is the most common malignant tumor of the head and neck. In Europe and the United States, it accounts for 2–3% of all malignancies [1]. In 2020, 377,713 people were diagnosed with lip cancer and OSCC worldwide, while 177,757 patients died, with a trend toward increasing numbers of patients under 50 years of age [2,3]. The large expansion of OSCC research and advances in diagnostic and therapeutic methods over the past 30 years have not resulted in a significant increase in the 5-year survival rate of patients, which is still about 55% [4]. Moreover, more than 40% of patients already have regional metastases at the time of disease diagnosis, and more than 60% of patients have tumors larger than 4 cm, indicating ineffective prevention of the disease. New strategies are needed to change the current uniform approach in treating all patients with the same clinical and pathohistologic features [5]. Treatment of patients should be based on proven biomarkers that provide the basis for individual differences in the genetic and biological behavior of tumors. Accumulation of mutations, chromosomal damage, and loss of cell control function result in histologic changes of normal oral epithelium into dysplasia, carcinoma in situ, and invasive OSCC [6]. Although the role of mEGFR in HNSCC is well established and numerous anti-EGFR drugs have been developed and are routinely used, poor response to therapy and resistance to therapy are frequently recorded, possibly due to the existence of nonclassical subcellular signaling of the Epidermal growth factor receptor (EGFR) pathway. Recent studies suggest that EGF, H2O2, UV radiation, therapeutic agents, and ionizing radiation may cause translocation of EGFR to the nucleus, where nuclear EGFR (nEGFR) interacts with various transcription factors (cyclin D1, ABCG2/BCRP, Aurora kinase A, COX-2, gene regulator c-Myc, iNOS) and acts on the activation of numerous genes involved in cell proliferation, tumor progression, and DNA repair [7–10]. Available literature indicates that overexpression of nEGFR in ovarian, breast, oropharyngeal, laryngeal, and esophageal cancers negatively affects disease prognosis and resistance to radiotherapy and chemotherapy, whereas its role in oral malignancies has not yet been investigated [8,11–16]. The above only confirms the complexity and scope of the network of signaling pathways mediated by EGFR activation that play an important role in cancer progression. The aim of this study is to use immunohistochemical methods to determine the expression of nEGFR in healthy oral mucosa, premalignant changes of the oral cavity (leukoplakia and erythroplakia), and OSCC, and to determine its influence on disease progression and clinical outcome in patients with OSCC. In addition, we analyzed the expression of markers of cell proliferation (Ki-67), cell cycle (mEGFR, p53, cyclin D1), and tumor stem cells (ABCG2) in the subjects' samples, plus their correlation with nEGFR expression.

2. Results

We analyzed the expression of nEGFR and other observed biomarkers (Ki-67, p53, cyclin D1, mEGFR, ABCG2) by immunohistochemical methods in 161 subjects divided into three groups: 59 subjects with healthy oral mucosa, 50 patients with premalignant changes (31 leukoplakias and 19 erythroplakias), and 52 patients with OSCC in all TNM stages. The demographic data of the groups of subjects are shown in Table 1.

Table 1. Demographic data of subjects included in the study.

Group of Subjects	Age (Years)	Gender	Number of Subjects
Control group with healthy oral mucosa	56.56 ± 11.97 54.28 ± 12.22 52.7 ± 11.84	♂32 ♀27	59
Patients with premalignant changes	64.22 ± 14.35 64.6 ± 9.92 63.9 ± 17.46	♂23 ♀27	50
Patients with Oral squamous cell carcinoma	55 ± 10.91 56 ± 10.87 54 ± 11.22	♂35 ♀17	52

2.1. *Results of Immunohistochemical Staining*

2.1.1. Expression of Ki-67 in Healthy Oral Mucosa, Premalignant Changes, and Invasive Oral Squamous Cell Carcinoma

The percentage of the Ki-67 proliferation index in the studied groups ranged from 0% to 81% with a mean expression value of 15.51 ± 14.87%. As expected, the percentage of Ki-67 proliferation index expression in the group of patients with OSCC is significantly higher (mean value 25.46 ± 19.22%) than in the group with healthy oral mucosa (mean value 8.93 ± 6.68%) and in the group of patients with premalignant changes (13 ± 10.99%). A statistically significant difference in the expression of the Ki-67 proliferation index was found between subjects with healthy oral mucosa and premalignant changes on the one hand and patients with OSCC on the other (p = 0.000001) (Figures 1 and 2).

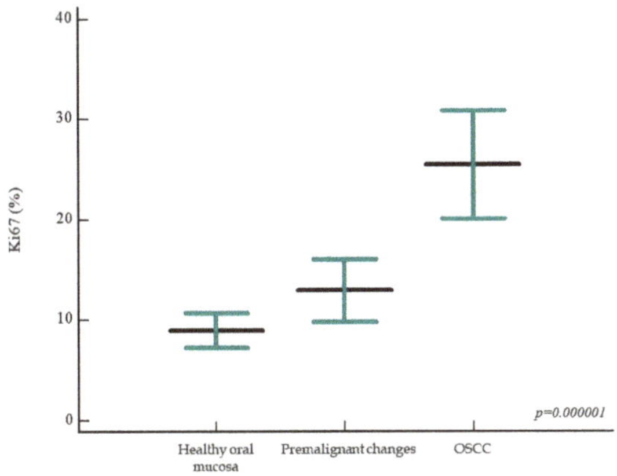

Figure 1. Percentage of Ki-67 proliferation index between analyzed patient groups. The percentage of Ki-67 proliferation index is significantly higher in the group of patients with OSCC than in individuals with healthy oral mucosa and premalignant changes ($p = 0.000001$); no statistically significant difference was found between the latter two groups. Horizontal lines indicate mean ± standard deviation; p, significance level in graph ANOVA.

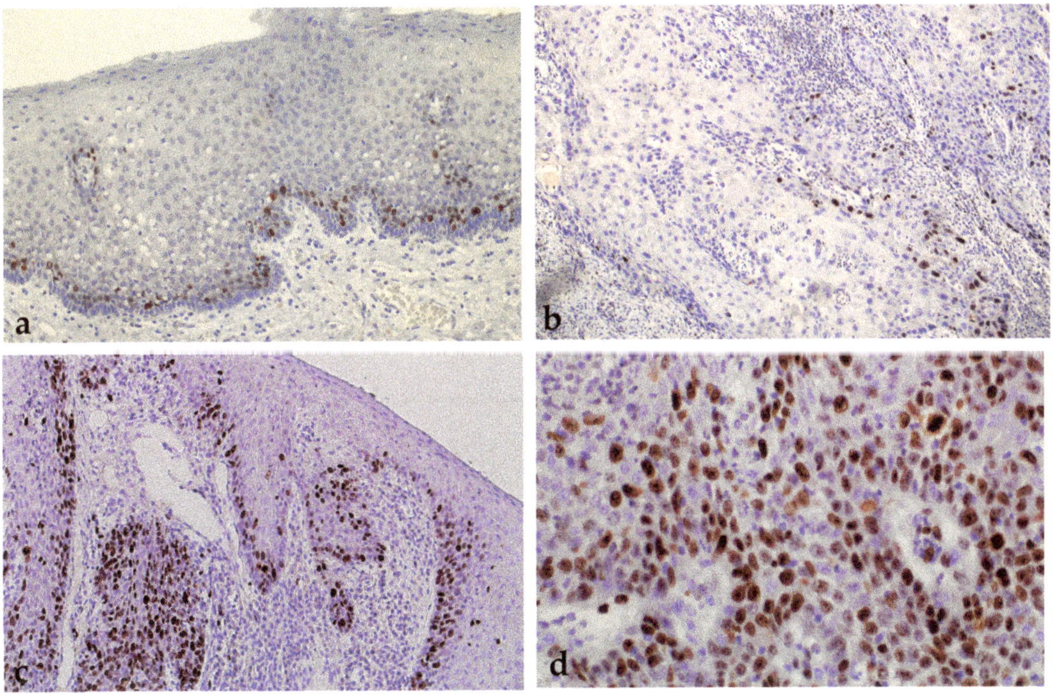

Figure 2. Oral erythroplakia with weak expression of Ki-67. Magnification 200× (**a**). OSCC showing a very low proliferation index. Magnification 100× (**b**). Immunohistochemical expression of Ki-67 in oral leukoplakia with moderate proliferation activity. Magnification 100× (**c**). OSCC with high proliferation activity with expression of Ki-67 in more than 30% of nuclei. Magnification 400× (**d**).

In the group of patients with premalignant changes, when comparing the percentage of Ki-67 proliferation index in relation to the presence of oral epithelial dysplasias, a statistically significant higher percentage of Ki-67 proliferation index was observed in the subgroup of high-grade dysplasias (median 18.87% with a range of 6% to 30.5%) compared with low-grade dysplasias (median 10.34% with a range of 1 to 20.6%) ($p = 0.005$).

2.1.2. Expression of p53 in Healthy Oral Mucosa, Premalignant Changes, and Invasive Oral Squamous Cell Carcinoma

When analyzing the expression of p53 protein, we found a statistically significant higher expression of the tested protein in the group of patients with premalignant changes and OSCC compared with the control group; also, a statistically significant difference was found between all analyzed groups ($p < 0.000001$) (Figures 3 and 4). When comparing the percentage of p53 protein expression in the dysplasia group by subgroup, no statistically significant difference was found ($p = 0.11$).

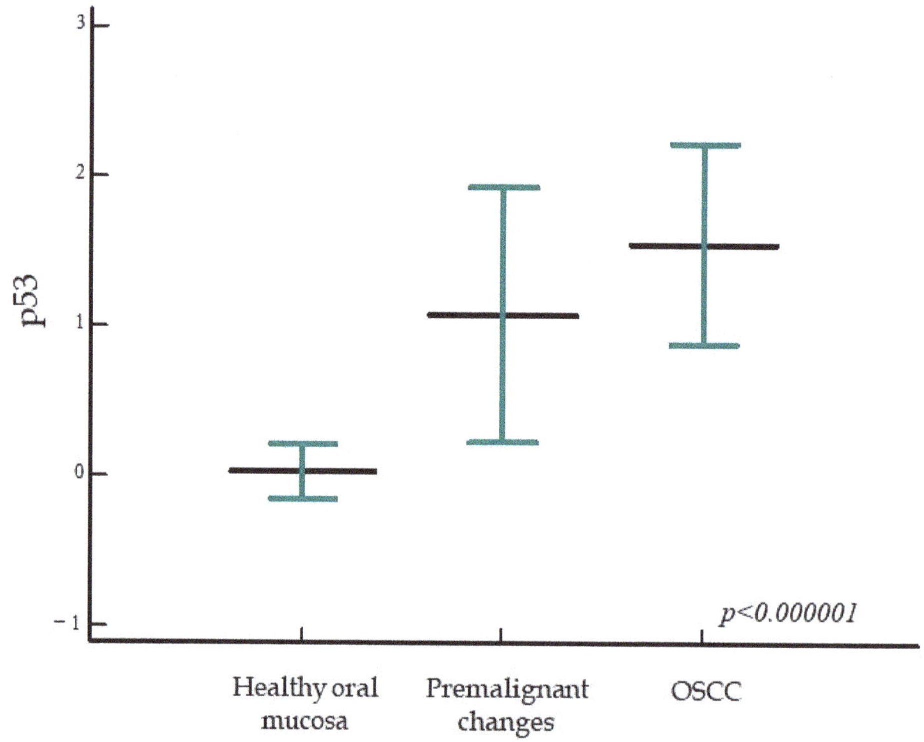

Figure 3. Expression of p53 protein in the studied groups. The percentage of p53 protein expression is significantly higher in the group of patients with premalignant changes and OSCC compared with subjects with healthy oral mucosa; moreover, a statistically significant difference was found between all studied groups ($p < 0.000001$). Horizontal lines indicate mean ± standard deviation; p, significance level is marked in Kruskal–Wallis graph.

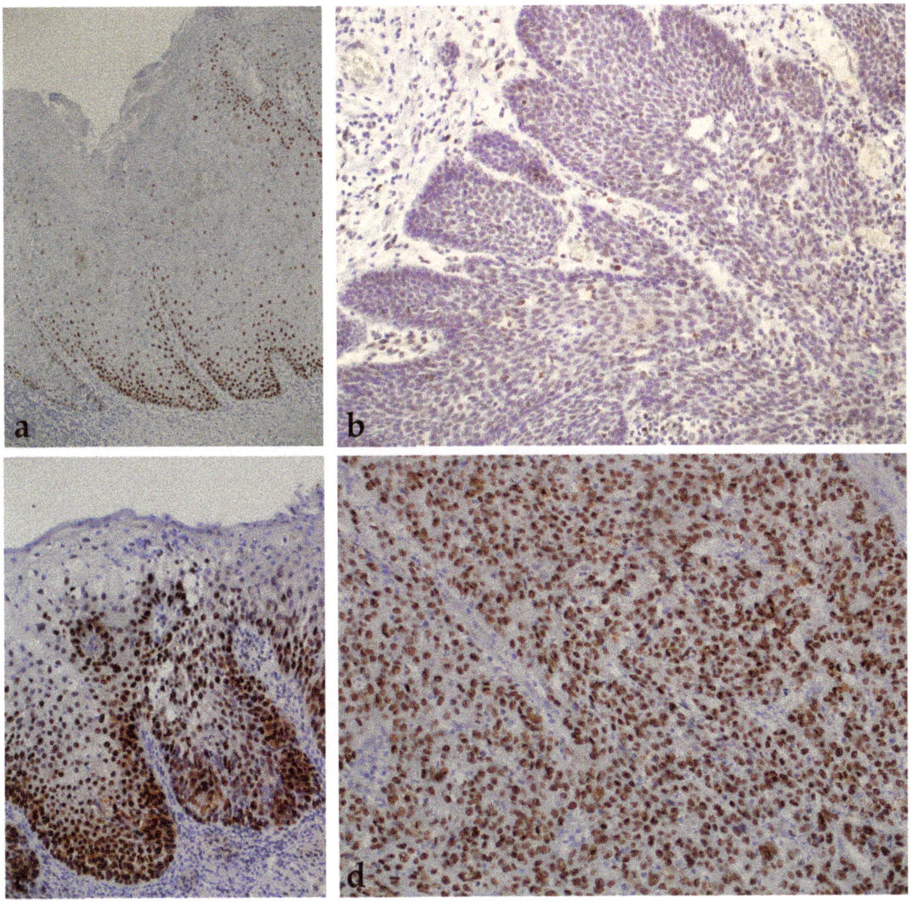

Figure 4. Moderate expression of p53 protein in oral leukoplakia according to the Allred scoring system (+). Magnification 100× (**a**). OSCC showing moderate p53 protein immunoreactivity according to the Allred scoring system (+). Magnification 200× (**b**). Oral erythroplakia with severe dysplasia and strong p53 protein expression in the dysplastic part of the affected epithelium according to the Allred scoring system (++). Magnification 200× (**c**). Strong immunohistochemical expression of p53 in OSCC according to the Allred scoring system (++). Magnification 200× (**d**).

2.1.3. Expression of Cyclin D1 in Healthy Oral Mucosa, Premalignant Changes, and Invasive Oral Squamous Cell Carcinoma

Analyzing the expression of cyclin D1, we found a statistically significant higher expression of the tested protein in the group of patients with premalignant changes and invasive OSCC compared to subjects with healthy oral mucosa; moreover, a statistically significant difference was found between all analyzed groups ($p < 0.000001$) (Figures 5 and 6). When comparing the percentage of cyclin D1 expression in the dysplasia group by subgroups, no statistically significant difference was found ($p = 0.18$).

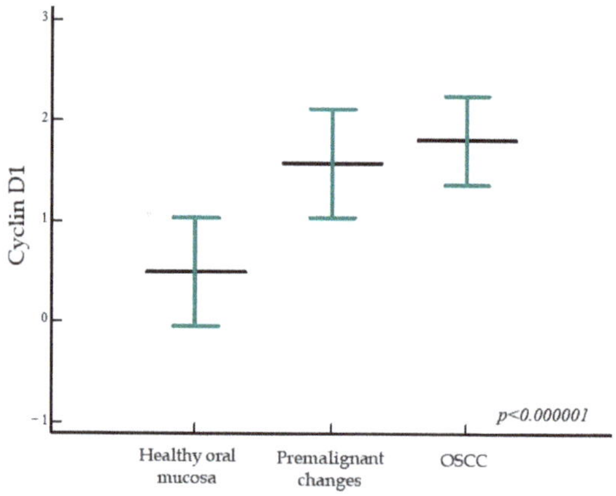

Figure 5. Cyclin D1 protein expression in the studied groups. The percentage of cyclin D1 protein expression is significantly higher in the group of patients with premalignant changes and OSCC compared with subjects with healthy oral mucosa; moreover, a statistically significant difference was found between all studied groups ($p < 0.000001$). Horizontal lines show mean ± standard deviation; p, significance level is marked on Kruskal–Wallis graph.

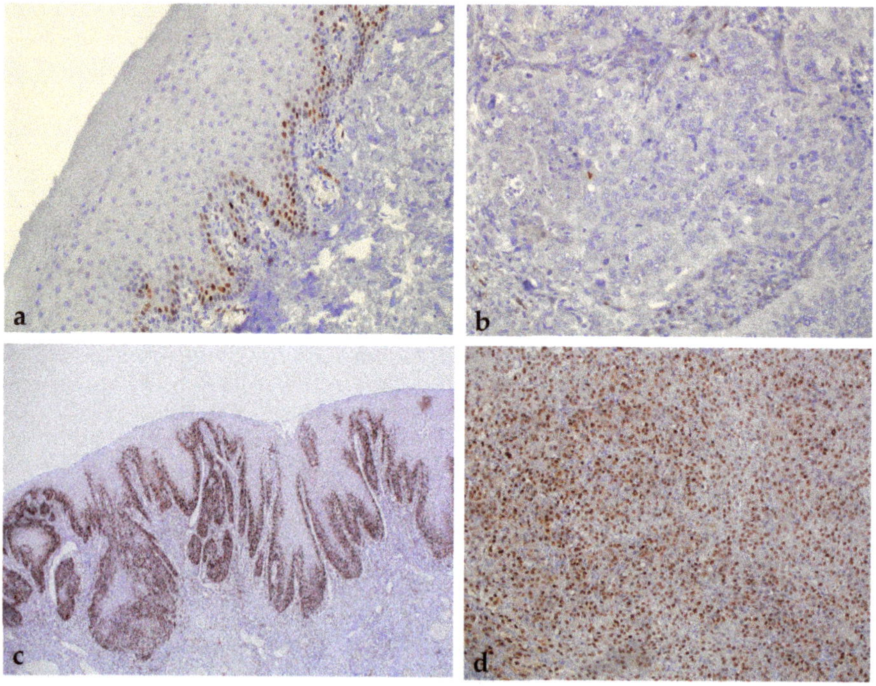

Figure 6. Oral leukoplakia with weak cyclin D1 protein expression according to the Allred scoring system (0). Magnification (**a**). OSCC without immunohistochemical expression of cyclin D1 according to the Allred scoring system (0). Magnification 200× (**b**). Strong immunohistochemical expression of cyclin D1 in oral leukoplakia with moderate dysplasia according to the Allred scoring system (++). Magnification 100× (**c**). OSCC with strong expression of cyclin D1 according to the Allred scoring system (++). Magnification 100× (**d**).

2.1.4. ABCG2 Expression in Healthy Oral Mucosa, Premalignant Changes, and Invasive Oral Squamous Cell Carcinoma

Analyzing the expression of ABCG2, we found a statistically significant higher expression of the tested protein in the group of patients with premalignant changes and OSCC compared to subjects with healthy oral mucosa; moreover, a statistically significant difference was found between all analyzed groups ($p < 0.000001$) (Figures 7 and 8). When comparing the percentage of ABCG2 expression in the group of dysplasias by subgroups, a statistically significant difference was found, i.e., ABCG2 expression is stronger in higher grade dysplasias ($p = 0.02$).

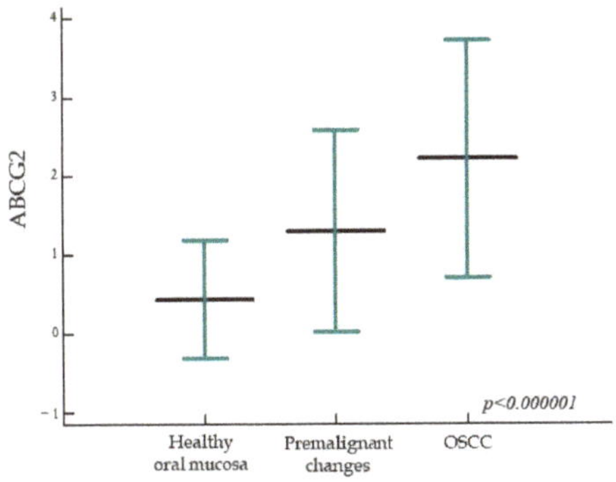

Figure 7. ABCG2 protein expression in the studied groups. The percentage of ABCG2 expression is significantly higher in the group of patients with premalignant changes and OSCC compared to subjects with healthy oral mucosa; moreover, a statistically significant difference was found between all studied groups ($p < 0.000001$). Horizontal lines indicate mean ± standard deviation; *p*, significance level is marked on Kruskal-Wallis graph.

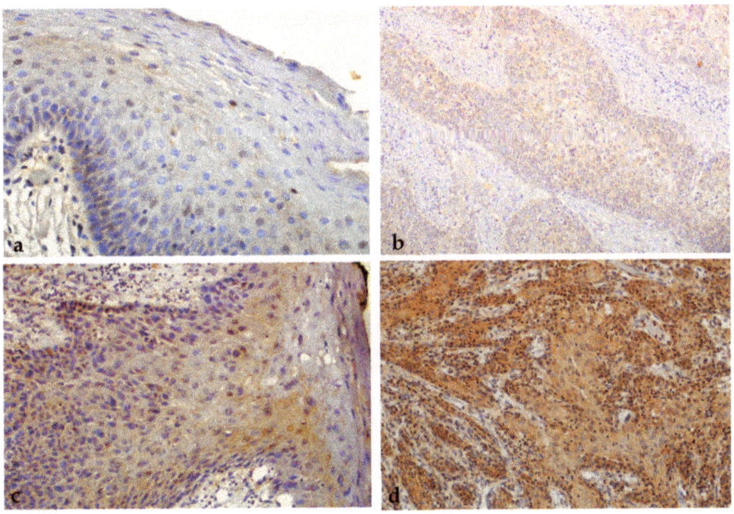

Figure 8. Moderate immunohistochemical expression of ABCG2 (++) in untransformed oral leukoplakia. Magnification 400× (**a**). Moderate immunohistochemical expression of ABCG2 (++) in OSCC. Magnification 200× (**b**). Strong immunohistochemical expression of ABCG2 (+++) in malignant transformed oral erythroplakia with severe epithelial dysplasia. Magnification 200× (**c**). Strong immunohistochemical expression of ABCG2 (+++) in OSCC. Magnification 200× (**d**).

2.1.5. Expression of nEGFR and mEGFR in Healthy Oral Mucosa, Premalignant Changes, and Invasive Oral Squamous Cell Carcinoma

In the control group, most samples (53/59) showed negative nEGFR expression (0), only 6 samples showed weaker expression of nEGFR (+), and moderate or strong expression (++/+++) was not found in any sample. Expression of mEGFR in the same group showed negative expression (0) in the largest number of samples (37/59), whereas weak expression of mEGFR (+) was present in 15 samples. Moderate expression of mEGFR (++) was detected in a smaller number of samples (7/59), while strong expression of mEGFR (+++) was not found in any sample (Figures 9–11).

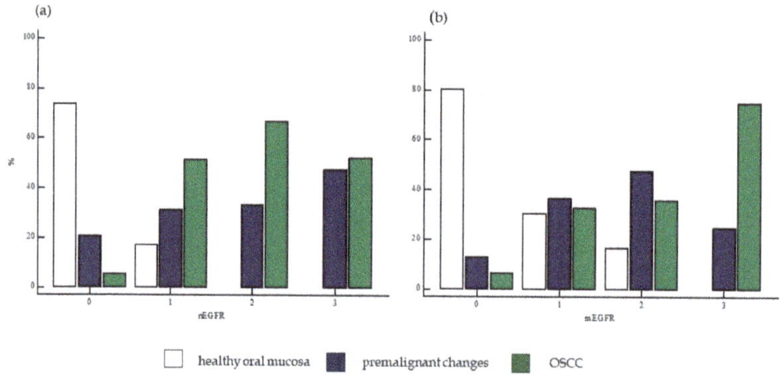

Figure 9. Expression of nEGFR and mEGFR between the studied groups of subjects. Comparisons of the expression of (**a**) nEGFR and (**b**) mEGFR between the groups of subjects analyzed showed statistical significance ($\chi^2 = 85.96$, $p < 0.0001$; $\chi^2 = 70.40$, $p < 0.0001$). Legend: nEGFR—nuclear EGFR; mEGFR—membrane EGFR; 0—negative, 1—weak expression, 2—moderate expression, 3—strong expression.

In the group of subjects with premalignant changes, a smaller number of samples (6/50) showed negative nEGFR (0), whereas the majority of subjects showed weak expression of nEGFR (+) (18/50) or moderate expression (++) (20/50). A smaller number of samples (6/50) showed strong expression of nEGFR (+++). Analysis of mEGFR revealed negative expression (0) in the majority of subjects (15/50), weak expression (+) in some subjects (11/50), and moderate expression (++) in a small number of subjects (4/50). Strong expression (+++) of mEGFR was detected in most samples (20/50) (Figures 9–11).

The strongest expression of both nEGFR and mEGFR was observed in the group of subjects with OSCC; nEGFR was moderately to strongly expressed in 30/50 samples (++/+++), and 22 samples had negative or weak expression (0/+). In 33/52 samples, mEGFR was moderately to strongly expressed (++/+++), and in 19 samples, expression was weak or negative (0/+) (Figures 9–11).

Comparisons of nEGFR and mEGFR expression between the groups of subjects analyzed showed statistical significance ($\chi^2 = 85.96$, $p < 0.0001$; $\chi^2 = 70.40$, $p < 0.0001$).

When the frequency of nEGFR expression was compared between the studied groups, a statistically significant difference was found in the expression of nEGFR in the different groups. The frequency of moderate (++) and strong nEGFR expression (+++) was significantly higher in the group of patients with OSCC and premalignant changes than in the group of healthy subjects ($\chi^2 = 49.85$, $p < 0.0001$). A difference in the expression of mEGFR was also observed in the different patient groups, with a significantly higher frequency of moderate (++) and strong expression of mEGFR (+++) in the group of patients with OSCC and premalignant changes compared with the group of healthy controls. ($\chi^2 = 34.05$, $p < 0.0001$) (Figure 12).

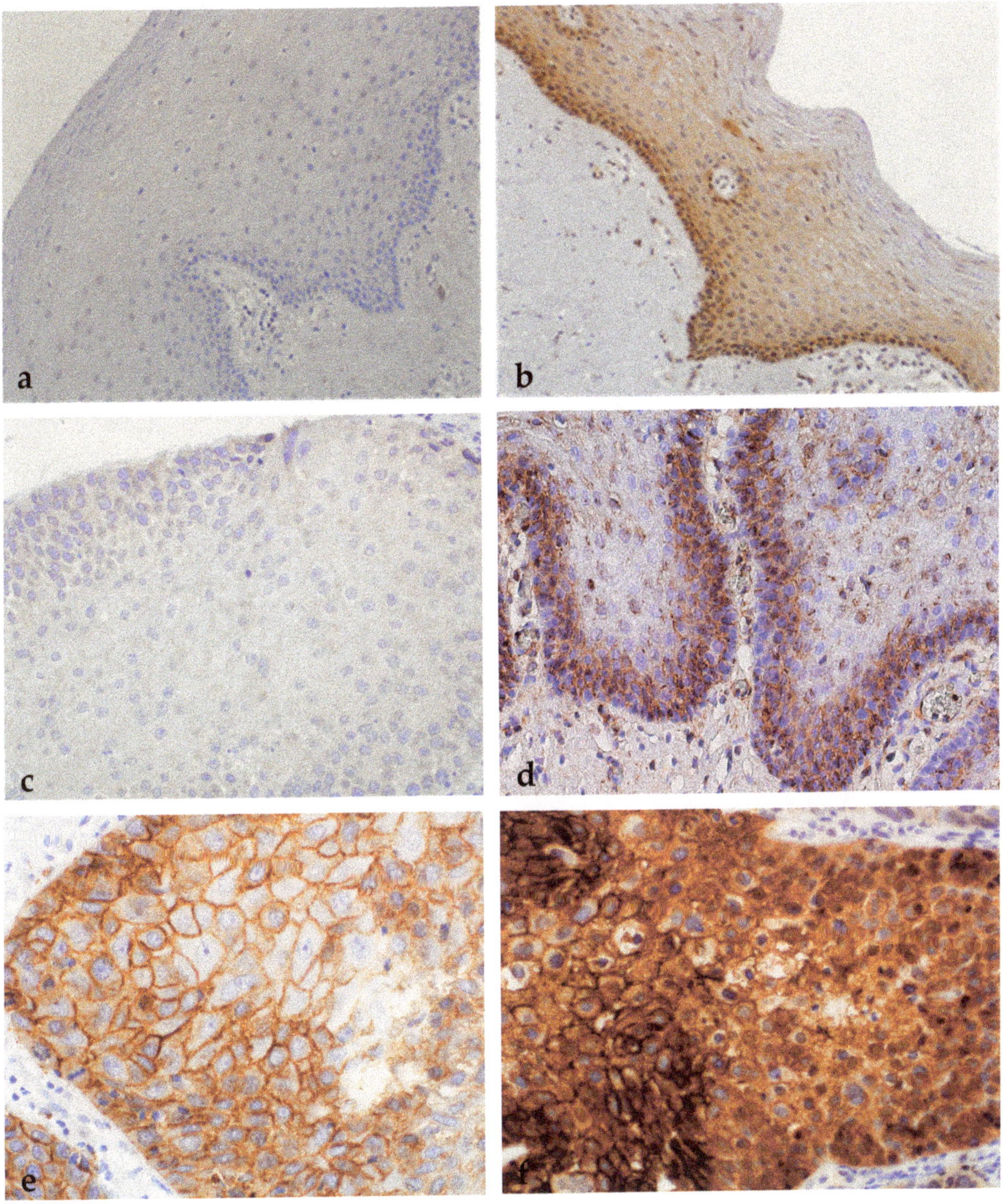

Figure 10. Immunohistochemical expression of mEGFR in healthy oral mucosa, oral premalignant changes, and OSCCs. (**a**) Negative expression of EGFR on the membrane of oral epithelium. (**b**) Moderate complete membrane staining of EGFR in oral mucosa (++). Magnification 200×. (**c**) Incomplete membrane staining of EGFR in more than 10% of cells in oral leukoplakia (+). (**d**) Moderate complete membrane staining of EGFR in oral leukoplakia (++). Magnification 400×. (**e**) Moderate complete membrane staining of EGFR in more than 10% of cells in OSCC (++). (**f**) Strong complete membrane staining in more than 10% of cells in OSCC (+++). Magnification 400×.

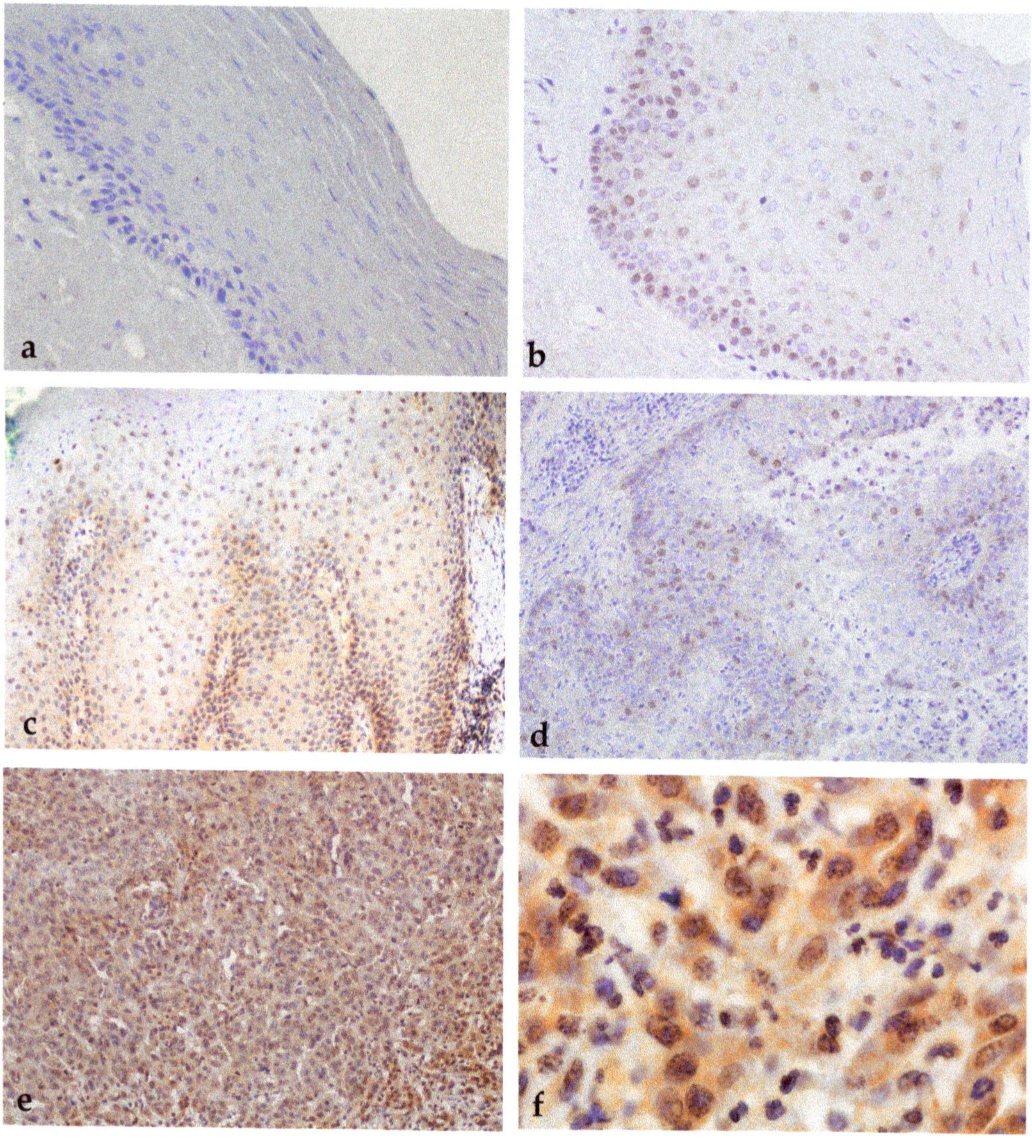

Figure 11. Immunohistochemical expression of nEGFR in healthy oral mucosa, oral premalignant changes, and OSCCs. (**a**) Negative immunohistochemical expression of nEGFR in healthy oral mucosa. Magnification 200×. (**b**) Oral leukoplakia with moderate dysplasia and weak expression of nuclear EGFR (+). Magnification 400×. (**c**) Oral erythroplakia with moderate expression of nuclear EGFR (++). Magnification 200×. (**d**) Weak expression of nEGFR in well-differentiated OSCC (+). (**e**) Strong nuclear staining for nEGFR in more than 35% of cells in moderately differentiated OSCC (+++). Magnification 200×. (**f**) Strong immunohistochemical staining for nEGFR in the nucleus and moderate staining for EGFR in the cytoplasm of OSCC. Magnification 1000×.

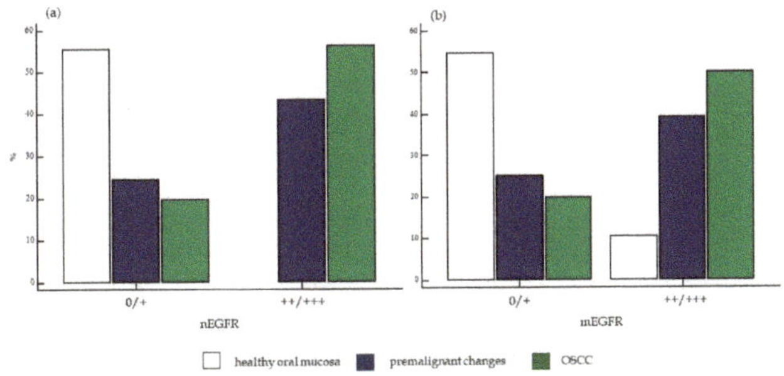

Figure 12. Presentation of the difference between weak and strong expression of nEGFR and mEGFR between the studied groups of subjects. Comparison of weak and strong expression of (**a**) nEGFR and (**b**) mEGFR between the analyzed groups of subjects revealed statistical significance ($\chi^2 = 49.85$, $p < 0.0001$; $\chi^2 = 34.05$, $p < 0.0001$). Legend: nEGFR—nuclear EGFR; mEGFR—membrane EGFR; 0—negative and weak expression, 1—moderate and strong expression.

2.1.6. Correlation of nEGFR Expression with mEGFR and Markers of Cell Cycle, Cell Proliferation, and Tumor Stem Cells in Healthy Oral Mucosa, Premalignant Changes, and Invasive Oral Squamous Cell Carcinoma

In the group of healthy subjects, the correlation of expression between the tested markers did not show statistically significant results, which are therefore not shown.

In the group of patients with premalignant changes, a statistically significant positive correlation was observed between nEGFR and Ki-67 ($\rho = 0.45$, $p = 0.001$), p53 ($\rho = 0.50$, $p = 0.0002$), cyclin D1 ($\rho = 0.42$, $p = 0.002$), mEGFR ($\rho = 0.54$, $p < 0.0001$) and ABCG2 ($\rho = 0.42$, $p = 0.002$). A statistically significant correlation was observed between mEGFR and Ki-67 ($\rho = 0.51$, $p = 0.0002$), p53 ($\rho = 0.50$, $p = 0.0002$), nEGFR ($\rho = 0.54$, $p < 0.0001$), cyclin D1 ($\rho = 0.38$, $p = 0.005$), and ABCG2 ($\rho = 0.49$, $p = 0.0003$).

In the group of patients with premalignant changes, a statistically significant positive correlation between the degree of dysplasia and nEGFR ($\rho = 0.60$, $p < 0.0001$), Ki-67 ($\rho = 0.42$, $p = 0.002$), p53 ($\rho = 0.50$, $p = 0.0002$), cyclin D1 ($\rho = 0.35$, $p = 0.01$), mEGFR ($\rho = 0.53$, $p = 0.0001$) was also detected, while ABCG2 showed no significant correlation ($\rho = 0.24$, $p = 0.10$).

Considering the association of nEGFR with cell analyzed markers in the OSCC group, a statistically significant positive correlation was observed between nEGFR and Ki-67 ($\rho = 0.31$, $p = 0.002$), p53 ($\rho = 0.30$, $p = 0.03$), and mEGFR ($\rho = 0.31$, $p = 0.02$), while the correlation with cyclin D1 ($\rho = 0.20$, $p = 0.16$) and ABCG2 ($\rho = 0.21$, $p = 0.12$) was not observed. A statistically significant correlation was observed between mEGFR and Ki-67 ($\rho = 0.34$, $p = 0.01$), p53 ($\rho = 0.37$, $p = 0.006$), and nEGFR ($\rho = 0.31$, $p = 0.02$), while the correlation with cyclin D1 ($\rho = 0.07$, $p = 0.62$) and ABCG2 ($\rho = -0.18$, $p = 0.19$) was not observed.

2.1.7. Association of Protein Expression of nEGFR and mEGFR and of Ki-67, p53, Cyclin D1, and ABCG2 with Clinicopathologic Parameters in Invasive Oral Squamous Cell Carcinoma

We analyzed the risk factors of alcohol and smoking, TNM stage of tumor, tumor localization, regional metastases, number of positive lymph nodes, histologic grade, lymphovascular invasion, perineural invasion (PNI), extranodal extension (ENE), margins, comorbidities, disease progression, HPV status, occurrence of another primary tumor, and death from the primary disease or another disease (Table 2). Statistical significance was found in the analysis of tumor sites in which expression of nEGFR and mEGFR was observed. No statistically significant difference was observed in the expression of nEGFR and mEGFR in relation to the other listed clinical data and pathohistological characteristics of the tumor. In the studied group of samples, the average tumor thickness was 7.5 ± 6.86 mm and the tumor size was 2.9 ± 1.39 cm.

Table 2. Associations of expression of investigated molecular biomarkers with clinical data and pathohistological features of tumors.

Molecular Biomarker	Ki-67			p53			Cyclin D1			ABCG2			nEGFR			mEGFR		
IHC scoring	≤30%	> 30%		0/+	++		0/+	++		0/+	++/+++		0/+	++/+++		0/+	++/+++	
Subject number	n = 30	n = 22		n = 9	n = 43		n = 9	n = 43		n = 9	n = 43		n = 22	n = 30		n = 19	n = 33	
harmful habits																		
none	0	8		3	9		3	10		4	9		7	8		6	7	
alcohol abuse	18	15	$\chi^2 = 0.359$, $p = 0.55$	9	25	$\chi^2 = 1.46$, $p = 0.48$	3	16	$\chi^2 = 2.20$, $p = 0.33$	4	15	$\chi^2 = 0.28$, $p = 0.59$	8	11	$\chi^2 = 9.71$, $p = 0.002$	6	13	$\chi^2 = 1.85$, $p = 0.60$
smoking	8	17		8	22		6	33		5	34		17	22		13	26	
both factors	8	15		8	22		2	15		3	14		8	11		6	13	
TNM disease stage																		
I	9	5		4	10		2	12		4	10		2	12		4	10	
II	7	5		4	8		2	10		3	9		8	4		5	7	
III	6	4	$\chi^2 = 2.02$, $p = 0.73$	1	9	$\chi^2 = 9.76$, $p = 0.28$	1	9	$\chi^2 = 5.48$, $p = 0.70$	0	10	$\chi^2 = 4.67$, $p = 0.32$	4	6	$\chi^2 = 14.58$, $p = 0.26$	3	7	$\chi^2 = 6.66$, $p = 0.88$
IV A	5	7		7	5		4	8		2	10		5	7		5	7	
IV B	3	1		2	2		0	4		0	4		3	1		2	2	
IV C	0	0		0	0		0	0		0	0		0	0		0	0	
histological tumor grade																		
1	18	10		9	19		6	22		6	22		14	14		10	16	
2	10	10	$\chi^2 = 1.08$, $p = 0.58$	7	13	$\chi^2 = 3.16$, $p = 0.53$	3	17	$\chi^2 = 3.47$, $p = 0.48$	3	17	$\chi^2 = 1.24$, $p = 0.53$	6	14	$\chi^2 = 6.2$, $p = 0.40$	6	14	$\chi^2 = 5.93$, $p = 0.43$
3	2	2		2	2		0	4		0	4		2	2		3	1	
lymphovascular invasion																		
absent	24	16	$p = 0.55$ *	14	26	$p = 0.53$ *	7	33	$p = 0.85$ *	9	31	$p = 0.07$ *	18	22	$p = 0.88$ *	15	25	$p = 0.78$ *
present	6	6		4	8		2	10		0	12		4	8		4	8	
perineural invasion																		
absent	16	12	$p = 0.93$ *	9	19	$p = 0.02$ *	6	22	$p = 0.54$ *	8	20	$p = 0.02$ *	12	16	$p = 0.25$ *	10	18	$p = 0.80$ *
present	14	10		9	15		3	21		1	26		10	14		9	15	
extranodal extension																		

Table 2. *Cont.*

Molecular Biomarker	Ki-67			p53			Cyclin D1			ABCG2			nEGFR			mEGFR		
absent	26	20	$p = 0.64$ *	15	31	$p = 0.67$	9	37	$p = 0.49$ *	9	37	$p = 0.23$	18	28	$p = 0.5$ *	18	19	$p = 0.25$ *
present	4	2		3	3		0	6		0	6		4	2		2	4	
disease progression																		
no	24	16	$p = 0.54$ *	12	28	$\chi^2 = 1.59$, $p = 0.66$	8	32	$p = 0.62$ *	9	31	$\chi^2 = 1.59$, $p = 0.07$	16	21	$p = 0.51$ *	14	26	$p = 0.66$ *
yes	6	6		6	6		1	11		0	12		6	6		5	7	
HPV status																		
negative	28	22	$p = 0.22$ *	16	34	$p = 0.11$	8	42	$p = 0.38$ *	9	41	$p = 0.51$ *	21	26	$p = 0.88$ *	17	33	$p = 0.19$ *
positive	2	0		2	0		1	1		0	2		1	1		2	0	
second primary tumor																		
no	27	16	$p = 0.11$ *	17	26	$p = 0.24$ *	7	36	$p = 0.75$ *	8	35	$p = 0.58$ *	18	23	$p = 0.35$ *	16	27	$p = 0.87$ *
yes	3	6		1	8		2	7		9	0		4	3		3	6	

* Fisher's exact test.

When comparing the relationship between the expression of Ki-67 proliferation index and clinicopathological features of patients with OSCC, no statistical significance was found.

When comparing the relationship between the expression of p53 protein and the clinicopathologic features of patients with OSCC, PNI and death from underlying diseases or other diseases were statistically significant. Tumors without PNI had a significantly higher frequency of p53 protein expression than tumors with PNI ($p = 0.02$).

When comparing the association of cyclin D1 expression with clinicopathologic features of patients with OSCC, no statistical significance was found.

When comparing the association of ABCG2 expression with clinicopathologic features of patients with OSCC, statistical significance was found for PNI, whereas no statistically significant differences were found for other parameters.

2.2. Survival Analysis

Only patients with OSCC were included in the survival analysis, and follow-up data were available for all patients. Patients' lifespan was followed from the time of diagnosis and/or surgery until last follow-up or death. All patients were treated surgically. The median follow-up time was 32.26 months with a range of 1 to 98 months. During the follow-up period, 18/52 patients died, of which 10 patients died from the underlying disease and 8 patients died from another cause of death and were censored in the analysis of experience. In addition, disease progression to a higher stage was observed in 12/52 patients during follow up. The median time to disease progression was 15 months with a range of 8 to 84 months.

For all biomarkers analyzed, the previously described cut-off values were used to divide patient groups into those with high or low expression of the tested proteins. In the analysis of survival, the influence of the parameters on overall survival was first determined by the Kaplan–Meier method, and the difference between survival curves was determined by the log-rank test.

When analyzing the influence of tumor clinicopathologic characteristics on overall patient survival, only a difference in survival between patient groups was found with respect to regional metastases ($p = 0.03$), lymphovascular invasion ($p = 0.04$), and the presence of a second primary tumor ($p = 0.01$) (Figure 13). Other previously described clinical and pathological features of the tumor had no effect on overall patient survival. It is important to note that the margin of the preparation, which has been shown to have an impact on overall experience, was negative in all samples and therefore was not statistically significant in this study for monitoring patient experience.

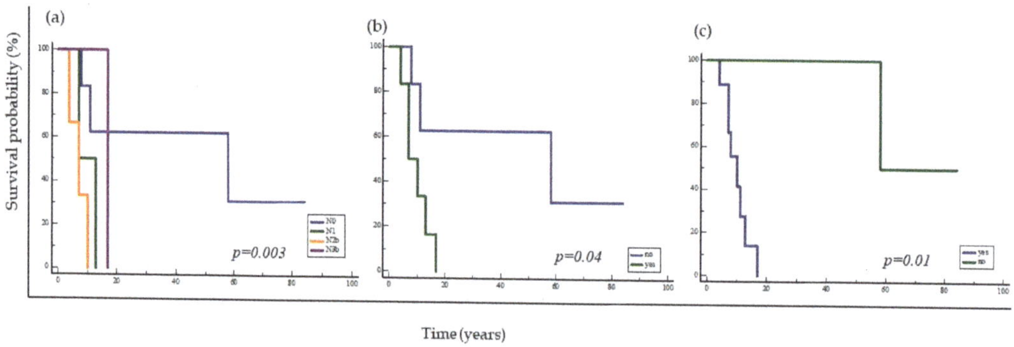

Figure 13. Kaplan–Meier survival curve considering the influence of clinicopathologic tumor characteristics in patients with OSCC. The curve shows significantly shorter survival of patients with higher N stage disease ($p = 0.003$) (**a**), lymphovascular invasion ($p = 0.04$) (**b**), and presence of a second primary tumor ($p = 0.01$) (**c**).

In addition, analysis of patients' overall survival based on the analyzed proteins showed a statistically significant association between nEGFR and survival ($p = 0.004$). Patients with moderate and strong expression of nEGFR (++/+++) in tumor tissue had significantly shorter overall survival compared to patients with negative and weak nEGFR (0/+) (Figure 14). This analysis revealed no difference in survival between patient groups with respect to expression of mEGFR, Ki-67, p53, cyclin D1, and ABCG2.

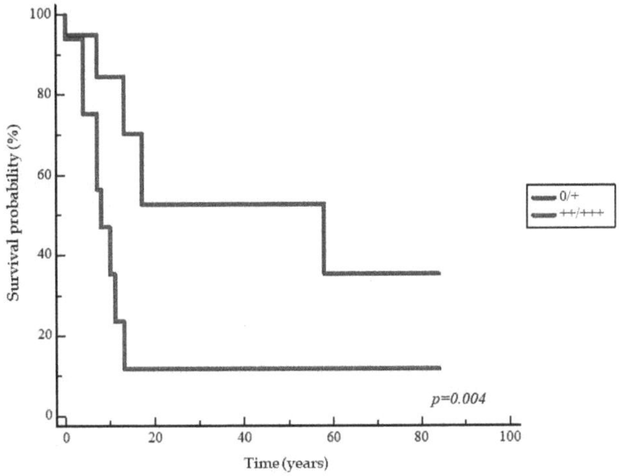

Figure 14. Kaplan–Meier survival curve in relation to nEGFR expression in patients with OSCC. The curve shows significantly shorter survival of patients with moderate and strong expression of nEGFR in tumor tissue ($p = 0.004$).

3. Discussion

Oral squamous cell carcinoma (OSCC) is the most common malignant tumor of the head and neck (HNSCC), i.e., the sixteenth most common cancer worldwide, with a relatively poor five-year survival rate of approximately 55%, despite significant advances in diagnostic and therapeutic procedures over the past 30 years [2,17]. Surgical resection of the tumor with or without neck dissection remains the method of choice in the treatment of OSCC. Adjuvant radiotherapy or chemoradiotherapy is performed depending on the pathohistological features of the tumor [1]. Although the presence of dysplasia in oral leukoplakia and oral erythroplakia is the most important prognostic factor for malignant transformation, the available diagnostic classifications of dysplasia have numerous shortcomings. One of the main reasons is the subjectivity of the observer and the resulting poor reproducibility of the diagnostic criteria, which has been confirmed by numerous studies showing a weak correlation between the degree of dysplasia and the malignant transformation of potentially malignant oral disorders (OPMD) [18–21]. Consequently, new biomarkers need to be found that can be used in routine practice to assess the risk of malignant transformation from premalignant changes in OSCC. Late detection of OSCC, the occurrence of locoregional disease recurrence, and metastatic disease are characterized by poor prognosis, and there is a need for the development of biomarkers for early detection of disease, more reliable prediction of disease prognosis, and selection of appropriate therapy [20]. The fact that patients with similar clinicopathologic features often have different disease progression, response to therapy, and treatment outcome points to the need to identify novel prognostic factors that more accurately determine the biologic behavior of tumors. Biomarkers of genomic instability could accurately measure the risk of malignant transformation from premalignant changes in OSCC and the risk of spread and metastasis of the primary tumor to regional lymph nodes and distant organs [19,22]. According to the results of this study, the mean age of patients with OSCC was 55.21 years, and the cancer occurred twice as often in men (67.3%; 35/52). The mean age of patients with premalignant changes was 64.22 years, and women were slightly more frequently affected (54%; 27/50). The distribution of age and sex in patients with OSCC depends on geographic location, and our data are consistent with those of European countries [23,24]. The most frequent localizations of premalignant changes and OSCC in the oral cavity were the tongue and the floor of the oral cavity (75%, 39/52 and 64%, and 32/50, respectively), which is consistent with the literature. The aforementioned areas have been shown to be predilection sites for premalignant changes and OSCC due to the deleterious effects of carcinogens that accumulate in the so-called salivary pool. For head and neck tumors, numerous diagnostic and prognostic markers have been investigated in clinical studies, but their clinical significance remains questionable [5,22]. Recent discoveries related to a completely new way of regulating cell proliferation and apoptosis through the independent action of EGFR in the nucleus of numerous tumors, such as ovarian, breast, oropharyngeal, laryngeal, and esophageal carcinoma, have been the basis for studying premalignant and malignant changes in the oral cavity, where the role of this receptor had not been previously elucidated [8,11–16]. In addition to nEGFR, we also analyzed the expression of markers of cell cycle and proliferation (Ki-67, cyclin D1, p53, mEGFR) and markers of tumor stem cells (ABCG2) involved in oral carcinogenesis. Ki-67 is considered one of the most important immunohistochemical markers of cell proliferation and aggressiveness of numerous tumors, such as breast, lung, prostate, cervical, soft tissue, and central nervous system tumors, and its excessive expression is a poor prognostic sign [25–27]. Although the results of studies on Ki-67 and HNSCC are conflicting, there are a larger number of studies indicating that overexpression of Ki-67 is associated with progression of OPMD and with a higher rate of locoregional recurrence as well as distant metastasis and worse OS, DFS, RFS, and MFS in patients with OSCC [28–31]. Moreover, expression in OSCC was inversely proportional to tumor differentiation. A statistically significant difference in the expression of Ki-67 was demonstrated between the groups of patients with OSCC on the one hand and subjects with premalignant changes and the control group on the other hand. In our study, the percentage proliferation index was significantly higher in the group of cancer patients compared with the healthy subjects and those with premalignant changes, whereas no statistically significant difference was demonstrated between the control group and the subjects with leukoplakia and erythroplakia. In the subjects with premalignant changes, the expression of Ki-67 increased statistically significantly with the progression of dysplasia ($p = 0.005$), which is consistent with data from the literature. Sharma, like us, demonstrated a positive correlation between Ki-67 expression and disease progression from low-grade dysplasia to high-grade dysplasia to OSCC in 65 subjects, 40 of whom had OSCC and 25 of whom had premalignant changes [32]. The increase in Ki-67 expression with progression of dysplasia in leukoplakias is the result of an observational study conducted by researchers from India in 2020 on 786 subjects with leukoplakia, of whom 126 had epithelial dysplasia, and 14 patients developed OSCC [33]. Similar results were also obtained by Dwivedi et al. [34]. Comparison of Ki-67 expression with clinicopathologic features of patients with OSCC did not reveal statistical significance. Birajdar's studies found increased expression of Ki-67 in poorly differentiated carcinomas compared with well-differentiated OSCC [35]. In our subject sample, we did not demonstrate a statistically significant association between Ki-67 expression and histologic differentiation of OSCC. The p53 protein is classified as a tumor suppressor protein, and due to its multiple roles in cellular homeostasis, it is classified as a central regulator of the genome. More than 50% of malignancies exhibit excessive p53 expression caused by p53 gene mutations and epigenetic alterations [36,37]. Numerous genetic analyzes have shown a high frequency of p53 gene mutations in the early stages of carcinogenesis in HNSCC (more than 70% of tumors) [38]. In our study, we found significantly higher expression in the group of subjects with OSCC and subjects with premalignant changes compared with the control group, and a statistically significant difference was also found between all analyzed groups. Considering the significant increase in p53 expression in premalignant changes compared with healthy mucosa and the evidence that expression correlates with malignant transformation of OPMD, as well as the small number of influences of p53 protein on patient experience, it is reasonable to assume that inactivation of this protein is crucial in the early phase of oral carcinogenesis. In our studies, the trend of increased expression of p53 is observed in advanced cancers compared with the early stages of the disease. A statistically significant association between p53 protein expression and clinicopathologic features of patients with OSCC was demonstrated for PNI and death from underlying disease or other diseases. OSCC without PNI had a significantly higher frequency of p53 expression than tumors without PNI ($p = 0.02$). The origin of PNI in head and neck tumors is still largely unknown due to the distinct molecular complexity of the process. It is known that the presence of PNI in HNSCC is a negative prognostic sign, and it is recommended that patients with OSSC and PNI receive postoperative adjuvant radiotherapy. The lack of studies investigating the impact of mutation and overexpression of p53 protein on the occurrence of PNI in patients with OSCC speaks to the complexity of the mechanism of nerve invasion itself. One of the signaling receptors on tumor cells associated with cell migration and PNI is Galanin receptors 2 (GALR2), which is thought to play a very important role in regulating PNI in HNSCC. Banerjee et al. induced cell lines from HNSCC to overexpress GALR2 and observed that this stimulated cell proliferation and tumor cell survival via activation of ERK and Akt in vitro and cell proliferation in vivo [39]. Thus, he proved that GALR2 receptor overexpression plays a protumoral role in HNSCC cells, whereas Kanazawa observed the opposite effect of GALR2 in patients with HNSCC and overexpression of p53 mutations [40]. According to our results, PNI occurred more frequently in advanced disease when the expression of p53 protein was also reduced, suggesting that the effect of p53 expression on the development of PNI is inversely proportional, and that p53 plays a much more important role in early carcinogenesis. Furthermore, the impact of p53 protein overexpression on overall survival of patients with OSCC is unknown. Khan failed to demonstrate a statistically significant correlation with clinicopathologic parameters in a sample of 29 OSCC [41]. In a prospective study by Ogmundsdóttir and colleagues on a sample of 144 subjects with premalignant (OL and lichen ruber planus) and malignant changes of the oral mucosa, they concluded that p53 gene mutations can persist in benign lesions of the oral mucosa for many years without developing malignant disease. Moreover, no association was found between p53 protein expression and OSCC recurrence or disease-related survival, whereas overall survival was shortened in patients overexpressing this protein [42]. Cyclin D1 regulates the cell cycle and plays an important role in tumorigenesis of numerous tumors, including OSCC. Cyclin D1 overexpression has been found in 32 to 88% of malignant tumors [43–45]. According to the results of numerous studies, cyclin D1 is considered a negative independent prognostic factor and biomarker for the aggressiveness of OSCC [46]. Huang demonstrated in 264 subjects with OSCC that overexpression of cyclin D1 was associated with higher tumor stage and poorly differentiated carcinomas, higher rate of regional metastases, and worse DFS and OS (282). In our study, we followed the dynamics of increased expression of cyclin D1 from normal mucosa to premalignant changes to OSCC demonstrating strong expression in 82.6% of tumors (43/52). Moharii et al. observed something similar in 75 patients with premalignant and malignant changes in the oral cavity [47]. We found no statistically significant difference in the dysplasia group in subjects with premalignant changes. When comparing the relationship between cyclin D1 expression and clinicopathologic features in patients with OSCC, no statistically significant differences were found, and there was no effect on the overall outcome. Numerous studies on OSCC have demonstrated the association between cyclin D1 expression and clinicopathologic and prognostic factors in patients with OSCC. Carlos de Vi-cente, Das, Gupta, and Guimaraes found higher expression of cyclin D1 in higher T-stage tumors, which was also confirmed by Zhao 2014 in his meta-analysis [48–51]. Wang and Liu found a statistically significant correlation between cyclin D1 expression and tumor thickness and depth of invasion (DOI) [52]. Many authors have demonstrated the increased expression of cyclin D1 in premalignant transformation and the positive dynamics of increased expression with the progression of dysplasia and progression to OSCC and disease progression. Numerous studies have also demonstrated the association between cyclin D1 expression and disease stage N, which was also confirmed by two meta-analyzes in 2014 and 2015 [53,54]. Interestingly, numerous authors such as Bov, Miyamoto, Lam, and Huang have found an increase in cyclin D1 expression with a decrease in tumor differentiation, i.e., an increase in the histological grade of the tumor [55,56]. The results of the present study suggest the opposite: the higher the histologic grade, the lower the expression of cyclin D1. Saawarn showed an increase in cyclin D1 expression with OSCC differentiation in 40 subjects, which is consistent with our observations [56]. Similar results were obtained by Angadi, Krishnapillai, and Das [57,58]. The relationship between cyclin D1 and the degree of tumor differentiation is controversial and has not yet been clarified. This discrepancy in results is partly explained by the use of different histologic criteria for determining cyclin D1 expression. Another explanation was provided by Woods and colleagues in a study of oral keratinocyte cell lines in which stimulation of cyclin D1 expression increased cell proliferation but did not block cell differentiation [59]. This suggests that cyclin D1 is able to directly affect transcriptional regulation of genes involved in oral keratinocyte differentiation independently of CDK. Therefore, Ohnishi concluded in 2014 that cyclin D1 is involved not only in cell proliferation but also in cell differentiation and prevention of cell death in OSCC [60]. Further studies are needed to investigate in detail the role of cyclin D1 in oral keratinocyte differentiation and whether it can modulate cell differentiation in OSCC toward less aggressive histological stages with better prognosis. Expression of the ABCG2 protein, also known as Breast Cancer Resistance Protein (BCRP), was recently discovered as a potential biomarker for the severity of OPMD and OSCC [61–63]. It is responsible for resistance to numerous drugs in many tumors and is one of the markers of tumor stem cells [64,65]. ABCG2 is overexpressed in the side population of tumor stem cells, which play an important role in oral carcinogenesis [66]. When we analyzed the expression of ABCG2, we found a statistically significant difference between the studied groups. The weakest expression of ABCG2 was detected in control mucosa, with an increase in immunoreactivity in the group of patients with premalignant changes and the highest expression of the protein in subjects with OSCC. We also demonstrated a significant increase in ABCG2 expression with progression of dysplasia in premalignant changes. A study by Shi et al. demonstrated the association between ABCG2 expression in oral lichen ruber planus and an increased risk of malignant transformation in a sample of 110 patients, whereas Feng confirmed the potential of ABCG2 in predicting malignant transformation by analyzing ABCG2 expression in healthy oral mucosa, premalignant changes, and oral cavity cancer in 8 cell lines and 189 subjects [62,63]. A detailed analysis of the sublocalization of ABCG2 immunoreactivity has not been described, although several papers mention the possible importance of intracellular localization of the protein. Several studies have observed membranous and nuclear expression of ABCG2 in malignant tumor cells, such as lung and laryngeal carcinomas and glioblastoma multiforme [67–69]. A possible novel role of ABCG2 within the nucleus as a transcriptional regulator involved in modulation of metastasis has been proposed in lung cancer [68]. In our samples, we observed immunoreactivity in the nucleus in addition to membrane and cytoplasmic expression of ABCG2. The main reason for the positive ABCG2 immunoreactivity in the different sublocalizations remains to be clarified in future studies. Analysis of the association between ABCG2 expression and clinicopathological features of OSCC revealed a statistically significant association with PNI ($p = 0.02$), while no statistically significant differences were found for the other parameters analyzed. The role of ABCG2 in OSCC is not known, and there are few studies in the available literature that have analyzed this role, mainly due to the resistance of OSCC to chemotherapy, following the findings related to breast cancer. Yanamoto et al. demonstrated that overexpression of ABCG2 in OSCC was associated with PNI, a higher rate of regional metastasis, and local recurrence in 89 subjects [70].

The concept of concomitant chemoradiotherapy, which includes the use of postoperative radiotherapy and cisplatin-based chemotherapy, has remained unchanged since its introduction in the 1960s [71]. Although a positive effect on locoregional disease control and survival has been demonstrated in patients with HNSCC, 5-year overall survival has not been significantly prolonged in advanced tumors and ranges from 30% to 60% [72]. The discovery of EGFR overexpression in numerous malignancies and its oncogenic effect on gene expression, cell proliferation, angiogenesis, apoptosis, cell motility and adhesion, and metastasis has led to the development of numerous drugs that inhibit its action. Given the overexpression of EGFR in more than 90% of head and neck tumors and the poorer survival of these patients, it was hypothesized that patients would benefit greatly from the use of anti-EGFR drugs [72]. Numerous inhibitors have been developed. The best known is cetuximab, a chimeric IgG1 monoclonal antibody that binds to the extracellular domain of the EGFR membrane and is approved in combination with radiotherapy for the treatment of advanced HNSCC and as monotherapy for locoregional recurrence and metastatic disease. In 2011, the FDA approved the use of cetuximab in combination with cisplatin-based chemotherapy and 5-FU to treat locoregional recurrence and metastatic disease. However, the fact that less than 20% of HNSCC respond to cetuximab and that concomitant use with chemoradiotherapy does not significantly improve disease outcomes in advanced disease is quite discouraging. Intensive work is being performed to identify possible causes of resistance to cetuximab in tumors with high EGFR expression [73,74]. One of the possible explanations for resistance is translocation of the receptor into the nucleus, which can be induced by irradiation, cetuximab, the effects of cisplatin, increased expression of EGFR ligands, and activation of the src kinase family [75]. This suggests that EGFR in the nucleus may influence the expression and transcription of numerous genes involved in tumorigenesis via other, as yet unknown, multiple downstream signaling pathways. Moreover, in addition to cetuximab, drugs have been developed that inhibit tyrosine kinase activity by binding to the intracellular domain of EGFR. Tyrosine kinase inhibitors (TKIs) such as gefitinib have shown limited clinical efficacy, responding in only 10% to 15% of patients with HNSCC. Less than 5% of HNSCC have EGFR mutations, which may partially explain the reported tumor resistance to TKIs [75]. Recent studies began to focus attention on the cellular sublocalization of EGFR, and it was found that this receptor can be overexpressed in the cytoplasm (cEGFR) as well as in the nucleus (nEGFR) in addition to the membrane, with potentially novel implications for the expression of numerous genes. These results indicate that there are still many unknowns in the action of EGFR that need to be investigated. There are few papers in the literature that have investigated the effects of cEGFR and nEGFR expression in HNSCC, and no single study focused on OSCC [16]. According to the available literature, this study is the first to investigate the expression and impact of nEGFR in premalignant and malignant changes of the oral cavity on malignant transformation and disease progression. A large number of studies have investigated the significance of EGFR overexpression by immunohistochemical methods in HNSCC, which represent a very large heterogeneous group of tumors with different biological behaviors [11–16,76]. Results are often contradictory, in part because of inconsistent quantification of immunohistochemical receptor expression, neglect of receptor expression in single cell compartments, and inclusion of different head and neck tumors in the studies.

Our results show a statistically significant difference in the expression of mEGFR and nEGFR between the studied groups ($p < 0.0001$) with an increase in moderate and strong expression and with the progression of genetic instabilities from the healthy control group, and premalignant changes to the OSCC. The results of this study regarding membrane expression of EGFR in premalignant and malignant changes are consistent with the available results from the literature. Mirza et al. found overexpression of mEGFR in 129 subjects in 51% of patients with premalignant changes and in 67% of patients with OSCC. Furthermore, they demonstrated that overexpression of mEGFR in patients with OSCC negatively affected 5-year OS and was associated with a higher risk of disease recurrence [77]. In 2018, Singala examined the expression of several molecular markers (EGFR, p53, c-erbB2) in 40 oral leukoplakias and 40 OSCC and also found a significant increase in EGFR expression with progression of premalignant changes in OSCC. They concluded that excessive co-expression of p53 and EGFR may indicate a higher risk of malignant transformation from leukoplakia to OSCC [78]. Ries reached similar conclusions when studying the malignant transformation of 98 leukoplakias, particularly emphasizing that expression of EGFR correlated more strongly with malignant transformation in relation to the degree of dysplasia [79]. Thus, the results of most studies on premalignant and malignant transformation of the oral cavity are consistent with the results of this study when we talk about the expression of mEGFR. In the available literature, there is no single study that investigated the expression of nuclear EGFR in premalignant and malignant transformation of the oral cavity, and therefore we cannot compare our results with the literature. A significant increase in the expression of both membrane and nuclear EGFR already in premalignant changes compared with the control group suggests that these two proteins play an important role in early oral carcinogenesis. When analyzing the correlation of nEGFR expression with mEGFR and markers of the cell cycle, cell proliferation and tumor stem cells in the studied groups, interesting results were found. In the group of patients with premalignant changes, a statistically significant positive correlation was observed between nEGFR and Ki-67, p53, cyclin D1, mEGFR, and ABCG2. Analysis of the correlation between the degree of dysplasia and the markers studied showed a statistically positive correlation with an increase in the degree of dysplasia and an increase in the expression of nEGFR, Ki-67, p53, cyclin D1, and mEGFR, whereas ABCG2, although not statistically significant, showed a visible positive trend. Similar observations of correlation between the studied cell cycle markers and tumor stem cells were demonstrated in patients with OSCC. A statistically significant positive correlation was observed between nEGFR and Ki67, p53, and mEGFR, whereas the correlation with cyclin D1 and ABCG2 was not observed but a positive trend was evident. A statistically significant correlation was observed between mEGFR and Ki67, p53, and nEGFR, whereas the correlation with cyclin D1 showed only a positive statistical trend. Cancer progression occurred in 12 patients with OSCC (23.1%), and 10 patients (19.2%) died as a result of OSCC. The correlation of the analyzed markers was not related to disease progression or death from OSCC. The above results of correlation of nEGFR with other markers studied cannot be compared with data from the literature because of the lack of studies that have investigated nEGFR in premalignant and malignant changes of the oral cavity. We can discuss the above results in the context of studies on other malignancies of the head and neck. Positive correlations between nEGFR and other investigated biomarkers in premalignant changes and dysplasias can be explained by the influence of EGFR on stimulating cell proliferation and blocking apoptosis, which has been confirmed in previous studies [7–11]. It is known that EGFR in the nucleus can activate transcription of cyclin D1 by binding to the promoter site of the CCND1 gene, which may explain the positive correlation between the aforementioned biomarkers. Blocking apoptosis is also possible by reducing CKI activity caused by mutations and overexpression of EGFR [7]. Ki-67 expression is closely related to cell proliferation and tumor cell growth, which is consistent with our results and the fact that an increase in Ki-67 expression is expected with the progression of dysplasia and OSCC. This was demonstrated by Jing et al. when they analyzed 396 samples of OSCC, oral dysplasia, and healthy oral mucosa [28]. Numerous studies have confirmed the high expression of the p53 gene in OSCC (54%, 75%, 95%, and 65%), and a trend toward increased expression with progression of premalignant changes in the oral cavity from hyperplasia to dysplasia to cancer has been noted [80–82]. Disruptive and nondisruptive mutations of the p53 protein result in impaired function of this protein with the inability to induce apoptosis in damaged cells. Liu demonstrated in hepatocellular carcinoma cell lines that nEGFR can affect cell apoptosis by stimulating the expression of SOS1, which then activates the HRAS/PI3K/AKT pathway, leading to nuclear translocation of p-AKT and Bcl-2. The interaction between p-AKT and ASPP2 facilitates the binding of BcL-2 to p53, leading to the release of p53 from the pro-apoptotic gene promoter. Activation of the HRAS/PI3K/AKT pathway by nEGFR-induced SOS1 also inhibits cisplatin-induced apoptosis [83]. In 2021, Marijić et al. examined the expression of mEGFR and nEGFR in laryngeal polyps, dysplasias, and squamous cell carcinomas, and confirmed a significantly higher frequency of strong nEGFR expression in cancer, dysplasias, and polyps, as well as strong expression of mEGFR in cancer and laryngeal dysplasias compared with polyps [16]. This was confirmed by our studies on premalignant changes and OSCC. In the group of subjects with OSSC, we observed a positive correlation of membrane and nuclear EGFR expression in agreement with the results of Psyrri et al. in oropharyngeal carcinomas [14]. Marijić demonstrated the inverse expression of mEGFR and nEGFR in squamous cell carcinomas of the larynx and concluded that only one EGFR signaling pathway, membrane or nuclear, controls further carcinogenesis in tumors [16]. The results of this study suggest that both EGFR signaling pathways influence carcinogenesis, possibly stimulating each other and possibly acting independently. One of the aims of this study was to analyze the expression level of nEGFR in relation to the studied clinical and pathological features of patients with OSCC. We did not find a single statistically significant association, which is similar to the results of Marijić and Psyria, on laryngeal and oral cavity cancer, whereas there are no comparable studies on the association between nEGFR and OSCC in the available literature [14,16]. When analyzing mEGFR in relation to the investigated clinicopathologic features of OSCC, we also did not find a single statistically significant correlation. Shahsavari failed to demonstrate any correlation between mEGFR expression and clinicopathologic features of OSCC, consistent with our findings [84]. In contrast, Costa et al. demonstrated the negative impact of EGFR on disease progression in individuals younger than 40 years, which contradicts our observations [85]. Abbas demonstrated an increase in mEGFR expression with an increasing histologic grade of the tumor in 30 OSCC and concluded that EGFR can be used as an indicator of tumor aggressiveness [86]. All of the aforementioned studies were performed on a small number of subjects, and there is a need for large multicenter studies that demonstrate the true relationship between membrane and nuclear EGFR expression and tumor clinicopathologic features.

In patients with OSSC, we additionally analyzed the impact of the investigated biomarkers and tumor clinicopathologic features on the overall patient experience. The median follow-up time of patients was 32.26 months. During this time, 18 patients died, ten of them from oral cavity cancer and the other eight from another cause unrelated to OSCC. Nine patients developed a second primary tumor during the follow-up period. Patients with OSCC who had regional disease, lymphatic invasion and the presence of a second primary tumor had significantly worse overall survival compared with patients without these features. According to the results of Brand's study of 594 patients with OSCC, the 1-year, 5-year, and 10 year cumulative risks of other primary tumors and disease recurrence were 17%, 30%, and 37%, respectively, and almost all locoregional disease recurrences occurred within the first 2 years after treatment. Other primary tumors significantly worsen the overall patient experience, making lifelong surveillance of patients with head and neck tumors extremely important because of the possible occurrence of other tumors in the oral cavity, which is genetically damaged by the accumulation of known risk factors. The lung and liver are the most common sites for other primary tumors outside the head and neck region, and it is occasionally necessary to screen with radiologic methods [87]. The presence of metastases in the regional lymph nodes decreases the survival rate of oral cavity cancer by 50% for each individual stage of disease. According to the TNM classification, the N stage of the disease is divided into four categories (N0-N3). The higher the N stage of the disease, the shorter the overall survival. In the presence of regional metastases, the patient is at least in the III stage of disease with a significantly reduced 5-year survival rate of about 51% compared with localized disease (stage I/ II), in which the survival rate is about 82% (1–2, 18). A Kaplan–Meier analysis of survival of patients with OSCC, depending on the expression of the markers studied, revealed a statistically significant shorter overall survival in patients with moderate and strong expression of nEGFR in tumor tissue compared to patients with weak expression. According to the available literature, these are the first results of a study investigating the impact of nEGFR expression in OSCC on overall patient survival (OS). Marijić demonstrated the negative impact of excessive expression of nEGFR on overall survival in laryngeal carcinomas, whereas Psyrri proved the same in oropharyngeal tumors [14,16]. Schmidt-Ullrich et al. demonstrated that irradiation of tumors leads to activation and internalization of EGFR in the nucleus [88]. Dittman demonstrated that EGFR and DNA-PK form a complex in the nucleus after irradiation, leading to increased DNA repair activity and acquired resistance to radiotherapy [89]. Treatment of carcinomas with cisplatin has also been shown to induce nuclear translocation of EGFR and increase resistance to chemotherapy [75]. This suggests that nEGFR plays an important role in DNA damage repair, which may explain the results of this study. In addition, we performed prognostic analyzes of clinicopathologic parameters for disease progression and death in OSCC. Alcohol consumption, clinical tumor stage, and PNI were found to be strong predictors of disease progression, whereas the presence of regional metastases, PNI, the number of positive lymph nodes, LVI, clinical tumor stage, and alcohol consumption were found to be strong predictors of death in patients with OSCC. The above observations are consistent with data from the literature [1,4,90].

Finally, the role of nEGFR in malignant tumors of the head and neck has not been adequately studied, whereas its role in premalignant and malignant changes in the oral cavity is unknown according to the available literature. The rapid increase in research related to the nuclear expression of EGFR was triggered by discoveries about the effects of this receptor on resistance to chemotherapy and radiotherapy. This demonstrates the complexity and inadequate knowledge of the signaling pathways mediated by EGFR. According to the available literature, this is the first study to investigate the impact of nEGFR expression in premalignant and malignant changes of the oral cavity and the negative impact on the overall experience of patients with OSCC. The above results suggest that nEGFR plays an important role in the development of OSCC. With readily available and convenient immunohistochemical methods, we can determine the expression of this receptor in the nucleus and widely apply it in clinical practice to more accurately determine the malignancy risk of precancerous lesions of the oral cavity compared with previous semiquantitative methods for determining dysplasia. Molecular quantification of the progression of premalignant changes in the oral mucosa would influence the type and extent of treatment and the frequency of patient follow-up. In OSCC resection, the application of molecular diagnostics could greatly alter the principles of tumor treatment by determining not only surgically or pathohistologically healthy margins but also the need for elective neck dissection or adjuvant treatment. Further studies in a large sample of subjects are needed to additionally and comprehensively investigate the role of nEGFR in OSCC and its interaction with membrane and cytoplasmic epidermal growth factor receptors. The only drawback we would cite to the use of nEGFR is the somewhat weaker visualization of the immunohistochemical response, as it is still an experimental antibody where the experience of the pathologist in reading is very important.

4. Materials and Methods

4.1. Patients

The study involved 161 patients treated at the Department of Maxillofacial Surgery, Dubrava University Hospital. They were divided into three groups: 50 patients with premalignant changes (leukoplakia and erythroplakia), 52 patients with invasive oral squamous cell carcinoma, and 59 subjects in the control group who had their mucosa removed due to non-tumour disease. All patients were followed for a period of at least 5 years. Inclusion criteria for patients were: clinically and pathohistologically verified premalignant change or OSCC; primary surgically-treated patients with OSCC; available pathohistological material for immunohistochemical analysis; available clinically and pathohistologically relevant data from medical history, hospital information system, clinical oncology database, and cancer registry of the Croatian Institute of Public Health. Patients previously treated for head and neck malignancy, patients with insufficient samples for immunohistochemical analysis, and patients with inadequate follow up or incomplete medical documentation were not included in this study.

4.2. Pathohistological Samples

Paraffin-embedded archival specimens from biopsies of premalignant changes (leukoplakia and erythroplakia), resected primary OSCC, and excised oral mucosal tissues with nonmalignant disease were used for this study. To confirm the diagnosis and to determine the adequacy of the quality and quantity of the pathohistological material, two pathologists from the Department of Pathology and Cytology of Dubrava University Hospital examined the subjects' specimens again separately. The specimens were first fixed in 10% buffered formalin (Kemika, Zagreb, Croatia), embedded in paraffin, cut into 3 to 4 µm thick sections, deparaffinized, and stained with hemalaun-eosin (HE).

4.3. Immunohistochemical Staining

In this study, 2–3 µm thick sections were prepared from the paraffin blocks and then dewaxed in a thermostat. To determine the expression of p53 and mEGFR proteins in the samples after deparaffinization, predigestion was performed in a thermobath (PT-link, DAKO, Glostrup, Denmark), followed by the use of "EnVision target Retrieval solution, High pH" (DAKO, Denmark), i.e., predigestion with exposure of epitopes by heat in a microwave oven with pH6 buffer to determine the expression of nEGFR and ABCG2 proteins. Immunohistochemical staining was performed using an automated immunohistochemical system (DAKO autostainer, DAKO, Denmark). For immunohistochemical staining, a "ready-to-use" p53 antibody (mouse monoclonal antibody, clone DO-7, DAKO, Denmark) was used with a 45-min incubation; an NCL-L EGFR antibody (Leica; Novocastra, Newcastle upon Tyne, UK) at dilution 1:50 with a 60-min incubation; an EGFR antibody (Thermo Fisher Scientific, Invitrogen, LSG Bioproduction, Waltham, M, USA), clone EGFR-1, at a dilution of 1:25 with a 90-min incubation; or ABCG2 antibody, clone B-1, at a dilution of 1:25 with a 90-min incubation. Immunohistochemical staining expression was detected by an indirect method using the EnVision detection kit (DAKO, Denmark). Subsequently, preparations were contrasted with hemalaun (1 min) and placed in an ascending series of alcohol (70–100%), and then in xylene and glass coverslip. Colon tissue served as a positive control for p53 and placental tissue for mEGFR, while paraffin-embedded breast tissue was used for nEGFR and ABCG2 according to the recommendations of the manufacturer of the antibodies tested.

For immunohistochemical analysis of cyclin D1 and Ki-67 expression, pre-digestion was performed in the Ventana BenchMark Ultra instrument (Roche Diagnostics, Basel, Switzerland) with thermostats and ULTRA Cell Conditioning Solution after deparaffinization. Immunohistochemical staining was performed using an automated immunohistochemical system. The optiViewUniversal DAB detection kit (Ventana Medical Systems) was used for visualization. Cyclin D1 antibody (rabbit monoclonal antibody, clone EP12, DAKO, Denmark) at a dilution of 1:75 with an incubation time of 12 min at a temperature of 37 °C and Ki67 antibody (mouse monoclonal antibody, clone MIB-1, DAKO, Denmark) at a dilution of 1:75 with an incubation time of 16 min at a temperature of 37 °C were both used for immunohistochemical staining. The resulting complex was visualized with hydrogen peroxide and the chromogen DAB, which forms a brown precipitate visible under the light microscope. This was followed by contrasting with hemalaun (1 min) and running through an ascending series of alcohol (70–100%), xylene, and coverslip. Paraffin-embedded tonsil tissue was used as a positive control for cyclin D1 and Ki-67.

4.4. Evaluation of Immunohistochemical Staining

In assessing cell proliferation index (Ki-67) expression, we relied on numerous papers in the literature that set the "cut-off" value at 30% of positively-stained nuclei. We classified lesions with more than 30% positive nuclei as highly proliferative, whereas lesions with less than 30% positive nuclei were classified as weakly to moderately proliferative [91].

Immunohistochemical expression of p53 and cyclin D1 was based on the Allred scoring system combining staining intensity and percentage of positively-stained nuclei [92]. Depending on the percentage of positively-stained nuclei, we divided expression into five categories. We labeled the lesions that did not have a single positively-stained nucleus with number 0 (negative lesions), the percentage of positive nuclei up to 1% with number 1, the percentage of positive nuclei from 1–10% with number 2, the percentage of positive nuclei from 10–33% with number 3, the percentage of positive nuclei from 34–66% with number 4, and number 5 if the lesions had more than 67% positively-stained nuclei. We also divided the intensity of staining into three categories, so that we assigned the number 0 as negative intensity of staining for lesions, in which not a single nucleus was stained under high magnification on the light microscope (×400); the number 1 was assigned for lesions with weak intensity of staining, where the staining is visible only at high magnification (×400); number 2 was assigned for lesions with moderate staining intensity, where the colored lesions are easily visible even at low magnification (×100); and number 3 or strong staining was assigned for lesions where the staining is clearly visible at low magnification. We divided the total sum of values for intensity of nuclear staining (0–3) and the percentage of positively-stained nuclei (0–5) of lesions into three groups: (0)—negative lesions or lesions with weak expression (sum 0–2); (+)—lesions with moderate growth (sum 3–5); and (++)—lesions with strong expression (sum 6–8). To evaluate the immunoreactivity of the ABCG2 protein with an experimental antibody, we used a scoring system previously described by Abdulmajeed [93]. This classification system combined the intensity of staining (0 = no staining to 4 = dark brown staining) and the percentage of positively-stained epithelial cells (0% = score 0; <25% = score 1; 25–49% = score 2; 50–74% = score 3; 75–100% = score 4), and lesions were classified into four groups: (0)—negative lesions; (+)—lesions with weak expression (sum 1–2); (++)—lesions with moderate expression (sum 3–5); and (+++)—lesions with strong expression (sum 6–8). We assessed membrane expression of EGFR according to the work of Cho EY et al.: (0)—no membrane staining or positivity in $\leq$10% of cells; (+) incomplete membrane staining in >10% of cells; (++) weak to moderately complete membrane staining in >10% of cells; and (+++) strong and complete membrane staining in >10% of cells [17]. To quantify nEGFR expression, we used the criteria described by Lo et al. We divided nEGFR immunoreactivity into four groups depending on the percentage of positive cells: (0) no nuclear staining; (+) 1–17% cells with positive nuclear staining; (++) 18–35% of cells with positive nuclear staining; and (+++) > 35% of cells with positive nuclear staining [8].

4.5. Statistical Analysis

Statistical processing of the data was performed with the statistical computer program MedCalc, version 12.5.0 (MedCalc Software, Ostend, Belgium; https://www.medcalc.org, accessed on 15 May 2021), and the results were presented in tables and graphs. Values of continuous variables are presented as mean $\pm$ standard deviation. Categorical (qualitative) data are presented in frequencies and percentages. Analysis of the distribution of the measured variables (Kolmogorov–Smirnov test) determines the difference in the distribution of each variable; the normality of the distribution varies from parameter to parameter, so the one-way ANOVA test (for data with normal distribution) and the nonparametric Kruskal–Wallis method were used to compare more than two groups of subjects. A Student–Newman–Keuls post hoc test was used to test for differences between groups. In addition, the nonparametric Mann–Whitney test was used. Associations (correlations) between individual parameters were examined using the Pearson test or the Spearman test and the regression model, depending on the normality of the data distribution. To test for differences in nominal variables, Fisher's exact test or the χ^2 test was used. In addition, the odds ratio with the confidence interval was calculated for each variable. The relationship between the expression of the analyzed biomarkers and the overall survival of the subjects was assessed by the Kaplan–Meier method, and the difference between the survival curves was determined by the log-rank test. The potential prognostic value of the analyzed biomarkers was determined with the ROC (Receiver Operating Characteristic) analysis. Test results were considered significant when $p \leq 0.05$.

5. Conclusions

The results of this study suggest a possibly important independent role of nEGFR in oral carcinogenesis. Our results point to the importance of identifying molecular markers that help us to identify the size of genetically altered and apparently healthy oral cavity mucosa and to distinguish high-risk patients with premalignant and malignant changes, which could have implications for changing the current treatment approach for these patients.

Author Contributions: Conceptualization, M.T. and I.L.; methodology, M.T., M.R., D.M. and I.L.; software, M.R.; validation, M.R., D.M. and I.L.; formal analysis, M.R.; investigation, M.T., M.R.; resources, I.L. and D.M.; data curation, M.T.; writing—original draft preparation, M.T. and M.R.; writing—review and editing, I.L. and D.M.; visualization, M.T., D.M. and M.R.; supervision, I.L. and D.M.; project administration, M.T. All authors have read and agreed to the published version of the manuscript.

Funding: This research received no external funding.

Institutional Review Board Statement: The study was conducted in accordance with the Declaration of Helsinki and approved by the Institutional Review Board of Dubrava University Hospital, Zagreb (2021/2202-06, 22 February 2021).

Informed Consent Statement: Informed consent was obtained from all subjects involved in the study.

Data Availability Statement: All data generated or analyzed during this study are included in this published article.

Conflicts of Interest: The authors declare no conflict of interest.

References

1. Shah, J.; Patel, S.; Singh, B. *Jatin Shah's Head and Neck Surgery and Oncology*, 4th ed.; Mosby: Maryland Heights, MI, USA, 2019.
2. Sung, H.; Ferlay, J.; Siegel, R.L.; Laversanne, M.; Soerjomataram, I.; Jemal, A.; Bray, F. Global Cancer Statistics 2020: GLOBOCAN Estimates of Incidence and Mortality Worldwide for 36 Cancers in 185 Countries. *CA Cancer J. Clin.* **2021**, *71*, 209–249. [CrossRef] [PubMed]
3. Patel, S.C.; Carpenter, W.R.; Tyree, S.; Couch, M.E.; Weissler, M.; Hackman, T.; Hayes, D.N.; Shores, C.; Chera, B.S. Increasing incidence of oral tongue squamous cell carcinoma in young white women, age 18 to 44 years. *J. Clin. Oncol.* **2011**, *29*, 1488–1494. [CrossRef] [PubMed]
4. Neville, B.W.; Day, T.A. Oral cancer and precancerous lesions. *CA Cancer J. Clin.* **2002**, *52*, 195–215. [CrossRef]
5. Budach, V.; Tinhofer, I. Novel prognostic clinical factors and biomarkers for outcome prediction in head and neck cancer: A systematic review. *Lancet Oncol.* **2019**, *20*, e313–e326. [CrossRef] [PubMed]
6. Hsieh, J.C.; Wang, H.-M.; Wu, M.-H.; Chang, K.-P.; Chang, P.-H.; Liao, C.-T., Liau, C.-T. Review of emerging biomarkers in head and neck squamous cell carcinoma in the era of immunotherapy and targeted therapy. *Head Neck* **2019**, *41* (Suppl. 1), 19–45. [CrossRef]
7. Lin, S.-Y.; Makino, K.; Xia, W.; Matin, A.; Wen, Y.; Kwong, K.Y.; Bourguignon, L.; Hung, M.-C. Nuclear localization of EGF receptor and its potential new role as a transcription factor. *Nature* **2001**, *3*, 802–808. [CrossRef] [PubMed]
8. Lo, H.-W.; Xia, W.; Wei, Y.; Ali-Seyed, M.; Huang, S.-F.; Hung, M.-C. Novel prognostic value of nuclear epidermal growth factor receptor in breast cancer. *Cancer Res* **2005**, *65*, 338–348. [CrossRef]
9. Hanada, N.; Lo, H.-W.; Day, C.-P.; Pan, Y.; Nakajima, Y.; Hung, M.-C. Co-regulation of B-Myb expression by E2F1 and EGF receptor. *Mol. Carcinog.* **2006**, *45*, 10–17. [CrossRef]
10. Hung, L.-Y.; Tseng, J.T.-C.; Lee, Y.-C.; Xia, W.; Wang, Y.-N.; Wu, M.-L.; Chuang, Y.-H.; Lai, C.-H.; Chang, W.-C. Nuclear epidermal growth factor receptor (EGFR) interacts with signal transducer and activator of transcription 5 (STAT5) in activating Aurora-A gene expression. *Nucleic Acids Res.* **2008**, *36*, 4337–4351. [CrossRef]
11. Hadžisejdić, I.; Mustać, E.; Jonjić, N.; Petković, M.; Grahovac, B. Nuclear EGFR in ductal invasive breast cancer: Correlation with cyclin-D1 and prognosis. *Mod. Pathol.* **2010**, *23*, 392–403. [CrossRef]
12. Kamio, T.; Shigematsu, K.; Sou, H.; Kawai, K.; Tsuchiyama, H. Immunohistochemical expression of epidermal growth factor receptors in human adrenocortical carcinoma. *Hum. Pathol.* **1990**, *21*, 277–282. [CrossRef]
13. Lipponen, P.; Eskelinen, M. Expression of epidermal growth factor receptor in bladder cancer as related to established prognostic factors, oncoprotein (c-erbB-2, p53) expression and long-term prognosis. *Br. J. Cancer* **1994**, *69*, 1120–1125. [CrossRef]
14. Psyrri, A.; Yu, Z.; Weinberger, P.M.; Sasaki, C.; Haffty, B.; Camp, R.; Rimm, D.; Burtness, B.A. Quantitative determination of nuclear and cytoplasmic epidermal growth factor receptor expression in oropharyngeal squamous cell cancer by using automated quantitative analysis. *Clin. Cancer Res.* **2005**, *11*, 5856–5862. [CrossRef]

15. Xia, W.; Wei, Y.; Du, Y.; Liu, J.; Chang, B.; Yu, Y.-L.; Huo, L.-F.; Miller, S.; Hung, M.-C. Nuclear expression of epidermal growth factor receptor is a novel prognostic value in patients with ovarian cancer. *Mol. Carcinog.* **2009**, *48*, 610–617. [CrossRef] [PubMed]
16. Marijić, B.; Braut, T.M.; Babarović, E.M.; Krstulja, M.M.; Maržić, D.; Avirović, M.M.; Kujundžić, M.M.; Hadžisejdić, I.M. Nuclear EGFR Expression Is Associated With Poor Survival in Laryngeal Carcinoma. *Appl. Immunohistochem. Mol. Morphol.* **2021**, *29*, 576–584. [CrossRef]
17. Cho, E.Y.; Choi, Y.-L.; Han, J.J.; Kim, K.-M.; Oh, Y.L. Expression and amplification of Her2, EGFR and cyclin D1 in breast cancer: Immunohistochemistry and chromogenic in situ hybridization. *Pathol. Int.* **2008**, *58*, 17–25. [CrossRef]
18. Parakh, M.K.; Ulaganambi, S.; Ashifa, N.; Premkumar, R.; Jain, A.L. Oral potentially malignant disorders: Clinical diagnosis and current screening aids: A narrative review. *Eur. J. Cancer Prev.* **2020**, *29*, 65–72. [CrossRef] [PubMed]
19. Elbehi, A.M.; Anu, R.; Ekine-Afolabi, B.; Cash, E. Emerging role of immune checkpoint inhibitors and predictive biomarkers in head and neck cancers. *Oral Oncol.* **2020**, *109*, 104977. [CrossRef] [PubMed]
20. Farah, C.S. Molecular, genomic and mutational landscape of oral leukoplakia. *Oral Dis.* **2021**, *27*, 803–812. [CrossRef] [PubMed]
21. Ranganathan, K.; Kavitha, L. Oral epithelial dysplasia: Classifications and clinical relevance in risk assessment of oral potentially malignant disorders. *J. Oral Maxillofac. Pathol.* **2019**, *23*, 19–27. [CrossRef] [PubMed]
22. Economopoulou, P.; De Bree, R.; Kotsantis, I.; Psyrri, A. Diagnostic Tumor Markers in Head and Neck Squamous Cell Carcinoma (HNSCC) in the Clinical Setting. *Front. Oncol.* **2019**, *9*, 827. [CrossRef] [PubMed]
23. Li, R.; Koch, W.M.; Fakhry, C.; Gourin, C.G. Distinct Epidemiologic Characteristics of Oral Tongue Cancer Patients. *Otolaryngol. Neck Surg.* **2013**, *148*, 792–796. [CrossRef] [PubMed]
24. Sarode, G.; Maniyar, N.; Sarode, S.C.; Jafer, M.; Patil, S.; Awan, K.H. Epidemiologic aspects of oral cancer. *Dis. Mon.* **2020**, *66*, 100988. [CrossRef] [PubMed]
25. Sorbye, S.W.; Kilvaer, T.K.; Valkov, A.; Donnem, T.; Smeland, E.; Al-Shibli, K.; Bremnes, R.M.; Busund, L.-T. Prognostic Impact of Jab1, p16, p21, p62, Ki67 and Skp2 in Soft Tissue Sarcomas. *PLoS ONE* **2012**, *7*, e47068. [CrossRef] [PubMed]
26. Josefsson, A.; Wikström, P.; Egevad, L.; Granfors, T.; Karlberg, L.; Stattin, P.; Bergh, A. Low endoglin vascular density and Ki67 index in Gleason score 6 tumours may identify prostate cancer patients suitable for surveillance. *Scand. J. Urol. Nephrol.* **2012**, *46*, 247–257. [CrossRef]
27. Ishihara, M.; Mukai, H.; Nagai, S.; Onozawa, M.; Nihei, K.; Shimada, T.; Wada, N. Retrospective analysis of risk factors for central nervous system metastases in operable breast cancer: Effects of biologic subtype and Ki67 overexpression on survival. *Oncology* **2013**, *84*, 135–140. [CrossRef]
28. Jing, Y.; Zhou, Q.; Zhu, H.; Zhang, Y.; Song, Y.; Zhang, X.; Huang, X.; Yang, Y.; Ni, Y.; Hu, Q. Ki-67 is an independent prognostic marker for the recurrence and relapse of oral squamous cell carcinoma. *Oncol. Lett.* **2019**, *17*, 974–980. [CrossRef]
29. Takkem, A.; Barakat, C.; Zakarea, S.; Zaid, K.; Najmeh, J.; Ayoub, M.; Seirawan, M.Y. Ki-67 Prognostic Value in Different Histological Grades of Oral Epithelial Dysplasia and Oral Squamous Cell Carcinoma. *Asian Pac. J. Cancer Prev.* **2018**, *19*, 3279–3286. [CrossRef]
30. Lopes, V.K.M.; de Jesus, A.S.; de Souza, L.L.; Miyahara, L.A.N.; Guimarães, D.M.; Pontes, H.A.R.; Pontes, F.S.C.; de Carvalho, P.L. Ki-67 protein predicts survival in oral squamous carcinoma cells: An immunohistochemical study. *Braz. Oral Res.* **2017**, *31*, e66. [CrossRef]
31. Xie, S.; Liu, Y.; Qiao, X.; Hua, R.-X.; Wang, K.; Shan, X.-F.; Cai, Z.-G. What is the Prognostic Significance of Ki-67 Positivity in Oral Squamous Cell Carcinoma? *J. Cancer* **2016**, *7*, 758–767. [CrossRef]
32. Sharma, S.; Maheshwari, V.; Narula, V.; Verma, S.; Jain, A.; Alam, K. Prognostic and Predictive Impact of Ki-67 in Premalignant and Malignant Squamous Cell Lesions of Oral Cavity. *Int. J. Head Neck Surg.* **2013**, *4*, 61–65. [CrossRef]
33. Mondal, K.; Mandal, R.; Sarkar, B.C. Importance of Ki-67 Labeling in Oral Leukoplakia with Features of Dysplasia and Carcinomatous Transformation: An Observational Study over 4 Years. *South Asian J. Cancer* **2020**, *9*, 099–104. [CrossRef]
34. Dwivedi, N.; Chandra, S.; Kashyap, B.; Raj, V.; Agarwal, A. Suprabasal expression of Ki-67 as a marker for the severity of oral epithelial dysplasia and oral squamous cell carcinoma. *Contemp. Clin. Dent.* **2013**, *4*, 7–12. [CrossRef]
35. Birajdar, S.S.; Radhika, M.; Paremala, K.; Gadivan, M.; Sudhakara, M.; Soumya, M. Expression of Ki-67 in normal oral epithelium, leukoplakic oral epithelium and oral squamous cell carcinoma. *J. Oral Maxillofac. Pathol.* **2014**, *18*, 169–176. [CrossRef]
36. Ozaki, T.; Nakagawara, A. Role of p53 in Cell Death and Human Cancers. *Cancers* **2011**, *3*, 994–1013. [CrossRef]
37. Renzi, A.; De Bonis, P.; Morandi, L.; Lenzi, J.; Tinto, D.; Rigillo, A.; Bettini, G.; Bellei, E.; Sabattini, S. Prevalence of p53 dysregulations in feline oral squamous cell carcinoma and non-neoplastic oral mucosa. *PLoS ONE* **2019**, *14*, e0215621. [CrossRef] [PubMed]
38. Tandon, S.; Tudur-Smith, C.; Riley, R.D.; Boyd, M.T.; Jones, T.M. A systematic review of p53 as a prognostic factor of survival in squamous cell carcinoma of the four main anatomical subsites of the head and neck. *Cancer Epidemiol. Biomark. Prev.* **2010**, *19*, 574–587. [CrossRef]
39. Banerjee, R.; Van Tubergen, E.A.; Scanlon, C.S.; Broek, R.V.; Lints, J.P.; Liu, M.; Russo, N.; Inglehart, R.C.; Wang, Y.; Polverini, P.J.; et al. The G protein–coupled receptor GALR2 promotes angiogenesis in head and neck cancer. *Mol. Cancer Ther.* **2014**, *13*, 1323–1333. [CrossRef] [PubMed]

40. Kanazawa, T.; Misawa, K.; Misawa, Y.; Maruta, M.; Uehara, T.; Kawada, K.; Nagatomo, T.; Ichimura, K. Galanin receptor 2 utilizes distinct signaling pathways to suppress cell proliferation and induce apoptosis in HNSCC. *Mol. Med. Rep.* **2014**, *10*, 1289–1294. [CrossRef] [PubMed]
41. Khan, Z.; Tiwari, R.P.; Mulherkar, R.; Sah, N.K.; Prasad, G.B.K.S.; Shrivastava, B.R.; Bisen, P.S. Detection of survivin and p53 in human oral cancer: Correlation with clinicopathologic findings. *Head Neck* **2009**, *31*, 1039–1048. [CrossRef]
42. Ögmundsdóttir, H.M.; Björnsson, J.; Holbrook, W.P. Role of TP53 in the progression of pre-malignant and malignant oral mucosal lesions. A follow-up study of 144 patients. *J. Oral Pathol. Med.* **2009**, *38*, 565–571. [CrossRef] [PubMed]
43. Baldin, V.; Lukas, J.; Marcote, M.J.; Pagano, M.; Draetta, G. Cyclin D1 is a nuclear protein required for cell cycle progression in G1. *Genes Dev.* **1993**, *7*, 812–821. [CrossRef]
44. Bartkova, J.; Lukas, J.; Strauss, M.; Bartek, J. Cyclin D1 oncoprotein aberrantly accumulates in malignancies of diverse histogenesis. *Oncogene* **1995**, *10*, 775–778. [PubMed]
45. Fu, M.; Wang, C.; Li, Z.; Sakamaki, T.; Pestell, R.G. Minireview: Cyclin D1: Normal and Abnormal Functions. *Endocrinology* **2004**, *145*, 5439–5447. [CrossRef]
46. Binabaj, M.M.; Bahrami, A.; Khazaei, M.; Ryzhikov, M.; Ferns, G.A.; Avan, A.; Hassanian, S.M. The prognostic value of cyclin D1 expression in the survival of cancer patients: A meta-analysis. *Gene* **2020**, *728*, 144283. [CrossRef]
47. Moharil, R.B.; Khandekar, S.; Dive, A.; Bodhade, A. Cyclin D1 in oral premalignant lesions and oral squamous cell carcinoma: An immunohistochemical study. *J. Oral Maxillofac. Pathol.* **2020**, *24*, 397. [CrossRef] [PubMed]
48. de Vicente, J.C.; Herrero-Zapatero, A.; Fresno, M.F.; López-Arranz, J.S. Expression of cyclin D1 and Ki-67 in squamous cell carcinoma of the oral cavity: Clinicopathological and prognostic significance. *Oral Oncol.* **2002**, *38*, 301–308. [CrossRef] [PubMed]
49. Gupta, S.; Khan, H.; Husain, N.; Misra, S.; Singh, N.; Negi, M. Prognostics of Cyclin-D1 expression with chemoradiation response in patients of locally advanced oral squamous cell carcinoma. *J. Cancer Res. Ther.* **2014**, *10*, 258–264. [CrossRef]
50. Guimaraes, E.; De Carli, M.; Sperandio, F.; Hanemann, J.; Pereira, A. Cyclin D1 and Ki-67 expression correlates to tumor staging in tongue squamous cell carcinoma. *Med. Oral Patol. Oral Cir. Bucal.* **2015**, *20*, e657–e663. [CrossRef]
51. Zhao, Y.; Yu, D.; Li, H.; Nie, P.; Zhu, Y.; Liu, S.; Zhu, M.; Fang, B. Cyclin D1 overexpression is associated with poor clinicopathological outcome and survival in oral squamous cell carcinoma in asian populations: Insights from a meta-analysis. *PLoS ONE* **2014**, *9*, e93210. [CrossRef]
52. Wang, L.; Liu, T.; Nishioka, M.; Aguirre, R.L.; Win, S.S.; Okada, N. Activation of ERK1/2 and cyclin D1 expression in oral tongue squamous cell carcinomas: Relationship between clinicopathological appearances and cell proliferation. *Oral Oncol.* **2006**, *42*, 625–631. [CrossRef]
53. Noorlag, R.; Van Kempen, P.M.W.; Stegeman, I.; Koole, R.; Van Es, R.J.J.; Willems, S.M. The diagnostic value of 11q13 amplification and protein expression in the detection of nodal metastasis from oral squamous cell carcinoma: A systematic review and meta-analysis. *Virchows Arch.* **2015**, *466*, 363–373. [CrossRef] [PubMed]
54. Huang, S.-F.; Cheng, S.-D.; Chuang, W.-Y.; Chen, I.-H.; Liao, C.-T.; Wang, H.-M.; Hsieh, L.-L. Cyclin D1 overexpression and poor clinical outcomes in Taiwanese oral cavity squamous cell carcinoma. *World J. Surg. Oncol.* **2012**, *10*, 40. [CrossRef] [PubMed]
55. Lam, K.Y.; Ng, I.O.L.; Yuen, A.P.W.; Kwong, R.L.W.; Wei, W. Cyclin D1 expression in oral squamous cell carcinomas: Clinicopathological relevance and correlation with p53 expression. *J. Oral Pathol. Med.* **2000**, *29*, 167–172. [CrossRef]
56. Saawarn, S.; Astekar, M.; Saawarn, N.; Dhakar, N.; Sagari, S.G. Cyclin D1 Expression and Its Correlation with Histopathological Differentiation in Oral Squamous Cell Carcinoma. *Sci. World J.* **2012**, *2012*, 978327. [CrossRef]
57. Angadi, P.V.; Krishnapillai, R. Cyclin D1 expression in oral squamous cell carcinoma and verrucous carcinoma: Correlation with histological differentiation. *Oral Surg. Oral Med. Oral Pathol. Oral Radiol. Endodontol.* **2007**, *103*, e30–e35. [CrossRef]
58. Mishra, R.; Das, B.R. Cyclin D1 expression and its possible regulation in chewing tobacco mediated oral squamous cell carcinoma progression. *Arch. Oral Biol.* **2009**, *54*, 917–923. [CrossRef] [PubMed]
59. Mallya, S.M.; Woods, M.; Pant, R. Cyclin D1 and cyclin D-dependent kinases enhance oral keratinocyte proliferation but do not block keratinocyte differentiation. *Int. J. Oncol.* **2010**, *37*, 1471–1475. [CrossRef] [PubMed]
60. Ohnishi, Y.; Watanabe, M.; Wato, M.; Tanaka, A.; Kakudo, K.; Nozaki, M. Cyclin D1 expression is correlated with cell differentiation and cell proliferation in oral squamous cell carcinomas. *Oncol. Lett.* **2014**, *7*, 1123–1127. [CrossRef]
61. Tamatani, T.; Takamaru, N.; Ohe, G.; Akita, K.; Nakagawa, T.; Miyamoto, Y. Expression of CD44, CD44v9, ABCG2, CD24, Bmi-1 and ALDH1 in stage I and II oral squamous cell carcinoma and their association with clinicopathological factors. *Oncol. Lett.* **2018**, *16*, 1133–1140. [CrossRef]
62. Shi, P.; Liu, W.; Zhou, Z.-T.; He, Q.-B.; Jiang, W.-W. Podoplanin and ABCG2: Malignant Transformation Risk Markers for Oral Lichen Planus. *Cancer Epidemiol. Biomark. Prev.* **2010**, *19*, 844–849. [CrossRef] [PubMed]
63. Feng, J.-Q.; Mi, J.-G.; Wu, L.; Ma, L.-W.; Shi, L.-J.; Yang, X.; Liu, W.; Zhang, C.-P.; Zhou, Z.-T. Expression of podoplanin and ABCG2 in oral erythroplakia correlate with oral cancer development. *Oral Oncol.* **2012**, *48*, 848–852. [CrossRef]
64. Diestra, J.E.; Scheffer, G.L.; Català, I.; Maliepaard, M.; Schellens, J.H.M.; Scheper, R.J.; Germà-Lluch, J.R.; Izquierdo, M.A. Frequent expression of the multi-drug resistance-associated protein BCRP/MXR/ABCP/ABCG2 in human tumours detected by the BXP-21 monoclonal antibody in paraffin-embedded material. *J. Pathol.* **2002**, *198*, 213–219. [CrossRef]
65. Mo, W.; Zhang, J.T. Human ABCG2: Structure, function, and its role in multidrug resistance. *Int. J. Biochem. Mol. Biol.* **2012**, *3*, 1–27.

66. Zhou, S.; Schuetz, J.D.; Bunting, K.D.; Colapietro, A.M.; Sampath, J.; Morris, J.J.; Lagutina, I.; Grosveld, G.C.; Osawa, M.; Nakauchi, H.; et al. The ABC transporter Bcrp1/ABCG2 is expressed in a wide variety of stem cells and is a molecular determinant of the side-population phenotype. *Nat. Med.* **2001**, *7*, 1028–1034. [CrossRef] [PubMed]
67. Bhatia, P.; Bernier, M.; Sanghvi, M.; Moaddel, R.; Schwarting, R.; Ramamoorthy, A.; Wainer, I.W. Breast cancer resistance protein (BCRP/ABCG2) localises to the nucleus in glioblastoma multiforme cells. *Xenobiotica* **2012**, *42*, 748–755. [CrossRef]
68. Liang, S.-C.; Yang, C.-Y.; Tseng, J.-Y.; Wang, H.-L.; Tung, C.-Y.; Liu, H.-W.; Chen, C.-Y.; Yeh, Y.-C.; Chou, T.-Y.; Yang, M.-H.; et al. ABCG2 Localizes to the Nucleus and Modulates CDH1 Expression in Lung Cancer Cells. *Neoplasia* **2015**, *17*, 265–278. [CrossRef]
69. Triaca, V.; Fico, E.; Rosso, P.; Ralli, M.; Corsi, A.; Severini, C.; Crevenna, A.; Agostinelli, E.; Rullo, E.; Riminucci, M.; et al. Pilot Investigation on p75ICD Expression in Laryngeal Squamous Cell Carcinoma. *Cancers* **2022**, *14*, 2622. [CrossRef] [PubMed]
70. Yanamoto, S.; Yamada, S.-I.; Takahashi, H.; Naruse, T.; Matsushita, Y.; Ikeda, H.; Shiraishi, T.; Seki, S.; Fujita, S.; Ikeda, T.; et al. Expression of the cancer stem cell markers CD44v6 and ABCG2 in tongue cancer: Effect of neoadjuvant chemotherapy on local recurrence. *Int. J. Oncol.* **2014**, *44*, 1153–1162. [CrossRef] [PubMed]
71. Cognetti, D.M.; Weber, R.S.; Lai, S.Y. Head and neck cancer: An evolving treatment paradigm. *Cancer* **2008**, *113*, 1911–1932. [CrossRef]
72. Kalyankrishna, S.; Grandis, J.R. Epidermal growth factor receptor biology in head and neck cancer. *J. Clin. Oncol.* **2006**, *24*, 2666–2672. [CrossRef]
73. Bauml, J.M.; Vinnakota, R.; Park, Y.A.; Bates, S.E.; Fojo, T.; Aggarwal, C.; Di Stefano, J.; Knepley, C.; Limaye, S.; Mamtani, R.; et al. Cisplatin versus cetuximab with definitive concurrent radiotherapy for head and neck squamous cell carcinoma: An analysis of Veterans Health Affairs data. *Cancer* **2019**, *125*, 406–415. [CrossRef]
74. Gillison, M.L.; Trotti, A.M.; Harris, J.; Eisbruch, A.; Harari, P.M.; Adelstein, D.J.; Jordan, R.C.K.; Zhao, W.; Sturgis, E.M.; Burtness, B.; et al. Radiotherapy plus cetuximab or cisplatin in human papillomavirus-positive oropharyngeal cancer (NRG Oncology RTOG 1016): A randomised, multicentre, non-inferiority trial. *Lancet* **2019**, *393*, 40–50. [CrossRef]
75. Burdick, J.S.; Chung, E.; Tanner, G.; Sun, M.; Paciga, J.E.; Cheng, J.Q.; Washington, K.; Goldenring, J.R.; Coffey, R.J. Treatment of Ménétrier's Disease with a Monoclonal Antibody against the Epidermal Growth Factor Receptor. *N. Engl. J. Med.* **2000**, *343*, 1697–1701. [CrossRef] [PubMed]
76. Sigismund, S.; Avanzato, D.; Lanzetti, L. Emerging functions of theEGFRin cancer. *Mol. Oncol.* **2018**, *12*, 3–20. [CrossRef]
77. Mirza, Y.; Ali, S.M.A.; Awan, M.S.; Idress, R.; Naeem, S.; Zahid, N.; Qadeer, U. Overexpression of EGFR in Oral Premalignant Lesions and OSCC and Its Impact on Survival and Recurrence. *Oncomedicine* **2018**, *3*, 28–36. [CrossRef]
78. Singla, S.; Singla, G.; Zaheer, S.; Rawat, D.S.; Mandal, A.K. Expression of p53, epidermal growth factor receptor, c-erbB2 in oral leukoplakias and oral squamous cell carcinomas. *J. Cancer Res. Ther.* **2018**, *14*, 388–393. [CrossRef]
79. Ries, J.; Vairaktaris, E.; Agaimy, A.; Bechtold, M.; Gorecki, P.; Neukam, F.W.; Nkenke, E. The relevance of EGFR overexpression for the prediction of the malignant transformation of oral leukoplakia. *Oncol. Rep.* **2013**, *30*, 1149–1156. [CrossRef]
80. Swaminathan, U.; Joshua, E.; Rao, U.K.; Ranganathan, K. Expression of p53 and Cyclin D1 in oral squamous cell carcinoma and normal mucosa: An Immunohistochemical study. *J. Oral Maxillofac. Pathol.* **2012**, *16*, 172–177. [CrossRef] [PubMed]
81. Kaur, J.; Srivastava, A.; Ralhan, R. Overexpression of p53 protein in betel- and tobacco-related human oral dysplasia and squamous-cell carcinoma in India. *Int. J. Cancer* **1994**, *58*, 340–345. [CrossRef] [PubMed]
82. Kerdpon, D.; Rich, A.M.; Reade, P.C. Expression of p53 in oral mucosal hyperplasia, dysplasia and squamous cell carcinoma. *Oral Dis.* **1997**, *3*, 86–92. [CrossRef]
83. Liu, K.; Jiang, T.; Ouyang, Y.; Shi, Y.; Zang, Y.; Li, N.; Lu, S.; Chen, D. Nuclear EGFR impairs ASPP2-p53 complex-induced apoptosis by inducing SOS1 expression in hepatocellular carcinoma. *Oncotarget* **2015**, *6*, 16507–16516. [CrossRef]
84. Ghorbanpour, M.; Shahsavari, F.; Miri, R. Expression of epidermal growth factor receptor in oral and esophageal squamous-cell carcinoma. *Dent. Res. J.* **2020**, *17*, 85. [CrossRef]
85. Costa, V.; Kowalski, L.; Coutinho-Camillo, C.; Begnami, M.; Calsavara, V.; Neves, J.; Kaminagakura, E. EGFR amplification and expression in oral squamous cell carcinoma in young adults. *Int. J. Oral Maxillofac. Surg.* **2018**, *47*, 817–823. [CrossRef] [PubMed]
86. Abbas, E.A.; Abdel-Aal, W.E.; Samy, A.A. Evaluation Of Transforming Growth Factor (Tgf-) And Epidermal Growth Factor Receptor (Egfr) Expression In Oral Squamous Cell Carcinoma. *Egypt. J. Hosp. Med.* **2002**, *7*, 168–176. [CrossRef]
87. Brands, M.T.; Smeekens, E.A.J.; Takes, R.P.; Kaanders, J.H.A.M.; Verbeek, A.L.M.; Merkx, M.A.W.; Geurts, S.M.E. Time patterns of recurrence and second primary tumors in a large cohort of patients treated for oral cavity cancer. *Cancer Med.* **2019**, *8*, 5810–5819. [CrossRef]
88. Schmidt-Ullrich, R.K.; Valerie, K.; Fogleman, P.B.; Walters, J. Radiation-induced autophosphorylation of epidermal growth factor receptor in human malignant mammary and squamous epithelial cells. *Radiat. Res.* **1996**, *145*, 81–85. [CrossRef]
89. Dittmann, K.; Mayer, C.; Fehrenbacher, B.; Schaller, M.; Raju, U.; Milas, L.; Chen, D.J.; Kehlbach, R.; Rodemann, H.P. Radiation-induced epidermal growth factor receptor nuclear import is linked to activation of DNA-dependent protein kinase. *J. Biol. Chem.* **2005**, *280*, 31182–31189. [CrossRef]
90. da Silva, L.A.B.; Lopes, M.L.D.D.S.; Sá, M.C.; Freitas, R.D.A.; Della Coletta, R.; da Silveira, E.J.D.; Miguel, M.C.D.C. Histopathologic grading and its relationship with outcome in oral tongue squamous cell carcinoma. *J. Oral Pathol. Med.* **2021**, *50*, 183–190. [CrossRef]

91. Elsheikh, S.; Green, A.R.; Aleskandarany, M.A.; Grainge, M.; Paish, C.E.; Lambros, M.B.K.; Reis-Filho, J.S.; Ellis, I.O. CCND1 amplification and cyclin D1 expression in breast cancer and their relation with proteomic subgroups and patient outcome. *Breast Cancer Res. Treat.* **2008**, *109*, 325–335. [CrossRef]
92. Zhang, Y.-Y.; Xu, Z.-N.; Wang, J.-X.; Wei, D.-M.; Pan, X.-L. G1/S-specific cyclin-D1 might be a prognostic biomarker for patients with laryngeal squamous cell carcinoma. *Asian Pac. J. Cancer Prev.* **2012**, *13*, 2133–2137. [CrossRef] [PubMed]
93. AbdulMajeed, A.A.; Dalley, A.J.; Farah, C.S. Putative cancer stem cell marker expression in oral epithelial dysplasia and squamous cell carcinoma. *J. Oral Pathol. Med.* **2013**, *42*, 755–760. [CrossRef] [PubMed]

International Journal of *Molecular Sciences*

MDPI

Article

Prognostic and Clinicopathological Significance of Epidermal Growth Factor Receptor (EGFR) Expression in Oral Squamous Cell Carcinoma: Systematic Review and Meta-Analysis

José Luis Cívico-Ortega [1,2], Isabel González-Ruiz [3], Pablo Ramos-García [1,2,*], David Cruz-Granados [1,2], Valerie Samayoa-Descamps [1,2] and Miguel Ángel González-Moles [1,2,*]

1 School of Dentistry, University of Granada, 18071 Granada, Spain; josecivico88@correo.ugr.es (J.L.C.-O.); dacruzgr@correo.ugr.es (D.C.-G.); vasamayoa@correo.ugr.es (V.S.-D.)
2 Instituto de Investigación Biosanitaria ibs.GRANADA, 18012 Granada, Spain
3 Hospital Universitario San Juan de Reus, CAP Marià Fortuny, 43204 Tarragona, Spain; isagonzru@gmail.com
* Correspondence: pabloramos@ugr.es (P.R.-G.); magonzal@ugr.es (M.Á.G.-M.)

Abstract: The aim of this systematic review and meta-analysis was to evaluate the current evidence in relation to the clinicopathological and prognostic significance of epidermal growth factor receptor (EGFR) overexpression in patients with oral squamous cell carcinoma (OSCC). We searched MEDLINE/PubMed, Embase, Web of Science, and Scopus for studies published before November 2022. We evaluated the quality of primary-level studies using the QUIPS tool, conducted meta-analyses, examined inter-study heterogeneity via subgroup analyses and meta-regressions, and performed small-study effects analyses. Fifty primary-level studies (4631 patients) met the inclusion criteria. EGFR overexpression was significantly associated with poor overall survival (hazard ratio [HR] = 1.38, 95% confidence intervals [CI] = 1.06–1.79, p = 0.02), N+ status (odds ratio [OR] = 1.37, 95%CI = 1.01–1.86, p = 0.04), and moderately–poorly differentiated OSCC (OR = 1.43, 95% CI = 1.05–1.94, p = 0.02). In addition, better results were obtained by the application of a cutoff point ≥10% tumor cells with EGFR overexpression (p < 0.001). In conclusion, our systematic review and meta-analysis supports that the immunohistochemical assessment of EGFR overexpression may be useful as a prognostic biomarker for OSCC.

Keywords: epidermal growth factor receptor; EGFR; oral cancer; prognosis; systematic review; meta-analysis

Citation: Cívico-Ortega, J.L.; González-Ruiz, I.; Ramos-García, P.; Cruz-Granados, D.; Samayoa-Descamps, V.; González-Moles, M.Á. Prognostic and Clinicopathological Significance of Epidermal Growth Factor Receptor (EGFR) Expression in Oral Squamous Cell Carcinoma: Systematic Review and Meta-Analysis. *Int. J. Mol. Sci.* **2023**, *24*, 11888. https://doi.org/10.3390/ijms241511888

Academic Editors: Marko Tarle and Ivica Lukšić

Received: 21 June 2023
Revised: 14 July 2023
Accepted: 18 July 2023
Published: 25 July 2023

1. Introduction

The global incidence of oral cancer is estimated to be 377,713 new cases per year, resulting in approximately 177,757 deaths, according to recent statistics from GLOBOCAN (IARC, WHO) [1]. Among all oral malignancies, oral squamous cell carcinoma (OSCC) accounts for approximately 90%, with a 5-year mortality rate approaching 50%. In the year 2000, Hanahan and Weinberg [2] introduced a set of distinctive characteristics that malignant neoplastic cells are expected to possess, irrespective of the tissue of tumor origin. This proposal has been designated as hallmarks of cancer, and was later updated and improved with new characteristics [3], which overall consist of sustaining proliferative signaling, evading growth suppressors, resistance to cell death, enabling replicative immortality, angiogenesis, activating invasion and metastasis, deregulating cellular energetics, and avoiding immune destruction, as well as two enabling characteristics, genome instability and mutation and tumor-promoting inflammation. The proposal of cancer hallmarks has had an enormous impact and influence on the scientific community and on the development of emerging lines of research in order to evaluate biomarkers in different cancers for diagnostic, prognostic, or treatment purposes. It should be noted, however, that limited evidence on the implications of these distinctive features in oral cancer is available to date [4].

Among these hallmarks of cancer, the ability of sustaining proliferative signaling is of remarkable relevance in oral oncogenesis [2,3], and in this regard, the epidermal growth factor receptor (EGFR) has received singular attention, having been extensively studied [5]. EGFR, also known as ErbB1/HER1, is the prototypical receptor of the EGFR tyrosine kinase receptors family, which also includes ErbB2/HER2/Neu, ErbB3/HER3, and ErbB4/HER4 [6]. The most recognized ligand of EGFR is EGF, although the receptor can also be activated by ligands such as TGF-α or HB-EGF, among others [7]. The preceding ligands appear to activate EGFR by the same mechanism of ligand binding, with receptor dimerization and recruitment of other signaling proteins [8]. The receptor can be constitutively activated by gene amplification or mutations, leading to a complex EGFR-mediated signal transduction with regulation of downstream molecular signaling pathways, being the most relevant MAPK (ras-Raf-MEK-Erk) and PI3K (PI3k-Akt-mTor) [9]. These pathways culminate in cell proliferation stimulating actions through the activation of transcription factors with upregulation of important oncogenes (*CCND1*/cyclin D1) among the most relevant [10,11]). EGFR overexpression has been considered a poor prognostic factor in cancers of the head and neck, esophagus, ovary, uterine cervix, and bladder through primary-level studies [12–16]. Moreover, the relevant oncogenic implications of EGFR have justified its consideration as a molecular target, cetuximab being the first monoclonal antibody to be approved by the FDA for the treatment of head and neck cancer [17].

Despite the relevance of EGFR, it seems surprising that there are no published evidence-based results through systematic reviews and meta-analyses specifically designed for oral cancer to date. Therefore, based on this background, our aim was to qualitatively and quantitatively evaluate the prognostic and clinicopathologic implications of EGFR overexpression in patients with OSCC.

2. Results

2.1. Results of the Literature Search

The flow diagram in Figure 1 depicts the process of identification, screening, and selection of primary-level studies. A total of 12,801 records were retrieved: 2415 from Embase, 5576 from Web of Science, 1618 from Scopus, and 3192 from PubMed. After duplicate removal, 6041 records were screened according to titles and abstracts, leaving a sample of 197 papers for full text evaluation (the studies excluded and their exclusion criteria were listed in the Supplementary Information). Finally, 50 primary-level studies meeting all eligibility criteria were included for qualitative evaluation and meta-analysis [18–67].

2.2. Study Characteristics

Table 1 summarizes the main characteristics of our study sample, and Table S2 (Supplementary Information) exhibits in detail the variables gathered from primary-level studies. These 50 studies, recruiting a total of 4631 patients (range: 9–429 patients), were published between 1988 and 2022. All studies were observational retrospective cohorts and applied immunohistochemistry in order to assess EGFR overexpression (n = 50, respectively). In relation to the experimental methods, the use of anti-EGFR antibodies was heterogeneous, the most used being Clone 31G7 (n = 6), Clone 2-18C9 (n = 5), D38B1 (n = 4), and Clone H11 (n = 4), with a dominant use of a cut point equal to 10% (n = 14) analyzed in the cell membrane (n = 29). A total of 16 studies processed their antibodies at dilutions <1:100, while 16 >1:100 and were incubated overnight (n = 12) or 1 h (n = 9), at 4 °C (n = 11) or room temperature (n = 9).

2.3. Qualitative Evaluation

The qualitative analysis was conducted using the QUIPS tool (Figure 2), which evaluates potential sources of bias in six domains:

Study participation. The risk of this bias was high in 78.00% of the reviewed studies, moderate in 16.00%, and low in 6.00%. Studies often did not report relevant data on the cohorts of oral cancer patients under study (e.g., alcohol and tobacco use, period and place of recruitment, etc.).

Study attrition. The risk of this bias was high in 42.00% of the studies, moderate in 2.00%, and low in 14.00%. The lack of reporting of essential data on patients' follow-up periods was also a common finding (total months, average periods, etc.).

Prognostic factor measurement. RoB was high in 44.00% of the studies, moderate in 14.00%, and low in 42.00%. Failure to report data important to the performance and repeatability of experimental methods (e.g., anti-EGFR antibodies, dilution, temperature, or incubation time) was frequent across the studies.

Outcome measurement. RoB was high in 14.29% of the studies, moderate in 28.57%, and low in 57.14%. Several studies do not clearly communicate the TNM staging system used, subject to periodic changes, or the clear definition of the survival endpoints under investigation, which are not standardized and currently lack international consensus.

Study confounding. RoB was high in 86.00% of the studies, moderate in 10.00%, and low in 4.00%. Relevant potentially confounding variables were frequently not taken into consideration in the study design, such as gender, age, or even relevant clinicopathological variables like histological grade or clinical stage with well-known prognostic value.

Statistical analysis and reporting. RoB was high in 76.00% of the studies, moderate in 4.00%, and low in 20.00%. Frequently, survival analyses did not report essential metrics such as hazards ratios with confidence intervals. More serious problems were linked to inappropriate statistical analyses, leading to erroneous results and conclusions.

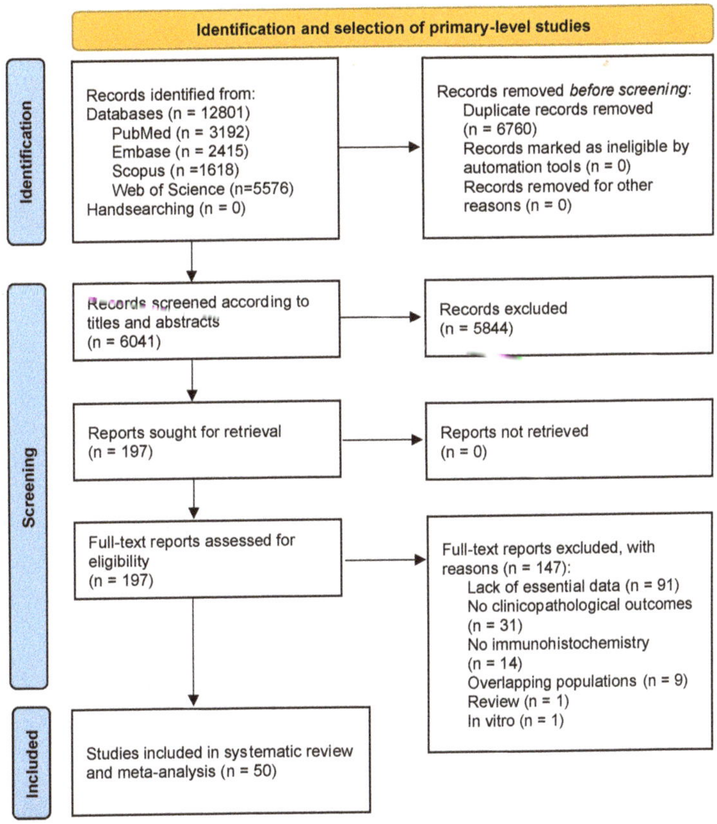

Figure 1. Flow diagram showing the identification and selection process of relevant studies, analyzing the prognostic and clinicopathological significance of EGFR overexpression in OSCC.

Table 1. Summarized study characteristics.

Summarized Characteristics of the Study Sample	
Total	50 studies
Year of publication	1988–2022
Total patients (range)	4631 (9—429)
Study design	
Retrospective cohort	50 studies
Experimental methods for EGFR expression determination	
Immunohistochemistry	50 studies
Anti-EGFR antibody	
Clone 31G7	6 studies
Clone 2-18C9	5 studies
Clone H11	4 studies
D38B1	4 studies
Clone 25	2 studies
Clone EP-22	2 studies
sc-03	2 studies
Ab-1	1 study
Ab-4	1 study
Clone 111.6	1 study
Clone 29.1	1 study
Clone 5B7	1 study
Clone SP9	1 study
E30	1 study
HPA018530	1 study
RPN 513	1 study
sc-003	1 study
Not reported	15 studies
Anti-EGFR antibody dilution	
>1:100	16 studies
<1:100	16 studies
Not reported	18 studies
Anti-EGFR antibody incubation time	
Overnight	12 studies
1 h	9 studies
Other	6 studies
Not reported	23 studies
Anti-EGFR antibody incubation temperature	
4 °C	11 studies
Room temperature	9 studies
Not reported	30 studies
Cut-off point	
>10	5 studies
10	14 studies
0	4 studies
Intensity-based	25 studies
Not reported	2 studies
Immunostaining pattern	
Membrane	29 studies
Membrane-cytoplasm	12 studies
Membrane-cytoplasm-nucleus	1 study
Not reported	8 studies
Geographical region	
Asian countries	20 studies
Non-Asian countries	30 studies

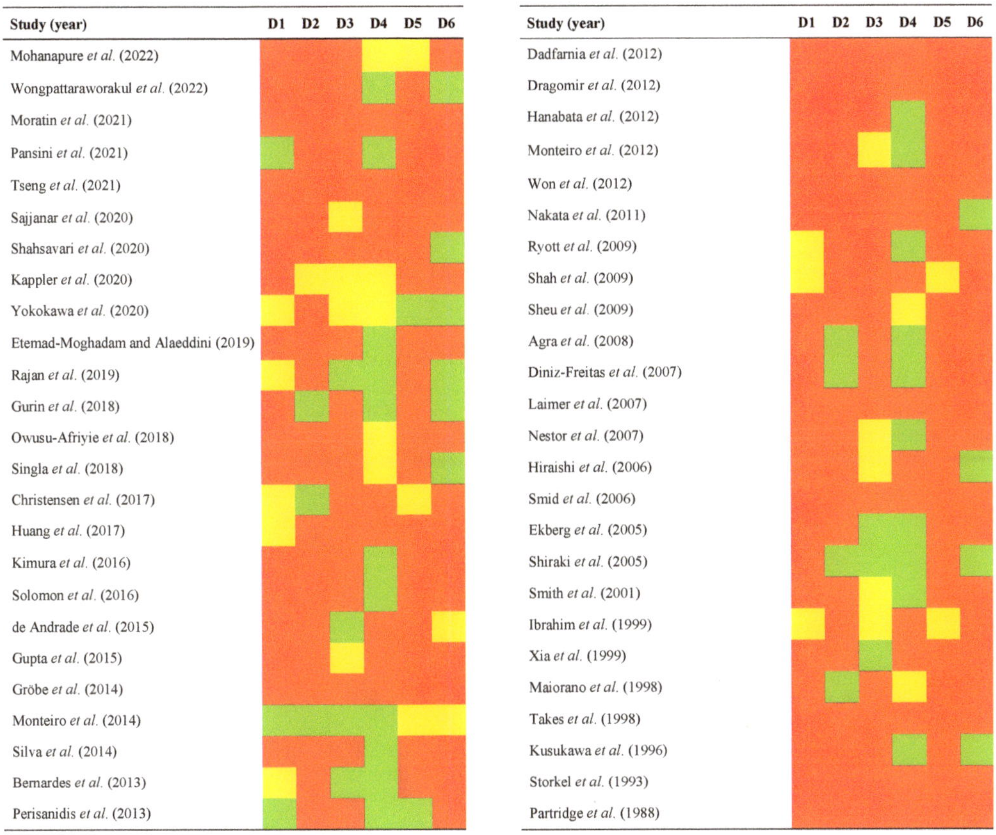

Figure 2. Quality plot graphically representing the risk of bias (RoB) across primary-level studies using a method specifically designed for systematic reviews and meta-analyses addressing questions on prognostic factor studies (i.e., Quality in Prognosis Studies -QUIPS- tool, developed by members of the Cochrane Prognosis Methods Group [68]). The following domains (D1–D6) were critically judged: D1, study participation; D2, study attrition; D3, prognostic factor measurement; D4, outcome measurement; D5, study confounding; and D6, statistical analysis/reporting. RoB was assessed for all domains throughout all studies and scored as potentially low (depicted as green color), moderate (yellow color), or high (red color) [18–67].

2.4. *Quantitative Evaluation (Meta-Analysis)*

2.4.1. Association between EGFR Overexpression and Prognostic Variables

Overall survival (OS). EGFR overexpression was significantly associated with a poor survival rate in patients with OSCC (HR = 1.38, 95%CI = 1.06–1.79, $p = 0.001$), and considerable statistical heterogeneity was present ($p < 0.001$, $I^2 = 77.7\%$) (Table 2, Figure 3). This result was derived from a meta-analyzed sample of 19 out of the 50 (38.00%) primary-level studies included in the present systematic review.

Table 2. Meta-analyses of prognostic and clinicopathological significance of EGFR overexpression in OSCC.

Meta-Analyses	No. of Studies	No. of Patients	Stat. Model	Wt	Pooled Data		Heterogeneity	
					ES (95% CI)	*p*-Value	P_{het}	I^2 (%)
SURVIVAL PARAMETERS								
Overall survival								
EGFR overexpression (all) [a]	19	2256	REM	D-L	HR = 1.38 (1.06–1.79)	0.02	<0.001	77.7
Subgroup analysis by geographical area [b]								
Asian	8	1053	REM	D-L	HR = 1.79 (0.89–3.58)	0.10	<0.001	84.2
Non-Asian	11	1203	REM	D-L	HR = 1.20 (0.95–1.52)	0.12	0.01	57.0
Subgroup analysis by anti-EGFR antibody dilution [b]								
>100	6	743	REM	D-L	HR = 1.56 (1.04–2.33)	0.03	<0.001	80.2
<100	6	689	REM	D-L	HR = 1.59 (1.21–2.11)	0.001	0.60	0.0
Not reported	7	824	REM	D-L	HR = 0.95 (0.44–2.03)	0.89	<0.001	85.3
Subgroup analysis by anti-EGFR antibody incubation time [b]								
1 h	1	208	—	—	HR = 2.75 (1.26–6.01)	0.01	—	0.0
Overnight	5	616	REM	D-L	HR = 0.86 (0.40–1.83)	0.70	<0.001	84.7
Other	4	506	REM	D-L	HR = 1.96 (0.93–4.10)	0.08	0.004	77.9
Not reported	9	926	REM	D-L	HR = 1.52 (1.04–2.22)	0.03	<0.001	73.8
Subgroup analysis by anti-EGFR antibody incubation temperature[b]								
4 °C	4	451	REM	D-L	HR = 0.79 (0.28–2.23)	0.65	<0.001	88.2
Room temperature	4	523	REM	D-L	HR = 2.93 (1.16–7.38)	0.02	0.004	77.5
Not reported	11	1282	REM	D-L	HR = 1.38 (1.04–1.82)	0.02	0.001	67.6
Subgroup analysis by anti-EGFR antibody [b]								
Clone 111.6	1	135	—	—	HR = 1.92 (0.95–3.86)	0.07	—	0.0
Clone 2-18C9	1	63	—	—	HR = 2.44 (0.66–8.96)	0.18	—	0.0
Clone 25	1	135	—	—	HR = 1.60 (0.97–2.64)	0.07	—	0.0
Clone 29.1	1	100	—	—	HR = 6.89 (0.88–53.97)	0.07	—	0.0
Clone 31G7	2	204	REM	D-L	HR = 2.12 (1.26–3.59)	0.005	0.51	0.0
Clone 5B7	1	77	—	—	HR = 2.71 (1.41–5.21)	0.003	—	0.0
Clone EP-22	1	120	—	—	HR = 0.15 (0.06–0.35)	<0.001	—	0.0
Clone H11	2	284	REM	D-L	HR = 1.33 (1.01–1.76)	0.05	0.76	0.0
D38B1	2	253	REM	D-L	HR = 2.05 (1.00–4.17)	0.05	0.26	22.0
E30	1	56	—	—	HR = 0.74 (0.38–1.44)	0.37	—	0.0
sc-003	1	111	—	—	HR = 18.67 (4.02–86.66)	<0.001	—	0.0
sc-03	1	140	—	—	HR = 1.65 (0.83–3.29)	0.15	—	0.0
Not reported	4	578	REM	D-L	HR = 0.99 (0–85–1.16)	0.93	0.31	15.5
Subgroup analysis by cut-off point [b]								
10	7	704	REM	D-L	HR = 1.62 (1.24–2.11)	<0.001	0.32	13.8
>10	3	320	REM	D-L	HR = 2.15 (0.07–61.90)	0.66	<0.001	94.0
Intensity-based	9	1232	REM	D-L	HR = 1.24 (0.95–1.63)	0.12	0.03	65.5
Subgroup analysis by immunostaining pattern [b]								
Membrane	10	1138	REM	D-L	HR = 1.31 (0.98–1.74)	0.07	0.001	67.0
Mixed membrane-cytoplasm	6	669	REM	D-L	HR = 2.02 (0.61–6.70)	0.25	<0.001	88.2
Not reported	3	449	REM	D-L	HR = 1.39 (0.97–2.01)	0.08	0.16	45.7
Subgroup analysis by overall risk of bias in primary-level studies [b]								
Low RoB	6	776	REM	D-L	HR = 1.83 (1.12–2.98)	0.02	<0.001	81.0
Moderate RoB	5	547	REM	D-L	HR = 0.79 (0.37–1.67)	0.53	<0.001	82.8
High RoB	8	933	REM	D-L	HR = 1.63 (1.14–2.31)	0.007	0.06	48.5
Univariable meta-regressions by study design and patients characteristics [c]								
Follow up (months, average)	6	1419	random-effects meta-regression		Coef = 0.000 (−0.032 to 0.032)	0.96 ±0.002 [d]	$het_{explained}$ = −64.29% [e]	
Sex (proportion of males, %)	18	2141	random-effects meta-regression		Coef = −0.010 (−0.056 to 0.036)	0.66 ±0.005 [d]	$het_{explained}$ = −13.93% [e]	
Age (years, mean)	16	1968	random-effects meta-regression		Coef = −0.003 (−0.108 to 0.102)	0.98 ±0.001 [d]	$het_{explained}$ = −14.39% [e]	

Table 2. *Cont.*

Meta-Analyses	No. of Studies	No. of Patients	Stat. Model	Wt	Pooled Data		Heterogeneity	
					ES (95% CI)	*p*-Value	P_{het}	I^2 (%)
SURVIVAL PARAMETERS								
Overall survival								
Clinical stage (proportion of stage-III/IV patients,%)	7	1032	random-effects meta-regression		Coef = −0.005 (−0.036 to 0.024)	0.56 ±0.005 [d]	het$_{explained}$ = −225.16% [e]	
Tobacco consumption (proportion of smokers, %)	9	12707	random-effects meta-regression		Coef = −0.008 (−0.032 to 0.016)	0.48 ±0.005 [d]	het$_{explained}$ = −13.06% [e]	
Areca nut/Betel quid consumption (proportion right chewers, %)	2	250	—		—	—	—	
Alcohol consumption (% of patients with positive habit)	5	660	random-effects meta-regression		Coef = −0.047 (−0.111 to 0.018)	0.25 ±0.004 [d]	het$_{explained}$ = 77.90% [e]	
Disease-free survival								
EGFR overexpression (all) [a]	19	2320	REM	D-L	HR = 1.22 (0.28–1.53)	0.08	<0.001	65.0
CLINICOPATHOLOGICAL CHARACTERISTICS								
T status								
EGFR overexpression (all) [a]	20	1565	REM	D-L	OR = 1.17 (0.72–1.90)	0.53	<0.001	65.0
N status								
EGFR overexpression (all) [a]	24	2040	REM	D-L	OR = 1.37 (1.01–1.86)	0.04	0.06	33.6
Clinical Stage								
EGFR overexpression (all) [a]	18	1456	REM	D-L	OR = 1.12 (0.68–1.84)	0.65	<0.001	65.2
Histological grade								
EGFR overexpression (all) [a]	25	1860	REM	D-L	OR = 1.43 (1.05–1.94)	0.02	0.14	23.8

Abbreviations: Stat., statistical; Wt, method of weighting; ES, effect size estimation; HR, hazard ratio; OR, odds ratio; CI, confidence intervals; REM, random-effects model; D-L, DerSimonian and Laird method; OSCC, oral squamous cell carcinoma; RoB, risk of bias; EGFR, epidermal growth factor receptor. [a]—Meta-analysis of aggregate (summary) data. [b]—Subgroup meta-analysis. [c]—Meta-regression analysis of the potential effect of study covariates on the association between EGFR overexpression and overall survival in OSCC. A meta-regression coefficient >0 indicates a greater impact of covariates on poor prognosis. [d]—*p*-value + standard error recalculated after 10,000 permutations based on Montecarlo simulations. [e]—Proportion of between-study variance explained (adjusted R^2 statistic) using the residual maximum likelihood (REML) method. A negative number for the proportion of heterogeneity explained reflects no heterogeneity explained.

Disease-free survival (DFS). Close to significant results were found between poor DFS and EGFR overexpression (HR = 1.22, 95%CI = 0.98–1.53, $p = 0.08$), and considerable statistical heterogeneity was also present ($p < 0.001$, $I^2 = 65.0\%$) (Table 2, Figure S15 in Supplementary Information).

2.4.2. Association between EGFR Overexpression and Clinicopathological Variables

Similar significant results were also found for EGFR overexpression with poor differentiated OSCCs (OR = 1.43, 95%CI = 1.05–1.94, $p = 0.02$) and with N+ status (OR = 1.37, 95%CI = 1.01–1.86, $p = 0.04$), only showing moderate heterogeneity was the last parameter ($p = 0.06$, $I^2 = 33.6\%$). On the other hand, EGFR overexpression was not significantly associated with a higher T status (OR = 1.17, 95%CI = 0.72–1.90, $p = 0.53$) or an advanced clinical stage (OR = 1.12, 95%CI = 0.68–1.84, $p = 0.65$) (Table 2, Figures S16–S19, in Supplementary Information).

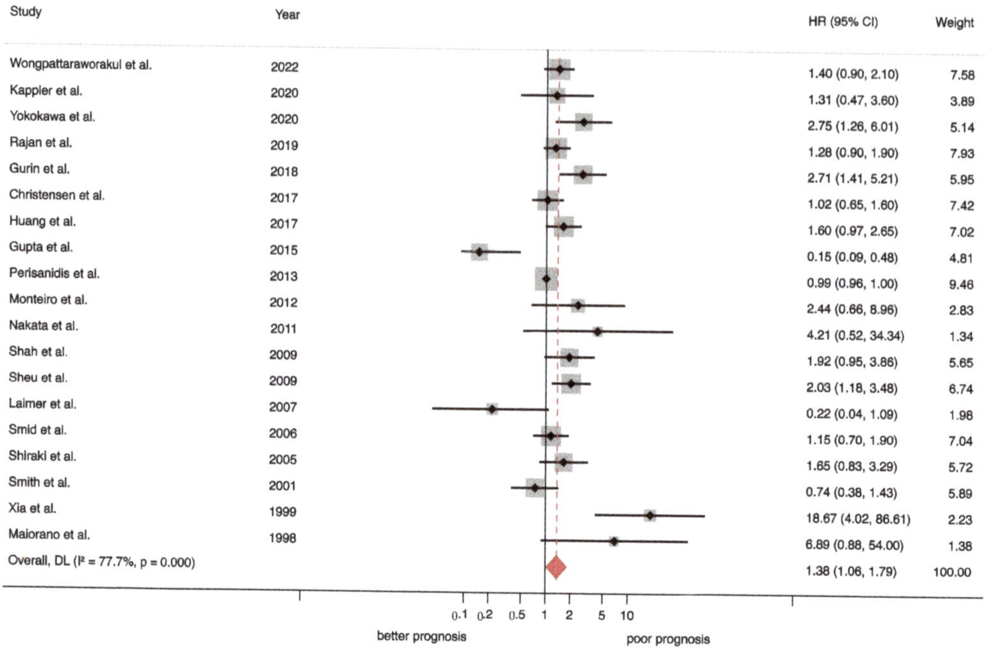

Figure 3. Forest plot graphically representing the meta-analysis on the association between EGFR overexpression and OS in patients with OSCC. Random-effects model, inverse-variance weighting (based on the DerSimonian and Laird method). A HR > 1 suggests that EGFR overexpression is associated with poor prognosis. Diamonds indicate the pooled HRs with their corresponding 95%CIs. Abbreviations: EGFR, epidermal growth factor receptor; OS, overall survival; OSCC, oral squamous cell carcinoma; HR, hazard ratio; CI, confidence intervals [19,23–25,28,34,40,42,43,45,48,51,53,55,56,59,65–67].

2.5. *Quantitative Evaluation (Secondary Analyses)*

Subgroup meta-analysis. The significant association found between EGFR overexpression and poor OS was also maintained by several subgroups after the stratified meta-analysis (anti-EGFR antibody dilution > 1:100: HR = 1.56, 95%CI = 1.04–2.33, $p = 0.03$; anti–EGFR antibody dilution < 1:100: HR = 1.59, 95%CI = 1.21–2.11, $p = 0.001$; room temperature incubation: HR = 2.93, 95%CI = 1.16–7.38, $p = 0.02$; anti–EGFR antibody Clone 31G7: HR = 2.12, 95% = 1.26–3.59, $p = 0.005$; anti–EGFR antibody Clone H11: HR = 1.33, 95%CI = 1.01–1.76, $p = 0.05$; anti–EGFR antibody D38B1: HR = 2.05, 95%CI = 1.00–4.17, $p = 0.05$; cut–off point of 10%: HR = 1.62, 95%CI = 1.24–2.11, $p < 0.001$, high RoB: HR = 1.63, 95%CI = 1.14–2.31, $p = 0.007$; low RoB: HR = 1.83, 95%CI = 1.12–2.98, $p = 0.02$) (Table 2, Figures S1–S8 in Supplementary Information).

Meta-regression analysis. The potential impact of additional study covariates, follow-up period, sex, age, clinical stage, and tobacco and alcohol consumption, on the association between OS and EGFR overexpression was also analyzed, and no significant differences were found ($p > 0.05$ for all covariates) (Table 2, Figures S9–S14 in Supplementary Information).

Analysis of small-study effects. Visual inspection analysis of the funnel plots' asymmetry and the statistical tests conducted for the same purpose confirmed the absence of small-study effects across clinicopathological variables (T status: $p_{Egger} = 0.51$, N status: $p_{Egger} = 0.26$; clinical stage: $p_{Egger} = 0.90$; histological grade: $p_{Egger} = 0.98$), while significant results were found for prognostic variables, where publication bias could not be ruled out (OS: $p_{Egger} = 0.03$, DFS: $p_{Egger} = 0.08$) (Figures S20–S25 in Supplementary Information).

3. Discussion

Our systematic review and meta-analysis on the prognostic implications of EGFR overexpression in oral cancer, conducted on 50 studies and 4631 patients, points out that there is an association with lower overall survival (HR = 1.38, 95%CI = 1.06–1.79, p = 0.02), higher probability of developing neck lymph node metastases (OR = 1.37, 95%CI = 1.01–1.86, p = 0.04), and higher risk of developing poorly differentiated tumors (OR = 1.43, 95% CI = 1.05–1.94, p = 0.02). Constitutive oncogenic activation of EGFR is the main mechanism for the acquisition of one of the essential hallmarks of oral cancer, i.e., the ability of tumor cells to maintain a sustained proliferation [2–4], which in turn conditions the cells to enter a state of genomic instability that facilitates the acquisition of new additive oncogenic alterations, new hallmarks, which will be clonally transmitted to their progeny. Constitutive activation of EGFR is essentially driven by gene amplification [6,69]; this leads to the formation of dimers between EGFR receptors in the cell membrane and the activation of pro-proliferative intracellular pathways, most notably MAPK and PI3K/Akt, leading to the activation of proliferative genes, essentially but not exclusively *CCND1*, which encodes the proliferation-stimulating protein cyclin D1 [10,11,70]. The oncogenic mechanism linked to the constitutive activation of EGFR is relevant in oral carcinogenesis, as it occurs in other human neoplasms in which, on average, 50–70% of malignant cells overexpress EGFR [6,17,69,71]. In our study, 56.39% of the tumors overexpressed EGFR. The frequency of activation of this oncogenic mechanism in oral carcinogenesis has justified that this protein is one of the few molecules selected as a therapeutic target in this neoplasm (cetuximab) [17]. However, despite its relevance, there is very little evidence-based information, in the form of systematic reviews and meta-analyses, on its prognostic implications [4]. There is only one systematic review and meta-analysis related to the prognostic implications of EGFR2 (ErbB2) overexpression in oral cancer, which reports its association with decreased survival and increased metastatic involvement of the neck lymph nodes [72]. Our meta-analysis, performed on the triple of studies and cases, shows similar results. The influence of EGFR overexpression on survival is obtained when 10% of EGFR+ tumor cells are used as a cut-off point, whereas cut-off points higher than 10% are not discriminative in this sense. This probably indicates that, once an oral carcinoma is established and developed, it is not the hyperproliferative state that is the essential driver of the acquisition of survival-worsening capabilities, but that others, such as the ability to invade and metastasize, resistance to cell death, etc., may then operate independently of the hyperproliferative state. Therefore, if this is so, how could the association found in our study, and in the previous meta-analysis [72], be explained, between EGFR overexpression and N+ status? We believe that this finding may depend on some emerging functions of cyclin D1 associated with invasion and thus with the metastatic capacity of a tumor. Our research group has recently reported [73] that cytoplasmic overexpression of cyclin D1 in oral tumor cells is significantly associated with invasive morphology and the development of actin-based protrusive structures lamellipodia and invadopodia through sequential EGFR-cyclin D1-CDK4/6-paxillin-Rac1 activation, this being an oncogenic pathway that links an essentially proliferative pathway (EGFR) with the increased metastatic capacity of tumor cells.

According to our critical qualitative/risk of bias (RoB) analysis, performed with the QUIPS tool [68] (developed by members of the Cochrane Prognostic Methods Group [74]), the studies presented a very similar design, but not all the same methodological rigor. As is usually found in observational studies, the main RoB source was associated with the lack of control of potentially confounding factors, which were not considered in the design or not integrated in the statistical analyses. Future studies should be better designed, correctly measuring and clearly reporting data related to essential clinical factors that were inconsistently published (e.g., tobacco and alcohol use). Important clinicopathologic or therapeutic variables with prognostic value were also not reported by primary-level studies, such as the number of surgical and non-surgical cases or the presence/absence of distant metastases. These variables sometimes are not published, or typically reported as aggregated data. Therefore, the influence of these covariates could not be quantitatively evaluated through meta-regressions or adjusted through subgroup meta-analyses. Consequently, as another recommendation of our systematic review, future studies should carefully report the clinicodemographical variables of interest, preferably via individual participant data, in order to increase the transparency and scientific quality of the published datasets. It should also be mentioned that in our RoB stratified subgroup meta-analysis, we found the largest effect size between worse survival and a higher methodological quality. This is an important fact that shows that the more carefully designed studies are able to better demonstrate the association between EGFR overexpression and poor prognosis in oral cancer. The methodological recommendations derived from the present systematic review are therefore strongly recommended in order to improve and standardize future research.

Some potential limitations of our systematic review and meta-analysis should also be discussed. First, a considerable statistical heterogeneity degree was observed in the meta-analysis on overall survival. Subsequent stratified meta-analyses revealed more homogeneous subgroups, indicating that potential explanatory sources of heterogeneity are inherent to the variability of experimental methods, singularly differences in anti-EGFR antibodies, cut-off points, and antibody dilutions. Second, the presence of publication bias could not be ruled out for all the variables investigated. Nevertheless, this is a real challenge hard to overcome in the current biomedical research era, where a model of publications of consistently positive results is firmly established [75]. Despite the above limitations, our study was carefully designed and developed following high methodological standards, and presents promising results, being the first meta-analysis to date specifically researching the prognostic implications of EGFR in oral cancer.

4. Materials and Methods

This systematic review and meta-analysis followed PRISMA and MOOSE reporting guidelines [76,77], and closely complied with the criteria of Cochrane Prognosis Methods Group [74] and Cochrane Handbook for Systematic Reviews of Interventions [78].

4.1. Protocol

To reduce bias risk and improve the transparency, accuracy, and integrity of this study, we previously registered the methodology protocol in the PROSPERO International prospective register of systematic reviews (www.crd.york.ac.uk/PROSPERO, registration number ID433551; accessed on 18 June 2023). The protocol is also consistent with the PRISMA-P Guidelines to ensure a strict approach [79].

4.2. Search Strategy

In order to perform the search, MEDLINE/Pubmed, Embase, Web of Science, and Scopus were the main databases employed. Only studies published before the search date (November 2022) were considered. The search was conducted by combining thesaurus terms used in databases (i.e., MeSH and EMTREE) with free terms, designed aiming to increase sensitivity and adapted to the syntax of each database consulted (Table S1 in Supplementary Information). We also manually examined the reference lists of the retrieved studies for additional relevant studies. All references are managed using Mendeley v1.17.10 software (Elsevier, Amsterdam, The Netherlands), and duplicate references were removed.

4.3. Eligibility Criteria

The following inclusion criteria were selected: original primary-level studies without restrictions by language, publication date, follow up periods, geographical area, age, or sex; evaluation of EGFR overexpression in OSCC; analysis of the association with at least one of the following prognostics and/or clinicopathological outcomes: overall survival (OS), disease-free survival (DFS), tumor size, N status, clinical stage, or histological grade. OS was defined as the time elapsed from the date of diagnosis/surgery to the date of death by any cause. DFS was defined as the time elapsed from diagnosis/surgery to the detection of locoregional or distant recurrence or to death without recurrence. Given the lack of international consensus standards to define survival endpoints in oncology research, any study using the terms OS/DFS was included, or by using other terms in compliance with our precedent definitions.

Studies meeting at least one of the following criteria were excluded: retracted articles, preclinical research (in vitro research or in vivo animal experimentation), case reports, editorials, letters, meeting abstracts, personal opinions, comments, book chapters, or secondary/tertiary-evidence level studies (systematic reviews, meta-analyses, scoping reviews, umbrella or overviews of reviews, etc.); squamous cell carcinomas from anatomic areas distinct to the oral cavity, and/or tumors of different histopathological lineage; no analysis of the main prognostic or clinicopathological outcomes of interest; lack or insufficient data for the estimation of statistical effect size metrics with their corresponding confidence intervals; and inter-study overlapping populations, determined by verifying the authors' names and affiliations, source of patients, and recruitment periods. To identify potential overlapping populations, the authors' names, affiliations, and recruitment period and settings were examined. In cases where the study was conducted by the same research group, we have included the most recent research, or the most complete data published.

4.4. Study Selection Process

A team of three blinded authors (JCO, DCG, and VSD) applied the eligibility criteria. A supervising author (PRG) was consulted to resolve any dissimilarities. Article selection was performed in two stages; the first stage consisted of screening the titles and abstracts of retrieved studies in an initial selection, and then reading the full text of selected papers, followed by excluding those that did not meet the inclusion criteria. The reviewers were first jointly trained and calibrated for the process of identifying and selecting studies for several screening rounds, achieving an excellent inter-rater reliability, as measured by calculating a Cohen's kappa statistic ($\kappa > 0.90$).

4.5. Data Extraction

After full text reading, authors independently extracted data from the selected articles and used a standardized data collection form using the software Excel (v.16/2018, Microsoft. Redmond, WA, USA). The extracted data sets were secondarily cross-checked together, with discrepancies resolved by consensus. Using the methods proposed by Luo et al. (2018) and Wan et al. (2014) [80,81], data expressed as medians, interquartile range, and/or maximum-minimum values were calculated and converted to means and standard deviation (SD). In cases where it was desirable to combine two or more different datasets expressed as means-standard deviation of subgroups into a single group, the Cochrane Handbook formula was applied [78]. Data were collected on first author, language and publication date, country, sample size, anatomical cancer subsite, sex and age of patients, tobacco use, areca nut and alcohol consumption, recruitment and follow-up period, experimental methods, and relative frequency of EGFR overexpression. Finally, the data necessary to analyze the clinicopathological outcomes was investigated.

4.6. Evaluation of Quality and Risk of Bias

The authors used the Quality in Prognosis Studies (QUIPS) tool (developed by members of the Cochrane Prognosis Methods Group [68]) to critically appraise the methodological quality and risk of bias of the studies at the primary level. The following six areas of potential bias were examined: (1) study participation; (2) study attrition; (3) prognostic factor measurement; (4) outcome measurement; (5) study confounding; and (6) statistical analysis/reporting. For each domain, the risk of bias was assessed as low, moderate, or high. Finally, to obtain an overall risk of bias score, an overall score was also estimated based on a method previously described by our research group [82–85].

4.7. Effect Measures

Odds ratios (OR) with their corresponding 95% confidence intervals (CI) were used as an effect measure for clinicopathological outcomes. EGFR overexpression was analyzed as a dichotomous categorical variable according to the scoring systems adopted by primary-level studies. Hazard ratios (HR) with 95%CI were used, due to the time-to-event nature, for the survival outcomes [86]. When authors directly reported HR and 95%CI, these were extracted from primary-level studies. If HR and/or 95%CI were not explicitly provided by the authors, we calculated them using standardized appropriated statistics [86,87]. If these results were only reported through survival curves, datasets were extracted from Kaplan-Meier curves with Engauge Digitizer 4.1 software (open-source digitizing software developed by M. Mitchell).

4.8. Synthesis Methods

The primary-level studies included in this systematic review reported different outcomes of interest. Thus, the number of studies and patients was variable for each meta-analysis performed for survival outcomes (overall survival and disease-free survival) and clinicopathological variables (T status, N status, clinical stage, and histological grade). Forest plots were constructed for these outcomes in order to display the results of individual studies, as well as the magnitude, precision, and direction of effects of pooled estimates derived from meta-analytical techniques. All meta-analyses were conducted using the inverse-variance method under a random-effects model (based on the DerSimonian and Laird method). This approach was *a priori* planned in our study protocol in order to account for the possibility that there are different underlying effects among study subpopulations (e.g., differences inherent to the variability of experimental methods, such as different anti-EGFR antibodies, dilutions, or incubation time). All analyses were run in the software Stata v. 16.1 (StataCorp, College Station, TX, USA).

The presence and extent of statistical heterogeneity was assessed using the χ^2-based Cochran's Q test. Given the low statistical power of Q-test, $p < 0.10$ was considered significant. We also applied the Higgins I^2 statistic to estimate what proportion of the variance in observed effects reflects the variation in true effects, rather than sampling error. The percentage of inter-study heterogeneity was quantified considering values of 50–75% as a moderate-to-high degree of inconsistency [88,89]. The possible causes of heterogeneity among studies were explored across subgroup meta-analyses and univariable random-effect meta-regression analyses using the restricted maximum likelihood (REML) method [90]. Due to the low number of observations reported by primary-level studies for secondary covariates included in meta-regressions, the *p*-values were re-calculated using a permutation test based on Monte Carlo simulations [91]. To obtain sufficient precision, the number of permutations was 10,000 [92]. Weighted bubble plots were also constructed to graphically represent the fitted meta-regression lines. Finally, in order to assess small-study effects, we planned to generate funnel plots [93] for meta-analyses. Furthermore, the Egger regression test was performed to statistically investigate the asymmetry of funnel plots (performing a linear regression of the effect estimates on their standard errors, weighting by 1/[variance of the effect estimate], considering a p_{Egger}-value < 0.10 as significant) [94].

5. Conclusions

In conclusion, our meta-analysis provides an evidence-based report that EGFR overexpression is a very frequent oncogenic mechanism in oral oncogenesis that is associated with a worse survival rate and a higher risk of developing lymph node metastases. Our results suggest that immunohistochemical detection of EGFR should be routinely included in the prognostic evaluation of patients with oral cancer, using 10% of EGFR+ tumor cells as a cut-off point to consider a positive case.

Supplementary Materials: The following supporting information can be downloaded at: https://www.mdpi.com/article/10.3390/ijms241511888/s1.

Author Contributions: Conceptualization, J.L.C.-O., I.G.-R., P.R.-G., D.C.-G., V.S.-D. and M.Á.G.-M.; methodology, J.L.C.-O., I.G.-R., P.R.-G., D.C.-G., V.S.-D. and M.Á.G.-M.; software, J.L.C.-O., I.G.-R., P.R.-G., D.C.-G., V.S.-D. and M.Á.G.-M.; validation, J.L.C.-O., I.G.-R., P.R.-G., D.C.-G., V.S.-D. and M.Á.G.-M.; formal analysis, J.L.C.-O., I.G.-R., P.R.-G., D.C.-G., V.S.-D. and M.Á.G.-M.; investigation, J.L.C.-O., I.G.-R., P.R.-G., D.C.-G., V.S.-D. and M.Á.G.-M.; resources, J.L.C.-O., I.G.-R., P.R.-G., D.C.-G., V.S.-D. and M.Á.G.-M.; data curation, J.L.C.-O., I.G.-R., P.R.-G., D.C.-G., V.S.-D. and M.Á.G.-M.; writing—original draft preparation, J.L.C.-O., I.G.-R., P.R.-G., D.C.-G., V.S.-D. and M.Á.G.-M.; writing—review and editing, J.L.C.-O., I.G.-R., P.R.-G., D.C.-G., V.S.-D. and M.Á.G.-M.; visualization, J.L.C.-O., I.G.-R., P.R.-G., D.C.-G., V.S.-D. and M.Á.G.-M.; supervision, M.Á.G.-M. and P.R.-G. All authors have read and agreed to the published version of the manuscript.

Funding: This research received no external funding.

Data Availability Statement: Data is contained within the article or supplementary material .

Acknowledgments: We would like to thank the research group CTS-392 (Plan Andaluz de Investigación, Junta de Andalucía, Spain).

Conflicts of Interest: The authors declare no conflict of interest.

References

1. Sung, H.; Ferlay, J.; Siegel, R.L.; Laversanne, M.; Soerjomataram, I.; Jemal, A.; Bray, F. Global Cancer Statistics 2020: GLOBOCAN Estimates of Incidence and Mortality Worldwide for 36 Cancers in 185 Countries. *CA Cancer J. Clin.* **2021**, *71*, 209–249. [CrossRef] [PubMed]
2. Hanahan, D.; Weinberg, R.A. The Hallmarks of Cancer. *Cell* **2000**, *100*, 57–70. [CrossRef] [PubMed]
3. Hanahan, D.; Weinberg, R.A. Hallmarks of cancer: The next generation. *Cell* **2011**, *144*, 646–674. [CrossRef] [PubMed]
4. González-Moles, M.Á.; Warnakulasuriya, S.; López-Ansio, M.; Ramos-García, P. Hallmarks of Cancer Applied to Oral and Oropharyngeal Carcinogenesis: A Scoping Review of the Evidence Gaps Found in Published Systematic Reviews. *Cancers* **2022**, *14*, 3834. [CrossRef]
5. Leemans, C.R.; Braakhuis, B.J.M.; Brakenhoff, R.H. The molecular biology of head and neck cancer. *Nat. Rev. Cancer* **2011**, *11*, 9–22. [CrossRef]
6. Yarden, Y.; Sliwkowski, M.X. Untangling THE ErbB signalling network. *Nat. Rev. Mol Cell Biol.* **2001**, *2*, 127–137. [CrossRef]
7. Schlessinger, J. Cell signaling by receptor tyrosine kinases. *Cell* **2000**, *103*, 211–225. [CrossRef]
8. Roepstorff, K.; Grandal, M.V.; Henriksen, L.; Knudsen, S.L.J.; Lerdrup, M.; Grøvdal, L.; Willumsen, B.M.; van Deurs, B. Differential effects of EGFR ligands on endocytic sorting of the receptor. *Traffic* **2009**, *10*, 1115–1127. [CrossRef]
9. Wee, P.; Wang, Z. Epidermal Growth Factor Receptor Cell Proliferation Signaling Pathways. *Cancers* **2017**, *9*, 52. [CrossRef]
10. Ramos-García, P.; González-Moles, M.Á.; González-Ruiz, L.; Ruiz-Ávila, I.; Ayén, Á.; Gil-Montoya, J.A. Prognostic and clinicopathological significance of cyclin D1 expression in oral squamous cell carcinoma: A systematic review and meta-analysis. *Oral Oncol.* **2018**, *83*, 96–106. [CrossRef]
11. Ramos-García, P.; Gil-Montoya, A.J.; Scully, C.; Ayén, A.; González-Ruiz, L.; Navarro-Triviño, F.J.; González-Moles, A.M. An update on the implications of cyclin D1 in oral carcinogenesis. *Oral Dis.* **2017**, *23*, 897–912. [CrossRef] [PubMed]
12. Humphreys, R.C.; Hennighausen, L. Transforming growth factor alpha and mouse models of human breast cancer. *Oncogene* **2000**, *19*, 1085–1091. [CrossRef]
13. Kawamata, H.; Kameyama, S.; Oyasu, R. In vitro and in vivo accelertration of the neoplastic phenotype of a low-tumorigenicity rat bladder carcinoma cell line by transfected transforming growth factor-α. *Mol. Carcinog.* **1994**, *9*, 210–219. [CrossRef] [PubMed]
14. Hirai, T.; Kuwahara, M.; Yoshida, K.; Kagawa, Y.; Hihara, J.; Yamashita, Y.; Toge, T. Clinical results of transhiatal esophagectomy for carcinoma of the lower thoracic esophagus according to biological markers. *Dis. Esophagus* **1998**, *11*, 221–225. [CrossRef]
15. Maurizi, M.; Almadori, G.; Ferrandina, M.G.; Distefano, M.; Romanini, M.E.; Cadoni, G.; Benedetti-Panici, P.; Paludetti, G.; Scambia, G.; Mancuso, S. Prognostic significance of epidermal growth factor receptor in laryngeal squamous cell carcinoma. *Br. J. Cancer* **1996**, *74*, 1253–1257. [CrossRef]
16. Nicholson, R.; Gee, J.M.; Harper, M. EGFR and cancer prognosis. *Eur. J. Cancer* **2001**, *37*, 9–15. [CrossRef]
17. Chong, C.R.; Jänne, P.A. The quest to overcome resistance to EGFR-targeted therapies in cancer. *Nat. Med.* **2013**, *19*, 1389–1400. [CrossRef] [PubMed]
18. Mohanapure, N.; Sinai Khandeparkar, S.; Saragade, P.; Gogate, B.; Joshi, A.; Mehta, S. Immunohistochemical study of epidermal growth factor receptor, human epidermal growth factor receptor 2/neu, p53, and Ki67 in oral squamous cell carcinoma. *J. Oral Maxillofac. Pathol.* **2022**, *26*, 127. [CrossRef]
19. Wongpattaraworakul, W.; Gibson-Corley, K.N.; Choi, A.; Buchakjian, M.R.; Lanzel, E.A.; Kd, A.R.; Simons, A.L. Prognostic Role of Combined EGFR and Tumor-Infiltrating Lymphocytes in Oral Squamous Cell Carcinoma. *Front Oncol.* **2022**, *12*, 885236. [CrossRef]
20. Etemad-Moghadam, S.; Alaeddini, M. Upregulation of ADAM10 in oral squamous cell carcinoma and its correlation with EGFR, neoangiogenesis and clinicopathologic factors. *J. Cranio-Maxillofac. Surg.* **2019**, *47*, 1583–1588. [CrossRef]

21. Singla, S.; Singla, G.; Zaheer, S.; Rawat, D.; Mandal, A. Expression of p53, epidermal growth factor receptor, c-erbB2 in oral leukoplakias and oral squamous cell carcinomas. *J. Cancer Res. Ther.* **2018**, *14*, 388. [CrossRef]
22. Owusu-Afriyie, O.; Owiredu, W.K.B.A.; Owusu-Danquah, K.; Larsen-Reindorf, R.; Donkor, P.; Acheampong, E.; Quayson, S.E. Expression of immunohistochemical markers in non-oropharyngeal head and neck squamous cell carcinoma in Ghana. *PLoS ONE* **2018**, *13*, e0202790. [CrossRef]
23. Gurin, D.; Slavik, M.; Hermanova, M.; Shatokhina, T.; Sana, J.; Kazda, T.; Selingerova, I.; Ahmad, P.; Smilek, P.; Horakova, Z.; et al. Prognostic impact of combined immunoprofiles in oropharyngeal squamous cell carcinoma patients with respect to AJCC 8th edition. *J. Oral Pathol. Med.* **2018**, *47*, 864–872. [CrossRef]
24. Huang, S.-F.; Chien, H.-T.; Chuang, W.-Y.; Lai, C.-H.; Cheng, S.-D.; Liao, C.-T.; Wang, H.-M. Epidermal growth factor receptor intron-1 CA repeat polymorphism on protein expression and clinical outcome in Taiwanese oral squamous cell carcinoma. *Sci. Rep.* **2017**, *7*, 4963. [CrossRef]
25. Christensen, A.; Kiss, K.; Lelkaitis, G.; Juhl, K.; Persson, M.; Charabi, B.W.; Mortensen, J.; Forman, J.L.; Sørensen, A.L.; Jensen, D.H.; et al. Urokinase-type plasminogen activator receptor (uPAR), tissue factor (TF) and epidermal growth factor receptor (EGFR): Tumor expression patterns and prognostic value in oral cancer. *BMC Cancer* **2017**, *17*, 572. [CrossRef]
26. Kimura, I.; Kitahara, H.; Ooi, K.; Kato, K.; Noguchi, N.; Yoshizawa, K.; Nakamura, H.; Kawashiri, S. Loss of epidermal growth factor receptor expression in oral squamous cell carcinoma is associated with invasiveness and epithelial-mesenchymal transition. *Oncol. Lett.* **2016**, *11*, 201–207. [CrossRef]
27. Solomon, M.C.; Vidyasagar, M.S.; Fernandes, D.; Guddattu, V.; Mathew, M.; Shergill, A.K.; Carnelio, S.; Chandrashekar, C. The prognostic implication of the expression of EGFR, p53, cyclin D1, Bcl-2 and p16 in primary locally advanced oral squamous cell carcinoma cases: A tissue microarray study. *Med. Oncol.* **2016**, *33*, 138. [CrossRef]
28. Gupta, S.; Khan, H.; Kushwaha, V.S.; Husain, N.; Negi, M.; Ghatak, A.; Bhatt, M. Impact of EGFR and p53 expressions on survival and quality of life in locally advanced oral squamous cell carcinoma patients treated with chemoradiation. *Cancer Biol. Ther.* **2015**, *16*, 1269–1280. [CrossRef]
29. de Andrade, A.L.D.L.; Ferreira, S.J.; Ferreira, S.M.S.; Ribeiro, C.M.B.; Freitas, R.D.A.; Galvão, H.C. Immunoexpression of EGFR and EMMPRIN in a series of cases of head and neck squamous cell carcinoma. *Pathol. Res. Pract.* **2015**, *211*, 776–781. [CrossRef]
30. Pansini, P.F.; Valle, I.B.D.; Damasceno, T.C.D.; de Abreu, P.M.; Có, A.C.G.; López, R.V.M.; Lenzi, J.; Rocha, R.M.; Souza, E.D.; Curado, M.P.; et al. Differential Expression of Potential Biomarkers of Oral Squamous Cell Carcinoma Development. *Head Neck Pathol.* **2021**, *15*, 1127–1136. [CrossRef]
31. Gröbe, A.; Eichhorn, W.; Fraederich, M.; Kluwe, L.; Vashist, Y.; Wikner, J.; Smeets, R.; Simon, R.; Sauter, G.; Heiland, M.; et al. Immunohistochemical and FISH analysis of EGFR and its prognostic value in patients with oral squamous cell carcinoma. *J. Oral Pathol. Med.* **2014**, *43*, 205–210. [CrossRef]
32. Silva, S.D.; Alaoui-Jamali, M.A.; Hier, M.; Soares, F.A.; Graner, E.; Kowalski, L.P. Cooverexpression of ERBB1 and ERBB4 receptors predicts poor clinical outcome in pN+ oral squamous cell carcinoma with extranodal spread. *Clin. Exp. Metastasis* **2014**, *31*, 307–316. [CrossRef]
33. Monteiro, L.S.; Ricardo, S.; Delgado, M.L.; Garcez, F.; do Amaral, B.; Lopes, C. Phosphorylated EGFR at tyrosine 1173 correlates with poor prognosis in oral squamous cell carcinomas. *Oral Dis.* **2014**, *20*, 178–185. [CrossRef]
34. Perisanidis, C.; Wrba, F.; Brandstetter, A.; Kornek, G.; Mitchell, D.; Seemann, R.; Selzer, E.; Ewers, R.; Filipits, M. Impact of epidermal growth factor receptor, mesenchymal–epithelial transition factor, and insulin-like growth factor receptor 1 expression on survival of patients with oral and oropharyngeal cancer. *Br. J. Oral Maxillofac. Surg.* **2013**, *51*, 234–240. [CrossRef]
35. Bernardes, V.F.; Gleber-Netto, F.O.; de Sousa, S.F.; Rocha, R.M.; de Aguiar, M.C.F. EGFR status in oral squamous cell carcinoma: Comparing immunohistochemistry, FISH and CISH detection in a case series study. *BMJ Open* **2013**, *3*, e002077. [CrossRef]
36. Dragomir, L.P.; Mărgăritescu, C.; Florescu, A.; Olimid, A.D.; Dragomir, M.; Popescu, M.R. The immunoexpression of EGFR and Her2/neu in oral squamous carcinoma. *Rom. J. Morphol. Embryol.* **2012**, *53*, 597–601.
37. Won, H.S.; Jung, C.-K.; Chun, S.H.; Kang, J.-H.; Kim, Y.-S.; Sun, D.-I.; Kim, M.-S. Difference in expression of EGFR, pAkt, and PTEN between oropharyngeal and oral cavity squamous cell carcinoma. *Oral Oncol.* **2012**, *48*, 985–990. [CrossRef]
38. Hanabata, Y.; Nakajima, Y.; Morita, K.; Kayamori, K.; Omura, K. Coexpression of SGLT1 and EGFR is associated with tumor differentiation in oral squamous cell carcinoma. *Odontology* **2012**, *100*, 156–163. [CrossRef]
39. Dadfarnia, T.; Mohammed, B.S.; Eltorky, M.A. Significance of Ki-67 and p53 immunoexpression in the differential diagnosis of oral necrotizing sialometaplasia and squamous cell carcinoma. *Ann. Diagn. Pathol.* **2012**, *16*, 171–176. [CrossRef]
40. Monteiro, L.S.; Diniz-Freitas, M.; Garcia-Caballero, T.; Warnakulasuriya, S.; Forteza, J.; Fraga, M. Combined cytoplasmic and membranous EGFR and p53 overexpression is a poor prognostic marker in early stage oral squamous cell carcinoma. *J. Oral. Pathol. Med.* **2012**, *41*, 559–567. [CrossRef]
41. Tseng, Y.-K.; Chen, C.-F.; Shu, C.-W.; Lee, C.-H.; Chou, Y.-T.; Li, Y.-J.; Liou, H.-H.; Cheng, J.-T.; Chen, C.-L.; Ger, L.-P.; et al. Effect of EGFR on SQSTM1 Expression in Malignancy and Tumor Progression of Oral Squamous Cell Carcinoma. *Int. J. Mol. Sci.* **2021**, *22*, 12226. [CrossRef]
42. Nakata, Y.; Uzawa, N.; Takahashi, K.-I.; Sumino, J.; Michikawa, C.; Sato, H.; Sonoda, I.; Ohyama, Y.; Okada, N.; Amagasa, T. EGFR gene copy number alteration is a better prognostic indicator than protein overexpression in oral tongue squamous cell carcinomas. *Eur. J. Cancer* **2011**, *47*, 2364–2372. [CrossRef]

43. Shah, N.G.; Trivedi, T.I.; Tankshali, R.A.; Goswami, J.V.; Jetly, D.H.; Shukla, S.N.; Shah, P.M.; Verma, R.J. Prognostic significance of molecular markers in oral squamous cell carcinoma: A multivariate analysis. *Head Neck* **2009**, *31*, 1544–1556. [CrossRef]
44. Ryott, M.; Wangsa, D.; Heselmeyer-Haddad, K.; Lindholm, J.; Elmberger, G.; Auer, G.; Lundqvist, E.; Ried, T.; Munck-Wikland, E. EGFR protein overexpression and gene copy number increases in oral tongue squamous cell carcinoma. *Eur. J. Cancer* **2009**, *45*, 1700–1708. [CrossRef]
45. Sheu, J.J.-C.; Hua, C.-H.; Wan, L.; Lin, Y.-J.; Lai, M.-T.; Tseng, H.-C.; Jinawath, N.; Tsai, M.-H.; Chang, N.-W.; Lin, C.-F.; et al. Functional genomic analysis identified epidermal growth factor receptor activation as the most common genetic event in oral squamous cell carcinoma. *Cancer Res.* **2009**, *69*, 2568–2576. [CrossRef]
46. Agra, I.M.G.; Carvalho, A.L.; Pinto CA, L.; Martins, E.P.; Gonçalves Filho, J.; Soares, F.A.; Kowalski, L.P. Biological Markers and Prognosis in Recurrent Oral Cancer After Salvage Surgery. *Arch. Otolaryngol. Neck Surg.* **2008**, *134*, 743. [CrossRef]
47. Nestor, M.; Ekberg, T.; Dring, J.; van Dongen, G.A.; Wester, K.; Tolmachev, V.; Anniko, M. Quantification of CD44v6 and EGFR Expression in Head and Neck Squamous Cell Carcinomas Using a Single-Dose Radioimmunoassay. *Tumor Biol.* **2007**, *28*, 253–263. [CrossRef]
48. Laimer, K.; Spizzo, G.; Gastl, G.; Obrist, P.; Brunhuber, T.; Fong, D.; Barbieri, V.; Jank, S.; Doppler, W.; Rasse, M.; et al. High EGFR expression predicts poor prognosis in patients with squamous cell carcinoma of the oral cavity and oropharynx: A TMA-based immunohistochemical analysis. *Oral Oncol.* **2007**, *43*, 193–198. [CrossRef]
49. Diniz-Freitas, M.; García-Caballero, T.; Antúnez-López, J.; Gándara-Rey, J.M.; García-García, A. Pharmacodiagnostic evaluation of EGFR expression in oral squamous cell carcinoma. *Oral Dis.* **2007**, *13*, 285–290. [CrossRef]
50. Hiraishi, Y.; Wada, T.; Nakatani, K.; Negoro, K.; Fujita, S. Immunohistochemical expression of EGFR and p-EGFR in oral squamous cell carcinomas. *Pathol. Oncol. Res.* **2006**, *12*, 87–91. [CrossRef]
51. Smid, E.J.; Stoter, T.R.; Bloemena, E.; Lafleur, M.V.M.; Leemans, C.R.; van der Waal, I.; Slotman, B.J.; Langendijk, J.A. The importance of immunohistochemical expression of EGFr in squamous cell carcinoma of the oral cavity treated with surgery and postoperative radiotherapy. *Int. J. Radiat. Oncol.* **2006**, *65*, 1323–1329. [CrossRef] [PubMed]
52. Moratin, J.; Mock, A.; Obradovic, S.; Metzger, K.; Flechtenmacher, C.; Zaoui, K.; Fröhling, S.; Jäger, D.; Krauss, J.; Hoffmann, J.; et al. Digital Pathology Scoring of Immunohistochemical Staining Reliably Identifies Prognostic Markers and Anatomical Associations in a Large Cohort of Oral Cancers. *Front Oncol.* **2021**, *11*, 712944. [CrossRef] [PubMed]
53. Shiraki, M.; Odajima, T.; Ikeda, T.; Sasaki, A.; Satoh, M.; Yamaguchi, A.; Noguchi, M.; Nagai, I.; Hiratsuka, H. Combined expression of p53, cyclin D1 and epidermal growth factor receptor improves estimation of prognosis in curatively resected oral cancer. *Mod. Pathol.* **2005**, *18*, 1482–1489. [CrossRef] [PubMed]
54. Ekberg, T.; Nestor, M.; Engström, M.; Nordgren, H.; Wester, K.; Carlsson, J.; Anniko, M. Expression of EGFR, HER2, HER3, and HER4 in metastatic squamous cell carcinomas of the oral cavity and base of tongue. *Int. J. Oncol.* **2005**, *26*, 1177–1185. [CrossRef]
55. Smith, B.D.; Smith, G.L.; Carter, D.; DiGiovanna, M.P.; Kasowitz, K.M.; Sasaki, C.T.; Haffty, B.G. Molecular marker expression in oral and oropharyngeal squamous cell carcinoma. *Arch. Otolaryngol. Head Neck Surg.* **2001**, *127*, 780–785.
56. Xia, W.; Lau, Y.K.; Zhang, H.Z.; Xiao, F.Y.; Johnston, A.D.; Liu, A.R.; Li, L.; Katz, R.L.; Hung, M.C. Combination of EGFR, HER-2/neu, and HER-3 is a stronger predictor for the outcome of oral squamous cell carcinoma than any individual family members. *Clin. Cancer Res.* **1999**, *5*, 1164–4174. [PubMed]
57. Ibrahim, S.O.; Lillehaug, J.R.; Johannessen, A.C.; Liavaag, P.G.; Nilsen, R.; Vasstrand, E.N. Expression of biomarkers (p53, transforming growth factor alpha, epidermal growth factor receptor, c-erbB-2/neu and the proliferative cell nuclear antigen) in oropharyngeal squamous cell carcinomas. *Oral Oncol.* **1999**, *35*, 302–313. [CrossRef] [PubMed]
58. Takes, R.P.; Baatenburg de Jong, R.J.; Schuuring, E.; Litvinov, S.V.; Hermans, J.; van Krieken, J.H. Differences in expression of oncogenes and tumor suppressor genes in different sites of head and neck squamous cell. *Anticancer Res.* **1998**, *18*, 4793–4800.
59. Maiorano, E.; Favia, G.; Maisonneuve, P.; Viale, G. Prognostic implications of epidermal growth factor receptor immunoreactivity in squamous cell carcinoma of the oral mucosa. *J. Pathol.* **1998**, *185*, 167–174. [CrossRef]
60. Kusukawa, J.; Harada, H.; Shima, I.; Sasaguri, Y.; Kameyama, T.; Morimatsu, M. The significance of epidermal growth factor receptor and matrix metalloproteinase-3 in squamous cell carcinoma of the oral cavity. *Eur. J. Cancer B Oral Oncol.* **1996**, *32B*, 217–221. [CrossRef]
61. Störkel, S.; Reichert, T.; Reiffen, K.A.; Wagner, W. EGFR and PCNA expression in oral squamous cell carcinomas—A valuable tool in estimating the patient's prognosis. *Eur. J. Cancer B Oral Oncol.* **1993**, *29B*, 273–277. [CrossRef] [PubMed]
62. Partridge, M.; Gullick, W.J.; Langdon, J.D.; Sherriff, M. Expression of epidermal growth factor receptor on oral squamous cell carcinoma. *Br. J. Oral Maxillofac. Surg.* **1988**, *26*, 381–389. [CrossRef] [PubMed]
63. Shahsavari, F.; Miri, R.; Ghorbanpour, M. Expression of epidermal growth factor receptor in oral and esophageal squamous-cell carcinoma. *Dent. Res. J.* **2020**, *17*, 85–91.
64. Sajjanar, M.; Sajjan, P.; Puranik, R.; Vanaki, S.; Jayanth, V.; Naik, P. "Analysis of immunohistochemical expression of epidermal growth factor receptor in oral squamous cell carcinoma using tissue microarray technology and whole sections:" A comparative study. *J. Oral Maxillofac. Pathol.* **2020**, *24*, 499. [CrossRef]
65. Kappler, M.; Dauter, K.; Reich, W.; Bethmann, D.; Schwabe, M.; Rot, S.; Wickenhauser, C.; Al-Nawas, B.; Eckert, A.W. Prognostic impact of cytoplasmatic EGFR upregulation in patients with oral squamous cell carcinoma: A pilot study. *Mol. Clin. Oncol.* **2020**, *13*, 1. [CrossRef] [PubMed]

66. Yokokawa, M.; Morita, K.; Oikawa, Y.; Kayamori, K.; Sakamoto, K.; Ikeda, T.; Harada, H. Co-expression of EGFR and MET has a synergistic effect on the prognosis of patients with oral squamous cell carcinoma. *J. Oral Pathol. Med.* **2020**, *49*, 235–242. [CrossRef]
67. Rajan, A.; Gibson-Corley, K.N.; Choi, A.B.; Ofori-Amanfo, G.K.; Eyck, P.T.; Espinosa-Cotton, M.; Sperry, S.M.; Simons, A.L. Impact of Nuclear Interleukin-1 Alpha and EGFR Expression on Recurrence and Survival Outcomes in Oral Squamous Cell Carcinomas. *J. Oncol.* **2019**, *2019*, 1–12. [CrossRef]
68. Hayden, J.A.; Côté, P.; Bombardier, C. Evaluation of the quality of prognosis studies in systematic reviews. *Ann. Intern. Med.* **2006**, *144*, 427–437.
69. Normanno, N.; De Luca, A.; Bianco, C.; Strizzi, L.; Mancino, M.; Maiello, M.R.; Carotenuto, A.; De Feo, G.; Caponigro, F.; Salomon, D.S. Epidermal growth factor receptor (EGFR) signaling in cancer. *Gene* **2006**, *366*, 2–16. [CrossRef]
70. Ramos-García, P.; González-Moles, M.Á.; Ayén, Á.; González-Ruiz, L.; Ruiz-Ávila, I.; Lenouvel, D.; Gil-Montoya, J.A.; Bravo, M. Asymmetrical proliferative pattern loss linked to cyclin D1 overexpression in adjacent non-tumour epithelium in oral squamous cell carcinoma. *Arch. Oral Biol.* **2019**, *97*, 12–17. [CrossRef]
71. Abd El-Rehim, D.M.; Pinder, S.E.; Paish, C.E.; Bell, J.A.; Rampaul, R.S.; Blamey, R.W.; Robertson, J.F.R.; Nicholson, R.I.; Ellis, I.O. Expression and co-expression of the members of the epidermal growth factor receptor (EGFR) family in invasive breast carcinoma. *Br. J. Cancer* **2004**, *91*, 1532–1542. [CrossRef]
72. Meng, Y.; Yang, P.; Ma, L.; Tarantino, G. Prognostic and clinical implications of c-erbB-2 expression in patients with oral cancer: A meta-analysis. *Medicine* **2020**, *99*, e20575. [CrossRef]
73. Ramos-García, P.; Bravo, M.; González-Ruiz, L.; González-Moles, M.Á. Significance of cytoplasmic cyclin D1 expression in oral oncogenesis. *Oral Dis.* **2018**, *24*, 98–102. [CrossRef] [PubMed]
74. Riley, R.D.; Ridley, G.; Williams, K.; Altman, D.G.; Hayden, J.; de Vet, H.C.W. Prognosis research: Toward evidence-based results and a Cochrane methods group. *J. Clin. Epidemiol.* **2007**, *60*, 863–865, author reply 865–866. [CrossRef]
75. Kyzas, P.A.; Denaxa-Kyza, D.; Ioannidis, J.P.A. Almost all articles on cancer prognostic markers report statistically significant results. *Eur. J. Cancer* **2007**, *43*, 2559–2579. [CrossRef]
76. Page, M.J.; McKenzie, J.E.; Bossuyt, P.M.; Boutron, I.; Hoffmann, T.C.; Mulrow, C.D.; Shamseer, L.; Tetzlaff, J.M.; Akl, E.A.; Brennan, S.E.; et al. The PRISMA 2020 statement: An updated guideline for reporting systematic reviews. *BMJ* **2021**, *372*, 71. [CrossRef]
77. Stroup, D.F.; Berlin, J.A.; Morton, S.C.; Olkin, I.; Williamson, G.D.; Rennie, D.; Moher, D.; Becker, B.J.; Sipe, T.A.; Thacker, S.B. Meta-analysis of observational studies in epidemiology: A proposal for reporting. *J. Am. Med. Assoc.* **2000**, *283*, 2008–2012. [CrossRef]
78. Higgins, J.P.; Green, S. *Cochrane Handbook for Systematic Reviews of Interventions: Cochrane Book Series*; Wiley and Sons: Hoboken, NJ, USA, 2008; pp. 1–649. [CrossRef]
79. Shamseer, L.; Moher, D.; Clarke, M.; Ghersi, D.; Liberati, A.; Petticrew, M.; Shekelle, P.; Stewart, L.A.; PRISMA-P Group. Preferred reporting items for systematic review and meta-analysis protocols (PRISMA-P) 2015: Elaboration and explanation. *BMJ* **2015**, *350*, g7647. [CrossRef]
80. Luo, D.; Wan, X.; Liu, J.; Tong, T. Optimally estimating the sample mean from the sample size, median, mid-range, and/or mid-quartile range. *Stat. Methods Med. Res.* **2018**, *27*, 1785–1805. [CrossRef]
81. Wan, X.; Wang, W.; Liu, J.; Tong, T. Estimating the sample mean and standard deviation from the sample size, median, range and/or interquartile range. *BMC Med. Res. Methodol.* **2014**, *14*, 135. [CrossRef]
82. González-Moles, M.Á.; Ayén, Á.; González-Ruiz, I.; De Porras-Carrique, T.; González-Ruiz, L.; Ruiz-Ávila, I.; Ramos-García, P. Prognostic and Clinicopathological Significance of FADD Upregulation in Head and Neck Squamous Cell Carcinoma: A Systematic Review and Meta-Analysis. *Cancers* **2020**, *12*, 2393. [CrossRef]
83. Ramos-García, P.; González-Moles, M.Á. Prognostic and Clinicopathological Significance of the Aberrant Expression of β-Catenin in Oral Squamous Cell Carcinoma: A Systematic Review and Meta-Analysis. *Cancers* **2022**, *14*, 479. [CrossRef]
84. Ramos-García, P.; González-Moles, M.Á.; Warnakulasuriya, S. Significance of p53 overexpression in the prediction of the malignant transformation risk of oral potentially malignant disorders: A systematic review and meta-analysis. *Oral Oncol.* **2022**, *126*, 105734. [CrossRef]
85. González-Moles, M.Á.; Moya-González, E.; García-Ferrera, A.; Nieto-Casado, P.; Ramos-García, P. Prognostic and Clinicopathological Significance of Telomerase Reverse Transcriptase Upregulation in Oral Cancer: A Systematic Review and Meta-Analysis. *Cancers* **2022**, *14*, 3673. [CrossRef]
86. Tierney, J.F.; Stewart, L.A.; Ghersi, D.; Burdett, S.; Sydes, M.R. Practical methods for incorporating summary time-to-event data into meta-analysis. *Trials* **2007**, *8*, 16. [CrossRef]
87. Parmar, M.K.; Torri, V.; Stewart, L. Extracting summary statistics to perform meta-analyses of the published literature for survival endpoints. *Stat. Med.* **1998**, *17*, 2815–2834. [CrossRef]
88. Higgins, J.P.T.; Thompson, S.G. Quantifying heterogeneity in a meta-analysis. *Stat. Med.* **2002**, *21*, 1539–1558. [CrossRef]
89. Higgins, J.P.T.; Thompson, S.G.; Deeks, J.J.; Altman, D.G. Measuring inconsistency in meta-analyses. *BMJ* **2003**, *327*, 557–560. [CrossRef]
90. Thompson, S.G.; Higgins, J.P.T. How should meta-regression analyses be undertaken and interpreted? *Stat. Med.* **2002**, *21*, 1559–1573. [CrossRef]

91. Higgins, J.P.T.; Thompson, S.G. Controlling the risk of spurious findings from meta-regression. *Stat. Med.* **2004**, *23*, 1663–1682. [CrossRef]
92. Kemp, A.W.; Manly, B.F.J. *Randomization, Bootstrap and Monte Carlo Methods in Biology*; CRC Press: Boca Raton, FL, USA, 2006; Volume 53. [CrossRef]
93. Sterne, J.A.C.; Sutton, A.J.; Ioannidis, J.P.A.; Terrin, N.; Jones, D.R.; Lau, J.; Carpenter, J.; Rücker, G.; Harbord, R.M.; Schmid, C.H.; et al. Recommendations for examining and interpreting funnel plot asymmetry in meta-analyses of randomised controlled trials. *BMJ* **2011**, *343*, d4002. [CrossRef]
94. Egger, M.; Davey Smith, G.; Schneider, M.; Minder, C. Bias in meta-analysis detected by a simple, graphical test. *BMJ* **1997**, *315*, 629–634. [CrossRef]

International Journal of *Molecular Sciences*

Article

Interaction between Cigarette Smoke and Human Papillomavirus 16 E6/E7 Oncoproteins to Induce SOD2 Expression and DNA Damage in Head and Neck Cancer

Diego Carrillo-Beltrán [1], Julio C. Osorio [2], Rancés Blanco [2], Carolina Oliva [2], Enrique Boccardo [3] and Francisco Aguayo [4,*]

1 Instituto de Bioquímica y Microbiología, Facultad de Ciencias, Universidad Austral de Chile, Valdivia 5090000, Chile; diego.carrillo@uach.cl
2 Laboratorio de Oncovirología, Programa de Virología, Instituto de Ciencias Biomédicas (ICBM), Facultad de Medicina, Universidad de Chile, Santiago 8380000, Chile
3 Department of Microbiology, Institute of Biomedical Sciences, University of Sao Paulo, Sao Paulo 05508-900, Brazil; eboccardo@usp.br
4 Departamento de Biomedicina, Facultad de Medicina, Universidad de Tarapacá, Arica 1000000, Chile
* Correspondence: fraguayog@academicos.uta.cl

Abstract: Even though epidemiological studies suggest that tobacco smoking and high-risk human papillomavirus (HR-HPV) infection are mutually exclusive risk factors for developing head and neck cancer (HNC), a portion of subjects who develop this heterogeneous group of cancers are both HPV-positive and smokers. Both carcinogenic factors are associated with increased oxidative stress (OS) and DNA damage. It has been suggested that superoxide dismutase 2 (SOD2) can be independently regulated by cigarette smoke and HPV, increasing adaptation to OS and tumor progression. In this study, we analyzed SOD2 levels and DNA damage in oral cells ectopically expressing HPV16 E6/E7 oncoproteins and exposed to cigarette smoke condensate (CSC). Additionally, we analyzed SOD2 transcripts in The Cancer Genome Atlas (TCGA) Head and Neck Cancer Database. We found that oral cells expressing HPV16 E6/E7 oncoproteins exposed to CSC synergistically increased SOD2 levels and DNA damage. Additionally, the SOD2 regulation by E6, occurs in an Akt1 and ATM-independent manner. This study suggests that HPV and cigarette smoke interaction in HNC promotes SOD2 alterations, leading to increased DNA damage and, in turn, contributing to development of a different clinical entity.

Keywords: cancer; head and neck; human papillomavirus; cigarette smoke; SOD2; DNA damage

Citation: Carrillo-Beltrán, D.; Osorio, J.C.; Blanco, R.; Oliva, C.; Boccardo, E.; Aguayo, F. Interaction between Cigarette Smoke and Human Papillomavirus 16 E6/E7 Oncoproteins to Induce SOD2 Expression and DNA Damage in Head and Neck Cancer. *Int. J. Mol. Sci.* **2023**, *24*, 6907. https://doi.org/10.3390/ijms24086907

Academic Editor: Marko Tarle

Received: 13 March 2023
Revised: 31 March 2023
Accepted: 2 April 2023
Published: 7 April 2023

1. Introduction

Head and neck cancers (HNCs) represent a global health problem which affected ~830,000 subjects in 2020 worldwide, causing the death of more than 50% of them [1]. This cancer originates from different anatomical locations, such as the oropharynx, larynx, hypopharynx, mouth, lips, palate, and tonsils. Late diagnosis is a common problem in this type of cancer, accompanied by regional and distal metastases that worsen the patient's prognosis [2]. The risk factors associated with HNC are smoking, frequent alcohol consumption, and high-risk human papillomavirus (HR-HPV) infection [3]. HR-HPV E6 and E7 oncoproteins can induce the degradation of the tumor suppressors p53 and pRb, respectively, contributing to cell immortalization and transformation [4,5]. HPV16 is the most frequent HR-HPV genotype detected in HNCs, with 90% prevalence in this tumor [6–8]. However, HR-HPV infection is not a sufficient condition for carcinogenesis, with additional co-factors being required. Even though epidemiological studies suggest that tobacco smoking and HR-HPV are mutually exclusive risk factors for HNCs, some subjects who develop this cancer are both HR-HPV positive and smokers, suggesting the possibility of interactions [9].

Cigarette smoke is considered one of the leading agents related to HNC, this single factor being the cause of 42% of deaths associated with this disease [10]. More than 70 compounds in cigarette smoke are considered carcinogenic and classified into two types, those that directly promote DNA damage and those that require to be metabolized by host enzymes to promote the damage [11]. Most epithelial cells in head and neck tissues can be directly exposed to cigarette smoke, favoring the possibility of functional interactions with HR-HPV [12]. Both cigarette smoke and HR-HPV are inducers of oxidative stress (OS) since they favor the production of reactive oxygen species (ROS) such as hydrogen peroxide, nitric oxide, and superoxide that alter the cellular redox balance [13–15]. These changes lead to modifications in gene expression to modulate redox-sensitive proteins, many of which have been involved in cancer [14,16,17]. The family of superoxide dismutase (SOD) catalyzes the dismutation of superoxide (O_2^-) into hydrogen peroxide (H_2O_2) and oxygen and is suggested to be a prognostic factors in HNC [18,19]. In particular, the manganese superoxide dismutase 2 (SOD2) protein has the highest antioxidant capacity in the mitochondria when compared to other SOD family members. Moreover, SOD2 is suggested to be a prognostic biomarker of oral cancer malignancy because SOD2 overexpression is associated with lymph node metastases [18]. However, the role of SOD2 in cancer is complex, as it presents a dichotomy. First, SOD2 downregulation can lead to O_2^- accumulation, which is associated with increased DNA damage and cell proliferation during tumorigenesis [20]. Conversely, SOD2 positive regulation goes hand in hand with an improvement in the elimination of O_2^- and intracellular H_2O_2 increase, which correlates with adaptation to OS and activation of signaling pathways involved in tumor progression [21–24]. Specifically, increased SOD2 levels have been described in smoker HNC subjects and hypopharyngeal cells expressing the HPV16 E6 oncoprotein [25,26].

In this study, we report for the first time that HPV16 E6 and E7 oncoproteins and cigarette smoke cooperate to regulate SOD2 levels and DNA damage in head and neck cancer cells. Furthermore, we report a positive correlation between SOD2 upregulation and HPV16 E6 expression at the transcriptional level in HNCs from Chilean patients.

2. Results

2.1. HPV16 E6 and E7 Promote SOD2 Expression in Oral Cells

Oral cells (SCC143) were transduced with the retroviral vectors pLXSNE6/E7 or pLXSN. E6 and E7 transcripts were detected only in those cells transduced with the pLXSNE6/E7 vector (Figure 1A). Furthermore, we compared the levels of E6 and E7 transcripts in SCC143 and UM-SCC-100 cells with those obtained from SiHa cells (cervical cancer cell line containing two copies of HPV16 per cell) (Figure 1B,C). We found that the levels of E6/E7 transcripts in transduced SCC143 cells were similar to those obtained in SiHa cells and therefore selected these cells for further assays. Subsequently, we analyzed the proliferative capacity of SCC143V and SCC143E6/E7 cells, using a BrdU assay to analyze DNA synthesis. This assay detected a significant increase in proliferative activity in SCC143E6/E7 cells, and this, in turn, is dependent on ATM activation (Figure 1D). Then, using an RTqPCR assay, we saw a significant increase in SOD2 transcripts in SCC143 E6/E7 cells (Figure 1E). Finally, using WB, we detected the levels of the P53, pRb, pATM, ATM, and SOD2 proteins. The results demonstrate the functional activity of E6 and E7 through the downregulation of P53 and pRb, respectively (Figure 1F). In addition, the upregulation of pATM and SOD2 by the HPV16 E6 and E7 oncoproteins was confirmed (Figure 1F). These data indicate that the HPV16 E6 and E7 oncoproteins are increasing SOD2 transcripts and protein levels from oral cells.

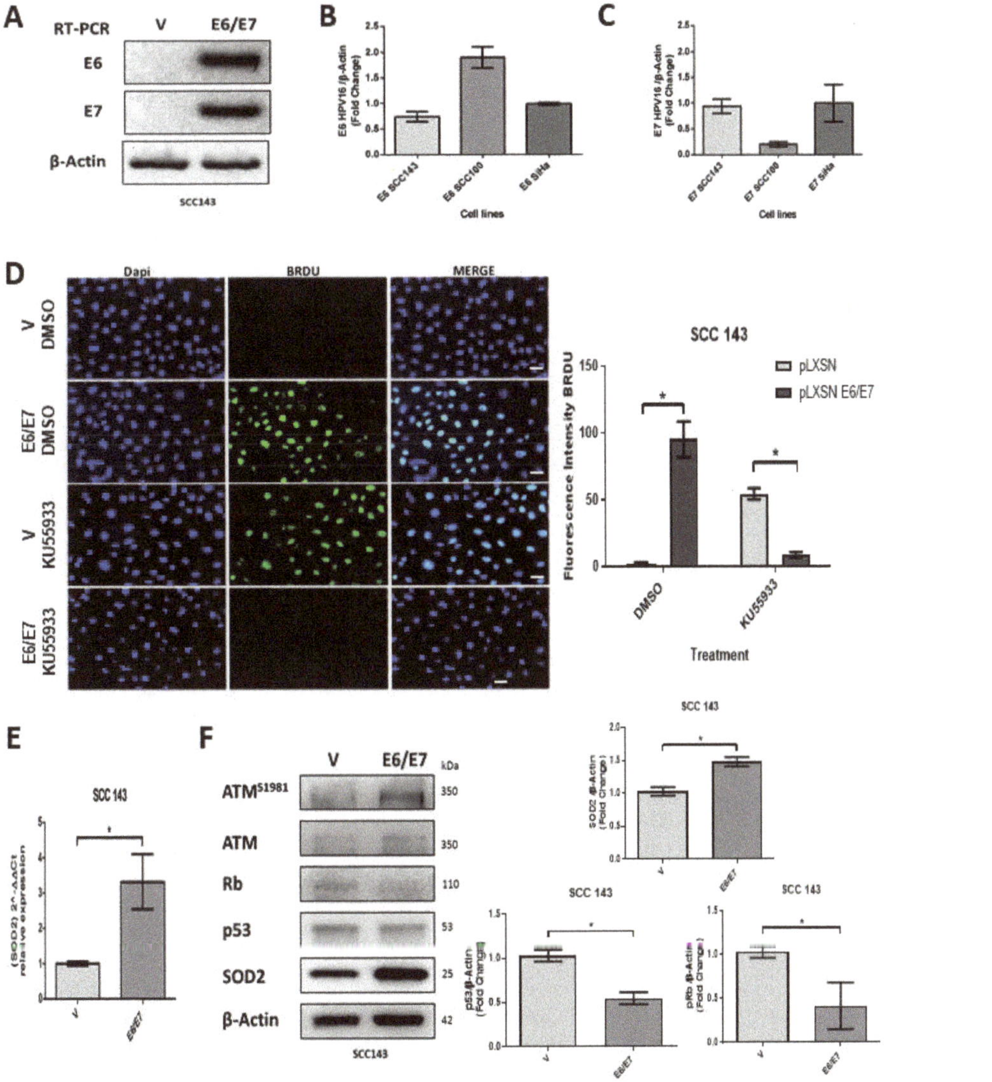

Figure 1. HPV16 E6/E7 induces SOD2 expression in oral cells. (**A**) HPV16 E6/E7 transcripts were evaluated by RT-PCR in SCC143V and SCC143E6/E7 cells; β-actin was used as the control. (**B**) E6 transcripts were assessed by RT-PCR in SiHa, SCC100E6/E7, and SCC143 E6/E7 cells and then normalized to the intensity of β-actin transcript. (**C**) E7 transcripts were assessed by RT-PCR in SiHa, SCC100E6/E7, and SCC143 E6/E7 cells, then normalized to the intensity of β-actin transcript. (**D**) BrdU assay to analyze DNA synthesis in SCC143V and SCC143 E6/E7 cells previously exposed to KU55933 (ATM) inhibitor. Scale bar: 10 μm. The graph represents fluorescence analysis performed with the fluorescence intensity. (**E**) The levels of SOD2 transcripts normalized by β-actin were evaluated by RT-qPCR in SCC143V and SCC143E6/E7 cells. (**F**) Western blot to evaluate ATM^{S1981}, ATM, Rb, p53, SOD2, and β-actin protein levels in SCC143V and SCC143E6/E7 cells. The graphs represent three independent Western blots for SOD2 pRb and p53 protein normalized by β-actin. Densitometric analyses were performed with ImageJ. Data are presented as the mean ± standard deviation (SD); average of three independent experiments, conducted in triplicate; * $p < 0.05$.

2.2. SOD2 Is Regulated by HPV16 E6 in an AKT1/ATM Independent Manner in Oral Cells

An assay with siRNA was performed to determine the relevant oncoprotein in the regulation of SOD2 levels. SCC143 E6/E7 cells were transfected with siRNA for E6 and E7 and scrambled control (SCR) for this assay. After 48 h post-transfection, SOD2 levels were analyzed by WB. In addition, WBs for p53 and pRb were included as indirect functionality control of the siRNAs. The results show p53 and pRb levels recovery when the E6 and E7 interferents are used, respectively. In addition, we detected that when using the E6 interferent of HPV16, the SOD2 levels decreased significantly (Figure 2A). On the other hand, we analyzed whether the increase in SOD2 levels was dependent on ATM activation, which is related to DNA damage repair and is activated by E6 and E7 oncoproteins. Therefore, SCC143 E6/E7 cells were treated with two concentrations of the specific inhibitor of ATM activation (KU55933) for 24 h. We observed no statistically significant differences in SOD2 levels when the inhibitor KU55933 was used (Figure 2B). In addition, we analyzed the role of PI3K/AKT signaling in SOD2 levels induced by HPV16 oncoproteins, as the extent of this pathway in SOD2 transcriptional regulation was previously reported [20]. Accordingly, SCC143 E6/E7 cells were treated with the PI3K-specific inhibitor (LY294002) for 24 h. Then we analyzed the levels of AKT, pAKT1S473, and SOD2 proteins by WB. First, we detected a decrease in the phosphorylated form of AKT1S473 when comparing SCC143 pLXSN with SCC143 pLXSN E6/E7, and there was no significant change in SOD2 levels when using the inhibitor LY294002 (Figure 2C). The data suggest that HPV16 E6 is relevant for inducing SOD2 levels in an ATM- and PI3K/AKT-independent manner.

2.3. HPV16 E6 and E7 Oncoproteins Together with CSC Induce an Increase in SOD2 Levels and DNA Damage in Oral Cells

Both cigarette smoke and HPV are risk factors for HNC and inducers of oxidative stress. Therefore, we hypothesize that HPV oncoproteins E6 and E7 and cigarette smoke may collaborate to induce SOD2 and genetic damage in oral cells. To assess this possible collaboration, we first evaluated non-toxic doses of CSCs in SCC 143 cells by using the MTS assay with different concentrations of the compound (Figure 3A). The results indicate the maximum non-lethal amount is 50 μg/mL of CSC. Then, to verify the functionality of the compound, we evaluated the cytochrome p450 (CYP1B1) transcript by RT-PCR and analyzed the activation of ERK and AKT1 by WB (Figure 3B,C). We observed a significant increase in the CYP1B1 transcript in SCC143 cells exposed to 10 μg/mL CSC. Moreover, CSC can upregulate the phosphorylated forms of ERK and AKT1 in SCC143 V and SCC143 E6/E7 cells. These data confirm the biological activity of CSC in this oral model. To determine the effect of HPV16 E6/E7 and CSC on SOD2 levels, SCC143 V and SCC143 E6/E7 cells were exposed to 10 and 50 ug/mL CSC for 24 h, using DMSO as a control (Figure 3D). The levels of pATM, ATM, Rb, and SOD2 proteins were then analyzed by WB. We observed a significant increase in SOD2 levels with 10 and 50 ug/mL CSC in both SCC143 V and SCC143 E6/E7 cells. However, a more substantial rise in SOD2 levels is observed in SCC143 E6/E7 cells with CSC at both concentrations. In addition, we detected a CSC-mediated increase in pATM and a CSC-mediated decrease in Rb protein (Figure 3A). The data suggest that both factors independently induce SOD2 levels, but CSC provides a more significant increase in SOD2 levels when HPV16 E6 and E7 are present. An immunofluorescence assay for Gamma-H2AX, a marker for single- and double-stranded DNA breaks, was performed to determine changes in genetic damage. In this way, SCC143 V and SCC143 E6/E7 cells were treated with 10 and 50 ug/mL of CSC for 24 h. Inhibitor KU55933 was included in this assay as a control to potentiate the damage induced by both factors. We observed that SCC143E6/E7 cells present a significant increase in the fluorescence intensity of Gamma-H2AX concerning the SCC143V. Furthermore, it can be seen that CSC induces a substantial increase in the fluorescence intensity of Gamma-H2AX compared to DMSO.

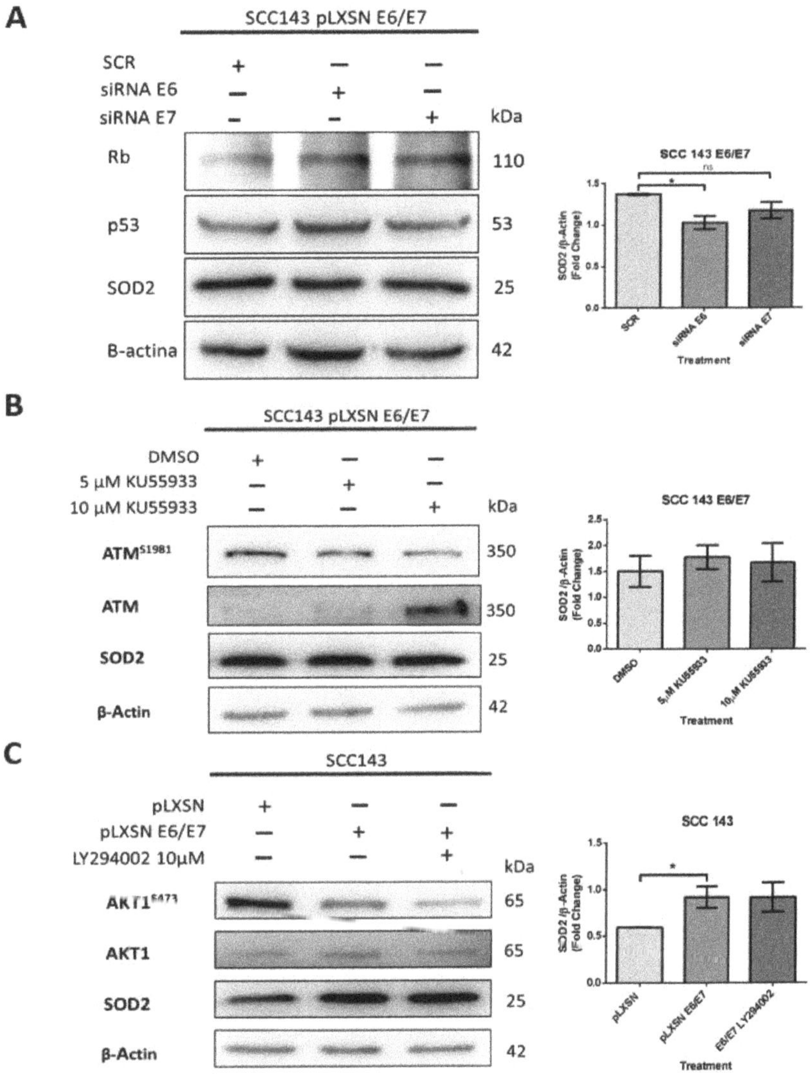

Figure 2. SOD2 is regulated by HPV16 E6 in an AKT1- and ATM-independent manner in oral cells. (**A**) Western blot performed for total protein extract of SCC143E6/E7 cells previously transfected with control siRNA (SCR), siRNA E6, or siRNA E7 (48 h) to evaluate Rb, p53, SOD2, and β-actin protein levels. (**B**) Western blot was performed with protein extracts from SCC143E6/E7 cells previously exposed to KU55933 (ATM) inhibitor for 24 h. The levels of total ATM, ATM^{S1981}, SOD2, and β-actin used as load control were analyzed. (**C**) Western blot was performed with protein extracts from SCC143E6/E7 cells previously exposed to LY294002 (PI3K) inhibitor for 24 h. The levels of total AKT1, AKT1^{S473}, SOD2, and β-actin were evaluated. The graphs represent three independent Western blots for SOD2 normalized by β-actin. Densitometric analyzes were performed with ImageJ. Data are presented as the mean ± standard deviation (SD); average of three independent experiments, conducted in triplicate; * $p < 0.05$; ns, not significant.

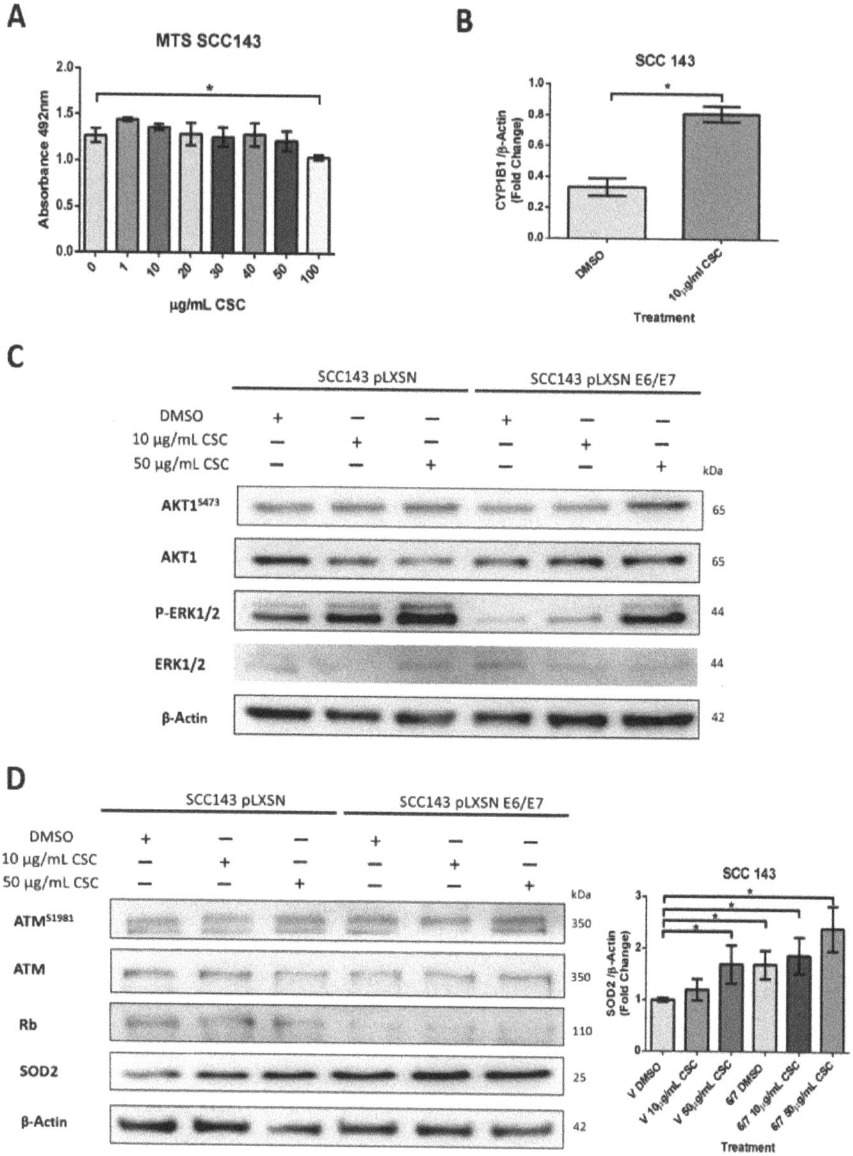

Figure 3. HPV16 E6/E7 oncoproteins and CSC increase SOD2 levels in oral cells. (**A**) MTS assay in SCC143 cells treated with CSC at different concentrations and incubated for 72 h. (**B**) CYP1B1 transcripts were evaluated by RT-PCR in SCC143 cells previously exposed to the inhibitor KU55933 (ATM) for 24 h. (**C**) Western blot performed for total protein extract of SCC143V and SCC143E6/E7 cells previously exposed to CSC for 24 h. The levels of total AKT1, AKT1^{S473}, ERK1/2, p-ERK1/2, and β-actin were evaluated. (**D**) Western blot performed for total protein extract of SCC143V and SCC143E6/E7 cells previously exposed to CSC for 24 h. The levels of total ATM, ATM^{S1981}, Rb, SOD2, and β-actin were evaluated. The graphs represent three independent Western blots for SOD2 normalized by β-actin. Densitometric analyzes were performed with ImageJ. Data are presented as the mean ± standard deviation (SD); average of three independent experiments, conducted in triplicate; * $p < 0.05$.

Furthermore, a more significant rise in Gamma-H2AX fluorescence intensity can be observed in CSC-treated SCC143E6/E7 cells. Upon exposing cells to ATM inhibitor and CSC, the fluorescence intensity increases due to the blockage of ATM-mediated repair (Figure 4). In summary, CSC with E6/E7 oncoproteins can individually induce SOD2 levels and genetic damage in oral cells. However, when both factors are present, the observed changes in SOD2 levels and genetic damage are enhanced.

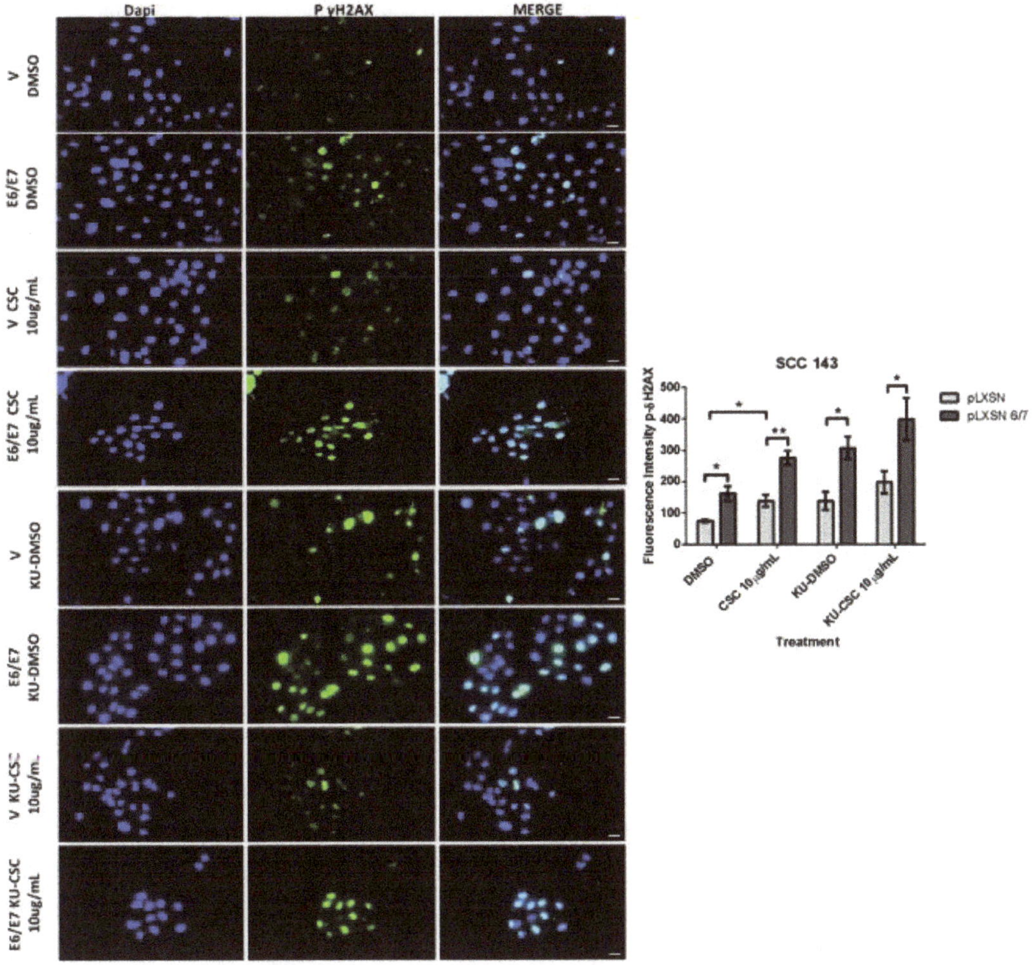

Figure 4. HPV16 E6/E7 oncoproteins and CSC increase DNA damage in oral cells. Indirect immunofluorescence (IFI) performed in SCC143V and SCC143E6/E7 cells previously exposed to CSC or CSC+ KU55933 (ATM) inhibitor for 24 h to evaluate γ-H2AX protein. Scale bar: 10 μm. The graph represents fluorescence analysis performed with the analysis of fluorescence intensity. Data are presented as the mean ± standard deviation (SD); average of three independent experiments, conducted in triplicate; * $p < 0.05$ and ** $p < 0.01$.

2.4. HPV16-Positive HNSCCs Correlate with Upregulation of SOD2 Transcripts

We evaluated the levels of SOD2 transcripts in 49 FFPE samples by RT-PCR. The cases were then distributed into three groups: HPV16 positive, HPV positive for another genotype, and HPV negative. When comparing the data of each group, we found statistically significant differences between the HPV-negative and the HPV16-positive samples (Figure 5A). Subsequently, we evaluated the E6 and E7 transcripts levels of the HPV16-positive samples. Considering these results, we distributed the data in groups of high or low levels of E6 or E7 transcripts. We detected that SOD2 levels correlate with high levels of E6 transcripts and not with E7 levels, presenting statistically significant differences between those samples that show differences in E6 transcript levels (Figure 5B). These data suggest that HPV16 E6 may be involved in SOD2 upregulation in HNC.

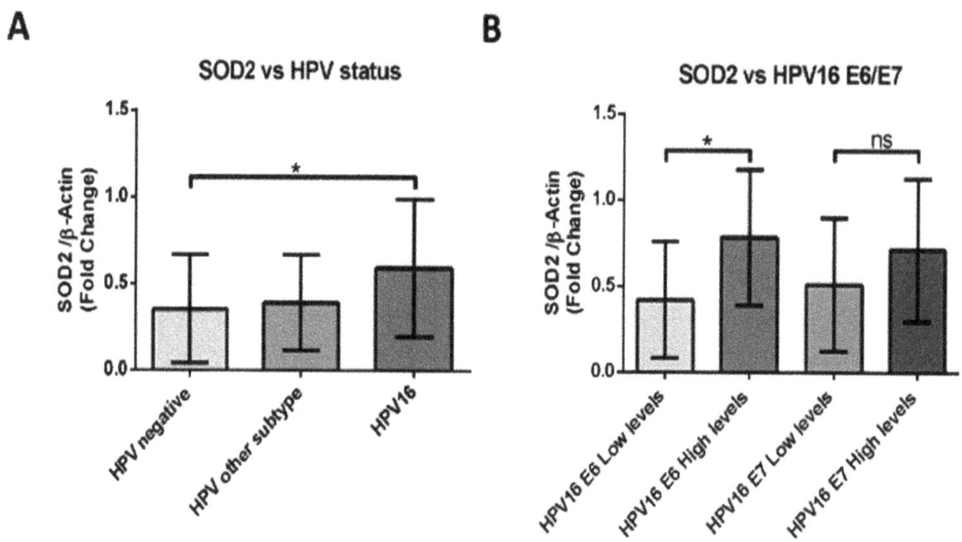

Figure 5. HPV16-positive HNSCCs correlate with upregulation of SOD2 transcripts. (**A**) SOD2 transcripts were evaluated by RT-PCR and normalized to β-actin transcript intensity. The sample data were separated into three groups: HPV negative, HPV16 positive, and other HPV genotypes. (**B**) The levels of the SOD2 transcript normalized by b-actin were evaluated by RT-PCR, according to the levels of HPV16 E6 or E7 transcripts. To generate these groups, the levels of E6 and E7 transcripts were evaluated in HPV16-positive samples, and they were stratified into high or low expression levels, considering the median of the data. Densitometric analyzes were performed by ImageJ software. Data are presented as the mean ± standard deviation (SD); average of three independent experiments, conducted in triplicate; * $p < 0.05$; ns, not significant.

On the other hand, we performed analyses with the UCSC Xena web source to analyze a functional and phenotypic correlational genomic dataset of head and neck tumors from the GDC TCGA database. In this context, we detected that SOD2 expression was increased only in oral floor cancer samples with a smoking history compared with HPV-negative oral floor cancer samples without a smoking history (Figure 6). Regarding the variables analyzed, we did not find the HPV genotype of the tumors positive for the virus.

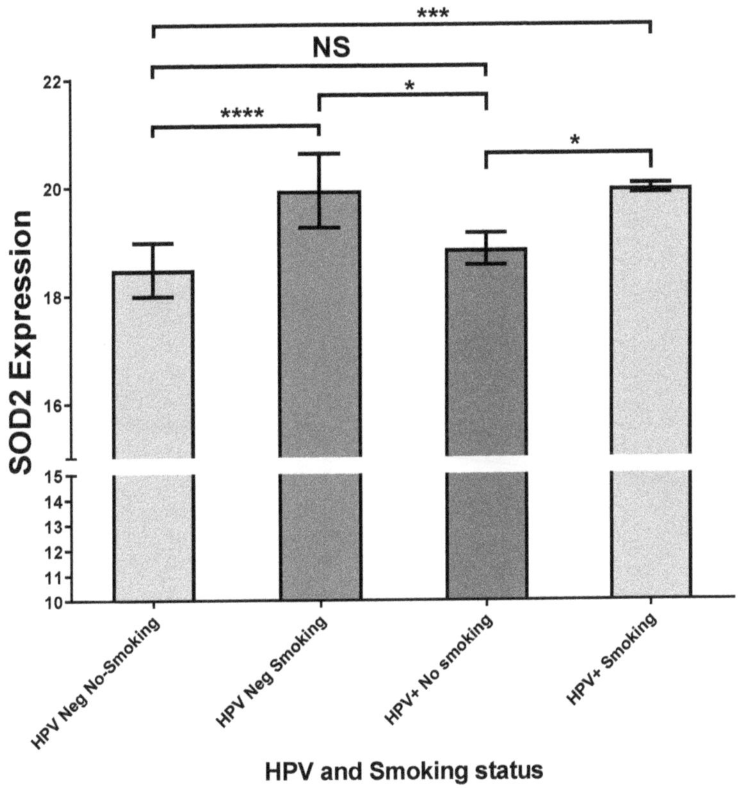

Figure 6. HPV positive and smoking since floor of mouth cancer present an up-expression of SOD2. Six hundred thirteen HNSSC samples were selected from the GDC TCGA Head and Neck Cancer Database, using the UCSC Xena web source. Twenty-eight HNSSC were selected under the following criteria: (1) HPV status information, (2) tobacco smoking history, (3) SOD2 expression, and (4) tumor primary site (floor of mouth); * $p < 0.05$, *** $p < 0.001$, **** $p < 0.0001$, NS, not significant.

3. Discussion

Cigarette smoke and HR-HPV are both potent inducers of carcinogenesis and tumor progression, modifying multiple pathways associated with the hallmarks of cancer [27–29]. Thus, both factors induce molecular signals through changes in gene expression of tumor suppressors and oncogenes in the cell [28,29]. In HNC, these molecular changes define the patient's clinical characteristics; thus, those HPV-positive tumors are defined as a different entity compared to cancers associated with cigarette smoke and alcohol [30]. Furthermore, inside HNC, the floor of the mouth is a common site for developing cancer with a high prevalence of HPV16 [31]. On the other hand, OSCC (posterolateral tongue and floor of mouth) is strongly associated with smoking history [32]. It is essential to consider the initiation of the tumor process since HPV-positive patients require other factors to generate cancer [33].

The reported prevalence of HPV in HNC depends on the anatomical origin; thus, the prevalence for the oropharynx is 25–85%; for the larynx, 20–25%; and for oral cancer, 24–32% [34–36]. We previously detected an HPV prevalence of 61.2% in oropharyngeal tumors and 11% in oral squamous cell carcinoma (OSCC) from Chile [7,37]. The HR-HPV genotype with the highest prevalence detected is HPV16, with 80% positivity in positive HPV samples, which is consistent with that reported by other authors [36,38]. Interestingly, via a transcript analysis, we detected a statistically significant increase in SOD2 only in

HPV16 positive cases when compared to HPV-negative cases. SOD2 expression studies in clinical models of tongue cancer have shown a significantly higher expression than in normal tissue samples. Furthermore, SOD2 expression was higher in late-stage (stages III and IV) than in early stage disease (stages I and II) [39]. During lung cancer chemotherapy, SOD2 overexpression increases resistance to the tyrosine kinase inhibitor anlotinib, used as a third line of treatment for patients with advanced NSCLC. Specifically, SOD2 promotes the inhibition of mitochondrial ROS production and the suppression of apoptosis [40]. In addition, SOD2 has a protective role against radiotherapy; it increases the malignant properties of tumor cells, such as invasion, migration, and anchorage-independent growth [19,41,42].

Termini L et al. demonstrated that the SOD2 protein was associated with the malignancy of cervical cancer (100% prevalence of HPV), considering it a possible biomarker of progression in this type of cancer [43]. However, by immunohistochemical analysis, Rabello S et al. suggested that the upregulation of SOD2 was independent of the presence of HPV16 and HPV18 in this type of cancer [44]. In this regard, when evaluating the E6 and E7 transcripts in the HNC samples, we observed a positive correlation between the levels of the HPV16 E6 transcript with the levels of SOD2, which in part reflects a possible relationship between the levels of SOD2 dependent on the expression of HPV16 E6. Along with the above, we detected the upregulation of SOD2 transcripts and protein in HPV16 E6, and E7 transduced oral cells. In addition, using siRNAs, we observed a dependence of SOD2 on the oncoprotein E6. In that sense, Cruz-Gregorio C et al. showed, in a hypopharyngeal cell model, that HPV16 E6 can promote mitochondrial metabolism, increasing mitochondrial protein levels, OS, and genetic damage [26].

We attempted to determine how HPV16-mediated SOD2 regulation occurs by evaluating the involvement of ATM and PI3K/AKT1. First, we analyzed whether ATM activation mediated by E6 and E7 oncoproteins could induce SOD2 levels since ATM is reportedly required for NF-κB-mediated SOD2 expression in the mammary epithelium [45]. However, we did not detect SOD2-level alterations in cells expressing HPV16 E6 and E7 oncoproteins when they were exposed to the KU55933 inhibitor. On the other hand, we analyzed the SOD2 dependence of the PI3K/AKT1 pathway in the SCC143E6/E7 model since it has been reported that this pathway can regulate transcription factors that bind to the SOD2 promoter, favoring its transcription, such as NF-κB and CREB [20,46,47]. However, we observed a decrease in $AKT1^{S473}$ levels when comparing CSCC143V and SCC143E6/E7 cells. Thus, as expected, we did not observe changes in SOD2 levels when cells were treated with LY294002. Interestingly, the decrease in pAKT1 has been associated with increased mitochondrial metabolism, favoring the expression of related proteins such as SOD2 [48]. In this regard, we hypothesize that the E6-mediated regulation of SOD2 is dependent on p53 downregulation. Previous studies show that p53 degradation allows the release of the transcription factor SP1, which maintains a binding site near the SOD2 promoter that is important in gene transcription [20,49].

Cigarette smoke cooperates with HR-HPV to promote cervical cancer progression [12,50,51]. However, studies that address the interaction of both components in HNC are scarce because epidemiological studies suggest that HR-HPV and tobacco are mutually exclusive factors for HNC development [12]. We previously reported that the interaction between cigarette smoke and HR-HPV induces DNA damage and increases E6 and E7 oncoproteins' expression in lung and cervical cancer models [52,53]. Other groups have determined that the interaction between cigarette smoke and HR-HPV can induce the expression of viral oncoproteins, favor viral infection and host genome integration, increase genetic damage, and modify the expression of relevant proteins in tumor progression, among other things [54–58]. Specifically, in OPSCC, positivity for HPV is a factor for good prognosis and better response to treatment [59]. However, through a retrospective study in patients with OPSCC who had exposure to cigarette smoke and were HPV positive, it was observed that the prognosis of the disease worsened, suggesting that this type of tumor is a new entity [60]. In the case of oral epithelium from US patients, it has been determined that those who have been exposed to tobacco are significantly associated with HPV16 infection [61].

Our results suggest that CSC induces the regulation of ERK1/2 and PI3K/AKT signaling pathways in oral cells independently of HPV16 E6 and E7 expression. In this regard, Si-Youngk et al. found that PI3K signaling levels do not change between smoking and non-smoking HPV-positive patients [62]. On the other hand, we detected that SOD2 levels and genetic damage are synergistically increased by HPV16 E6/E7 and CSC in oral cells. In this regard, SOD2 has been reported to be independently induced by cigarette smoke and HPV E6 and E7 oncoproteins [26,63]. The cigarette smoke/HPV cooperation may increase H_2O_2-mediated OS, increasing genetic damage and metastasis initiation [64,65]. We understand that, in this study, we did not find the underlying molecular mechanism of SOD2 regulation by HPV/cigarette smoke. We also know that it needs to be replicated in more head and neck cell models and in an in vivo model to demonstrate the mechanisms involved. Regarding the clinical samples analyzed in this study, it should be noted that they are from the oropharynx. In future research, other anatomical locations of the head and neck would have to be added. Future studies may molecularly address how this regulation occurs and the phenotypic changes that may be promoted by the synergistically induced regulation of SOD2 by CSC and HPV E6/E7.

Cigarette smoke and HPV16 are factors involved in the development and progression of cancer. Therefore, these factors may interact in head and neck epithelial cells and promote changes associated with cellular malignancy. Understanding how HPV/cigarette smoke cooperation can alter head and neck cells can allow us to predict the molecular changes associated with HNC induced by both factors. The data from this study suggest that the upregulation of SOD2 levels is mainly mediated by the HPV16 E6 oncoprotein in HNC. We show, in a model, the data found in this study (Figure 7). Furthermore, this is the first report of the cooperation between cigarette smoke and the HPV16 E6 and E7 oncoproteins inducing sod2 levels and genetic damage in oral cells. Finally, we hypothesize that the genetic damage caused by the collaboration of both factors may favor neoplastic development or favor tumor progression through the positive regulation of SOD2. Further determination of the combined effects of risk factors may provide new insights to improve the management of patients with HNC.

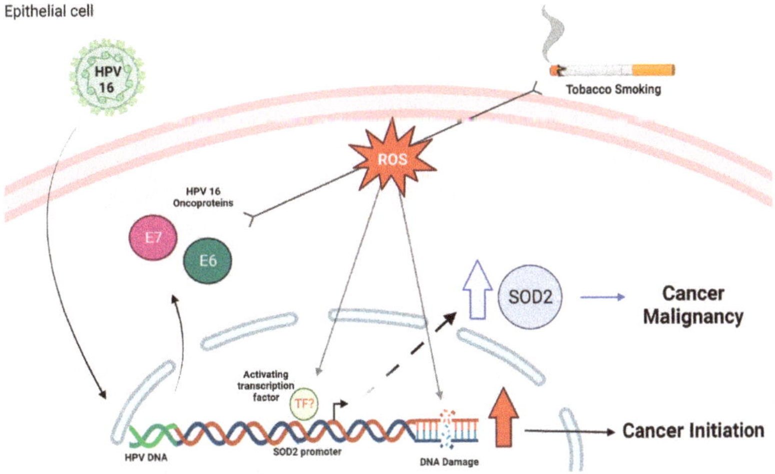

Figure 7. Proposed model of cigarette smoke and HPV16 interaction in HNSCC cells. HPV 16 E6 and E7 oncoproteins collaborate with cigarette smoke to increase genetic damage and SOD2 overexpression, promoting cancer initiation and malignancy, respectively. Created by BioRender.com. We allow the use of this image for educational use.

4. Materials and Methods

4.1. Cell Lines, Culture and Transductions

The SCC143 cell line (floor of mouth squamous cell carcinoma) and the UM-SCC-100 (Head and neck squamous cell carcinoma) cell line were obtained from the University of Pittsburgh [66]. GP + envAM-12 (CRL-9641™) retrovirus packaging cells were kindly donated by Dr. Enrique Boccardo, Institute of Biomedical Sciences, University of Sao Paulo, Sao Paulo, Brazil. Cells were incubated in Dulbecco's Modified Eagle Medium (DMEM) (Gibco, Carlsbad, CA, USA) supplemented with 10% fetal bovine serum (FBS) (Hyclone, Fremont, CA, USA), with antibiotics (100 units/mL penicillin and 100 g/mL streptomycin), and maintained at 37 °C in a 5% CO_2 atmosphere. For the subculture, cells were incubated with trypsin for 3–5 min and maintained with a new medium containing FBS (Hyclone, Fremont, CA, USA). SiHa (HTB-35™) cervical carcinoma cells were obtained from the American Type Culture Collection (ATCC; Manassas, VA, USA) and cultured in RPMI-1640 basal medium (Gibco, Carlsbad, CA, USA) supplemented with 10% heat-inactivated fetal bovine serum (FBS) (Hyclone, Fremont, CA, USA), 100 U/mL penicillin, 100 g/mL streptomycin, and 0.25 μg/mL amphotericin B (Gibco, Carlsbad, CA, USA). Cells were tested for mycoplasma contamination. Plasmids pLXSN and pLXSNHPV16E6/E7 were kindly donated by Dr. Massimo Tommasino, from the International Agency for Research on Cancer (IARC), Lyon, France. Retroviral transduction was performed with GP + envAM-12 packaging cells previously transfected with pLXSN or pLXSNHPV16E6/E7 plasmids for 24 h at 37 °C in an atmosphere containing 5% CO_2 with lipofectamine 2000 (Invitrogen, Carlsbad, CA, USA), according to the manufacturer's instructions. SCC143 cells and UM-SCC-100 were stably transduced and were then selected by 0.3 mg/mL Geneticin (GIBCO, Carlsbad, CA, USA).

4.2. Viability Assays (MTS)

SCC143 cells 5×10^3 were grown in 96-well plates. After 24 h, cells were treated with cigarette smoke condensate (CSC) prepared from 1R4F reference (Murty Pharmaceutical, Lexington, KY, USA). A stock solution of 40 mg/mL was prepared, and the maximum working solution that did not affect the viability of the cells was 50 μg/mL and was incubated for 72 h. Viability was measured using the CellTitter 96® aqueous non-radioactive cell proliferation assay kit (Promega, Madison, WI, USA), from which 20 μL of the reagent was added to each well, and the cells were incubated for 3 h. Finally, the absorbance was measured at 490 nm.

4.3. Real-Time Polymerase Chain Reaction (qPCR)

The qPCR was realized in a AriaMx Real-Time apparatus (Agilent, Santa Clara, CA, USA) in a 25 μL final volume. The components for qPCR were as follows: 12.5 μL 2X SYBR Green Mastermix (Bioline, London, UK), 7.5 μL nuclease-free water, and 1 μL cDNA template. The thermocycling conditions were as follows: 94 °C for 30 s, 58 °C for 20 s, and 72 °C for 20 s, for a total of 40 cycles. The relative copy number of each sample was calculated through the $2^{-\Delta\Delta Ct}$ method. All reactions were performed in triplicate.

4.4. Western Blot

Protein lysates obtained from SCC143 empty vector and E6/E7-transduced cells were extracted with RIPA 1X lysis buffer (Abcam, Cambridge, UK) containing protease and phosphatase inhibitor cocktail (Roche, Basel, Switzerland). Suspensions were centrifuged at 14,000× g for 15 min at 4 °C. The protein concentration was quantified with the PierceTM BCA protein assay kit (Thermo Scientific, Rockford, IL, USA). Next, 25 μg of total protein was loaded per well and separated by SDS-PAGE on 12% gels. Proteins were then transferred by electroblotting to Hybond-P ECL membranes (Amersham, Piscataway, NJ, USA), using a pH 8.3 Tris-glycine transfer buffer (20 mM Tris, 150 mM glycine, and 20% methanol) and a Trans–Blot® SD semi–dry electrophoretic transfer cell (Bio-Rad, Hercules, CA, USA). Membranes were blocked in 5% bovine serum albumin/0.5% Tween-20 in

Tris-buffered saline pH 7.6 (TBS) for 1 h at room temperature (RT) and then incubated overnight at 4 °C with primary antibodies against p53 (BD554294) (BD PharmigenTM, San Diego, CA, USA), pRb (ab24), pATM (ab36810), ATM (ab78), (Abcam, Cambridge, UK), pAKT1S473 (4060S) (Cell Signaling, Danver, MA, USA), β-actin (SC47778), SOD2 (SC 137254), AKT1(SC5298). ERK (SC514302), pERK (SC136521) (Santa Cruz Biotechnology, Inc., Dallas, TX, USA), and 1:1000 in TBS/Tween 20 (TBS–T20). After three washes in TBS–T20, the membranes were incubated either with Anti-Mouse IgG (BD Pharmingen; BD Biosciences, Heidelberg, Germany) or Anti-Rabbit IgG (Santa Cruz Biotechnology, Inc., Dallas, TX, USA) conjugated to HRP, diluted 1:1000 in BSA 5% blocking buffer for 1 h at RT. Membranes were washed three times for 15 min and revealed with the ClarityTM Western ECL detection reagent (Bio-Rad, Hercules, CA, USA) on a (ChemiDocTM Bio-Rad), according to manufacturer's instructions.

4.5. Immunofluorescence

Transduced cells were grown to confluence in treated coverslips in 24-well plate, washed twice with 1× PBS (pH 7.4), dried, and then incubated for 5 min with cold acetone/methanol. Next, cells were incubated with 3% bovine serum albumin (BSA) for 1 h at room temperature, followed by incubation with a primary monoclonal anti-specific protein antibody diluted in 1× PBS (1:50), according to the manufacturer's instructions. The fixed cells were washed three times for 5 min at room temperature and incubated with a secondary fluorescein isothiocyanate (FITC) (Santa Cruz biotechnology, Dallas, TX, USA). After three washes with 1× PBS, cells were incubated for 15 min with DAPI (Thermo Fisher Scientific, Waltham, MA, USA) and finally visualized in a fluorescence microscope.

4.6. Tissue Samples

We used previously collected 49 formalin-fixed, paraffin-embedded (FFPE) Oropharyngeal squamous-cell carcinomas (OPSCC) obtained between 2009 and 2020 from the José Joaquín Aguirre Clinical Hospital [37], University of Chile (Santiago, Chile). Each case was analyzed by a histopathologist. This study was approved by the Board of Directors of the Ethics Committee of the Hospital Clínico José Joaquín Aguirre, Universidad de Chile (Number 47-2019). The samples were characterized previously by Oliva C. et al., reporting a 61.2% (30/49) positivity for HPV [37]. HPV16 is the most prevalent genotype with 80% (24/30), followed by HPV6 with 10% (3/30), HPV33 with 6.7% (2/30), and HPV18 with 3.3% (1/30) [37].

4.7. FFPE RNA Extraction, cDNA Conversion, and RT-PCR

RNA purification was carried out using the High Pure RNA paraffin kit (Roche), following the manufacturer's instructions. The RNA obtained was suspended in 30 μL of RNA paraffin kit elution buffer and stored at −80 °C until use. The cDNA was prepared with 100 ng of purified RNA, RNAsin 1 U/μL (Promega, USA), 1× buffer TR (Promega, USA), 10 μg/μL random primers (Promega, USA), 20 U/μL MMLV (Promega, USA), and 2 mM dNTPs in a final volume of 20 μL. MMLV negative controls were included. The reaction mixture was incubated at 37 °C for 1 h and stored at −20 °C. RT-PCR was carried out using the primers of Table 1. β-actin mRNA levels were used for normalization of RNA expression. The amplification conditions were 94 °C for 5 min, followed by 33 cycles of denaturation at 95 °C for 45 s, annealing at 56 °C for 40 s, and extension at 72 °C for 45 s, with a final extension for 5 min at 72 °C. For semi-quantitative analysis, ImageJ software version 1.52a (National Institutes of Health, Bethesda, MD, USA) was used.

4.8. Gene Expression Analysis and Statistical Analysis

The UCSC Xena web source did allow us to explore functional genomic data sets and correlational genomic and phenotypic variables. We selected 613 HNSSC samples from GDC TCGA Head and Neck Cancer Database. We selected only 28 HNSSC that met the following criteria: (1) HPV status information, (2) tobacco-smoking history, (3) SOD2 expression, and (4) tumor primary site (floor of mouth).

Table 1. Primer list.

Primer	Forward 5′-3′	Reverse 5′-3′	Size (bp)
E6 small 16	CTGCAAGCAACAGTTACTGCGA	TCACACACTGCATATGGATTCCC	96
E7 small 16	CAATATTGTAATGGGCTCTGTCC	ATTTGCAACCAGAGACAACTGAT	120
PCO3/PCO4	ACACAACTGTGTTCACTAG	CAACTTCATCCACGTTCACC	110
GP5+/GP6+	TTTGTTACTGTGGTAGATATCAC	GAAAAATAAACTTAAATCATATTC	155
SOD2	GCCCTGGAACCTCACATCAAC	CAACGCCTCCTGGTACTTCTC	111
b-actin	CCACACAGGGGAGGTGATAG	CCACACAGGGGAGGTGATAG	115

A Mann–Whitney test was used to compare the means between two groups. Comparisons between multiple groups were performed using one-way ANOVA and Tukey's post hoc test. All statistical tests were performed as two-sided and considered significant at a p-value < 0.05. Statistical analyses were run using the GraphPad Prism 6 software.

Author Contributions: D.C.-B., E.B., R.B. and F.A. contributed to the study design and data interpretation and discussion; D.C.-B., J.C.O., R.B., C.O. and F.A. contributed to experiments, analysis of clinical samples, manuscript writing, and data interpretation; C.O. contributed to clinical specimens and data collection and analysis. All authors have read and agreed to the published version of the manuscript.

Funding: This study was supported by FONDECYT Postdoctoral Grant #3220237 (D.C.-B.), FAPESP 2010/20002-0 (E.B.), FAPESP 2019/26065-8 (E.B.) and Fondecyt #1221033 (F.A.)

Institutional Review Board Statement: This study was approved by the Board of Directors of the Ethics Committee of the Hospital Clínico José Joaquín Aguirre, Universidad de Chile (Number 47-2019).

Informed Consent Statement: This study obtained bioethics approval Number 47-2019 of the Ethics Committee of the Hospital Clínico José Joaquín Aguirre, Universidad de Chile. Patient consent was waived because it is a retrospective study and only the health professional in charge had access to the patient's data.

Data Availability Statement: Supporting data can be obtained through direct communication with the corresponding author Francisco Aguayo.

Conflicts of Interest: The authors declare no conflict of interest.

References

1. Chow, L.Q.M. Head and Neck Cancer. *N. Engl. J. Med.* **2020**, *382*, 60–72. [CrossRef]
2. Hsieh, C.Y.; Lin, C.C.; Huang, Y.W.; Chen, J.H.; Tsou, Y.A.; Chang, L.C.; Fan, C.C.; Lin, C.Y.; Chang, W.C. Macrophage secretory IL-1beta promotes docetaxel resistance in head and neck squamous carcinoma via SOD2/CAT-ICAM1 signaling. *JCI Insight* **2022**, *7*. [CrossRef]
3. Argiris, A.; Karamouzis, M.V.; Raben, D.; Ferris, R.L. Head and neck cancer. *Lancet* **2008**, *371*, 1695–1709. [CrossRef] [PubMed]
4. Scheffner, M.; Werness, B.A.; Huibregtse, J.M.; Levine, A.J.; Howley, P.M. The E6 oncoprotein encoded by human papillomavirus types 16 and 18 promotes the degradation of p53. *Cell* **1990**, *63*, 1129–1136. [CrossRef] [PubMed]
5. Heck, D.V.; Yee, C.L.; Howley, P.M.; Munger, K. Efficiency of binding the retinoblastoma protein correlates with the transforming capacity of the E7 oncoproteins of the human papillomaviruses. *Proc. Natl. Acad. Sci. USA* **1992**, *89*, 4442–4446. [CrossRef] [PubMed]
6. Tumban, E. A Current Update on Human Papillomavirus-Associated Head and Neck Cancers. *Viruses* **2019**, *11*, 922. [CrossRef]
7. Reyes, M.; Rojas-Alcayaga, G.; Pennacchiotti, G.; Carrillo, D.; Munoz, J.P.; Pena, N.; Montes, R.; Lobos, N.; Aguayo, F. Human papillomavirus infection in oral squamous cell carcinomas from Chilean patients. *Exp. Mol. Pathol.* **2015**, *99*, 95–99. [CrossRef] [PubMed]
8. Hubbers, C.U.; Akgul, B. HPV and cancer of the oral cavity. *Virulence* **2015**, *6*, 244–248. [CrossRef]
9. Munoz, J.P.; Gonzalez, C.; Parra, B.; Corvalan, A.H.; Tornesello, M.L.; Eizuru, Y.; Aguayo, F. Functional interaction between human papillomavirus type 16 E6 and E7 oncoproteins and cigarette smoke components in lung epithelial cells. *PLoS ONE* **2012**, *7*, e38178. [CrossRef]

10. Chen, X.; Mims, J.; Huang, X.; Singh, N.; Motea, E.; Planchon, S.M.; Beg, M.; Tsang, A.W.; Porosnicu, M.; Kemp, M.L.; et al. Modulators of Redox Metabolism in Head and Neck Cancer. *Antioxid. Redox Signal.* **2018**, *29*, 1660–1690. [CrossRef]
11. Tang, M.S.; Lee, H.W.; Weng, M.W.; Wang, H.T.; Hu, Y.; Chen, L.C.; Park, S.H.; Chan, H.W.; Xu, J.; Wu, X.R.; et al. DNA damage, DNA repair and carcinogenicity: Tobacco smoke versus electronic cigarette aerosol. *Mutat. Res./Rev. Mutat. Res.* **2022**, *789*, 108409. [CrossRef] [PubMed]
12. Aguayo, F.; Munoz, J.P.; Perez-Dominguez, F.; Carrillo-Beltran, D.; Oliva, C.; Calaf, G.M.; Blanco, R.; Nunez-Acurio, D. High-Risk Human Papillomavirus and Tobacco Smoke Interactions in Epithelial Carcinogenesis. *Cancers* **2020**, *12*, 2201. [CrossRef] [PubMed]
13. Ames, B.N.; Gold, L.S. Endogenous mutagens and the causes of aging and cancer. *Mutat. Res.* **1991**, *250*, 3–16. [CrossRef]
14. De Marco, F. Oxidative stress and HPV carcinogenesis. *Viruses* **2013**, *5*, 708–731. [CrossRef] [PubMed]
15. Lin, W.J.; Jiang, R.S.; Wu, S.H.; Chen, F.J.; Liu, S.A. Smoking, alcohol, and betel quid and oral cancer: A prospective cohort study. *J. Oncol.* **2011**, *2011*, 525976. [CrossRef]
16. Carrillo, D.; Munoz, J.P.; Huerta, H.; Leal, G.; Corvalan, A.; Leon, O.; Calaf, G.M.; Urzua, U.; Boccardo, E.; Tapia, J.C.; et al. Upregulation of PIR gene expression induced by human papillomavirus E6 and E7 in epithelial oral and cervical cells. *Open Biol.* **2017**, *7*, 170111. [CrossRef]
17. Carrillo-Beltran, D.; Munoz, J.P.; Guerrero-Vasquez, N.; Blanco, R.; Leon, O.; de Souza Lino, V.; Tapia, J.C.; Maldonado, E.; Dubois-Camacho, K.; Hermoso, M.A.; et al. Human Papillomavirus 16 E7 Promotes EGFR/PI3K/AKT1/NRF2 Signaling Pathway Contributing to PIR/NF-kappaB Activation in Oral Cancer Cells. *Cancers* **2020**, *12*, 1904. [CrossRef] [PubMed]
18. Kurokawa, H.; Sakimoto, M.; Yamashita, Y.; Murata, T.; Kajiyama, M. Manganese superoxide dismutase (Mn-SOD) correlates with prognosis of patients with oral squamous cell carcinoma. *Fukuoka Igaku Zasshi* **1998**, *89*, 321–327.
19. Noh, J.K.; Woo, S.R.; Yun, M.; Lee, M.K.; Kong, M.; Min, S.; Kim, S.I.; Lee, Y.C.; Eun, Y.G.; Ko, S.G. SOD2- and NRF2-associated Gene Signature to Predict Radioresistance in Head and Neck Cancer. *Cancer Genom. Proteom.* **2021**, *18*, 675–684. [CrossRef] [PubMed]
20. Kim, Y.S.; Gupta Vallur, P.; Phaeton, R.; Mythreye, K.; Hempel, N. Insights into the Dichotomous Regulation of SOD2 in Cancer. *Antioxidants* **2017**, *6*, 86. [CrossRef]
21. Dhar, S.K.; Tangpong, J.; Chaiswing, L.; Oberley, T.D.; St Clair, D.K. Manganese superoxide dismutase is a p53-regulated gene that switches cancers between early and advanced stages. *Cancer Res.* **2011**, *71*, 6684–6695. [CrossRef] [PubMed]
22. Connor, K.M.; Hempel, N.; Nelson, K.K.; Dabiri, G.; Gamarra, A.; Belarmino, J.; Van De Water, L.; Mian, B.M.; Melendez, J.A. Manganese superoxide dismutase enhances the invasive and migratory activity of tumor cells. *Cancer Res.* **2007**, *67*, 10260–10267. [CrossRef] [PubMed]
23. Liu, Z.; Li, S.; Cai, Y.; Wang, A.; He, Q.; Zheng, C.; Zhao, T.; Ding, X.; Zhou, X. Manganese superoxide dismutase induces migration and invasion of tongue squamous cell carcinoma via H_2O_2-dependent Snail signaling. *Free Radic. Biol. Med.* **2012**, *53*, 44–50. [CrossRef]
24. Talarico, M.C.R.; Nunes, R.A.L.; Silva, G.A.F.; Costa, L.; Cardoso, M.R.; Esteves, S.C.B.; Zanatta Sarian, L.O.; Zeferino, L.C.; Termini, L. High Expression of SOD2 Protein Is a Strong Prognostic Factor for Stage IIIB Squamous Cell Cervical Carcinoma. *Antioxidants* **2021**, *10*, 724. [CrossRef] [PubMed]
25. Lee, D.J.; Lee, H.M.; Kim, J.H.; Park, I.S.; Rho, Y.S. Heavy alcohol drinking downregulates ALDH2 gene expression but heavy smoking up-regulates SOD2 gene expression in head and neck squamous cell carcinoma. *World J. Surg. Oncol.* **2017**, *15*, 163. [CrossRef]
26. Cruz-Gregorio, A.; Aranda-Rivera, A.K.; Aparicio-Trejo, O.E.; Coronado-Martinez, I.; Pedraza-Chaverri, J.; Lizano, M. E6 Oncoproteins from High-Risk Human Papillomavirus Induce Mitochondrial Metabolism in a Head and Neck Squamous Cell Carcinoma Model. *Biomolecules* **2019**, *9*, 351. [CrossRef]
27. Pfeifer, G.P.; Denissenko, M.F.; Olivier, M.; Tretyakova, N.; Hecht, S.S.; Hainaut, P. Tobacco smoke carcinogens, DNA damage and p53 mutations in smoking-associated cancers. *Oncogene* **2002**, *21*, 7435–7451. [CrossRef]
28. Sobus, S.L.; Warren, G.W. The biologic effects of cigarette smoke on cancer cells. *Cancer* **2014**, *120*, 3617–3626. [CrossRef]
29. Pal, A.; Kundu, R. Human Papillomavirus E6 and E7: The Cervical Cancer Hallmarks and Targets for Therapy. *Front. Microbiol.* **2019**, *10*, 3116. [CrossRef]
30. Gillison, M.L.; D'Souza, G.; Westra, W.; Sugar, E.; Xiao, W.; Begum, S.; Viscidi, R. Distinct risk factor profiles for human papillomavirus type 16-positive and human papillomavirus type 16-negative head and neck cancers. *J. Natl. Cancer Inst.* **2008**, *100*, 407–420. [CrossRef]
31. Lerman, M.A.; Almazrooa, S.; Lindeman, N.; Hall, D.; Villa, A.; Woo, S.B. HPV-16 in a distinct subset of oral epithelial dysplasia. *Mod. Pathol.* **2017**, *30*, 1646–1654. [CrossRef] [PubMed]
32. Schmidt, B.L.; Dierks, E.J.; Homer, L.; Potter, B. Tobacco smoking history and presentation of oral squamous cell carcinoma. *J. Oral Maxillofac. Surg.* **2004**, *62*, 1055–1058. [CrossRef]
33. Smith, E.M.; Rubenstein, L.M.; Haugen, T.H.; Hamsikova, E.; Turek, L.P. Tobacco and alcohol use increases the risk of both HPV-associated and HPV-independent head and neck cancers. *Cancer Causes Control* **2010**, *21*, 1369–1378. [CrossRef] [PubMed]
34. Wittekindt, C.; Wagner, S.; Sharma, S.J.; Wurdemann, N.; Knuth, J.; Reder, H.; Klussmann, J.P. HPV—A different view on Head and Neck Cancer. *Laryngo-Rhino-Otologie* **2018**, *97*, S48–S113. [CrossRef] [PubMed]

35. Wurdemann, N.; Wagner, S.; Sharma, S.J.; Prigge, E.S.; Reuschenbach, M.; Gattenlohner, S.; Klussmann, J.P.; Wittekindt, C. Prognostic Impact of AJCC/UICC 8th Edition New Staging Rules in Oropharyngeal Squamous Cell Carcinoma. *Front. Oncol.* **2017**, *7*, 129. [CrossRef]
36. Saraiya, M.; Unger, E.R.; Thompson, T.D.; Lynch, C.F.; Hernandez, B.Y.; Lyu, C.W.; Steinau, M.; Watson, M.; Wilkinson, E.J.; Hopenhayn, C.; et al. US assessment of HPV types in cancers: Implications for current and 9-valent HPV vaccines. *J. Natl. Cancer Inst.* **2015**, *107*, djv086. [CrossRef] [PubMed]
37. Oliva, C.; Carrillo-Beltran, D.; Boettiger, P.; Gallegos, I.; Aguayo, F. Human Papillomavirus Detected in Oropharyngeal Cancers from Chilean Subjects. *Viruses* **2022**, *14*, 1212. [CrossRef]
38. Michaud, D.S.; Langevin, S.M.; Eliot, M.; Nelson, H.H.; Pawlita, M.; McClean, M.D.; Kelsey, K.T. High-risk HPV types and head and neck cancer. *Int. J. Cancer* **2014**, *135*, 1653–1661. [CrossRef] [PubMed]
39. Liu, X.; Wang, A.; Lo Muzio, L.; Kolokythas, A.; Sheng, S.; Rubini, C.; Ye, H.; Shi, F.; Yu, T.; Crowe, D.L.; et al. Deregulation of manganese superoxide dismutase (SOD2) expression and lymph node metastasis in tongue squamous cell carcinoma. *BMC Cancer* **2010**, *10*, 365. [CrossRef]
40. Li, S.; Cao, C.; Huang, Z.; Tang, D.; Chen, J.; Wang, A.; He, Q. SOD2 confers anlotinib resistance via regulation of mitochondrial damage in OSCC. *Oral Dis.* **2022**. [CrossRef]
41. Jung, C.H.; Kim, E.M.; Song, J.Y.; Park, J.K.; Um, H.D. Mitochondrial superoxide dismutase 2 mediates gamma-irradiation-induced cancer cell invasion. *Exp. Mol. Med.* **2019**, *51*, 1–10. [CrossRef] [PubMed]
42. Yun, M.; Choi, A.J.; Lee, Y.C.; Kong, M.; Sung, J.Y.; Kim, S.S.; Eun, Y.G. Carbonyl reductase 1 is a new target to improve the effect of radiotherapy on head and neck squamous cell carcinoma. *J. Exp. Clin. Cancer Res.* **2018**, *37*, 264. [CrossRef]
43. Termini, L.; Filho, A.L.; Maciag, P.C.; Etlinger, D.; Alves, V.A.; Nonogaki, S.; Soares, F.A.; Villa, L.L. Deregulated expression of superoxide dismutase-2 correlates with different stages of cervical neoplasia. *Dis. Markers* **2011**, *30*, 275–281. [CrossRef]
44. Rabelo-Santos, S.H.; Termini, L.; Boccardo, E.; Derchain, S.; Longatto-Filho, A.; Andreoli, M.A.; Costa, M.C.; Lima Nunes, R.A.; Lucci Angelo-Andrade, L.A.; Villa, L.L.; et al. Strong SOD2 expression and HPV-16/18 positivity are independent events in cervical cancer. *Oncotarget* **2018**, *9*, 21630–21640. [CrossRef] [PubMed]
45. Dyer, L.M.; Kepple, J.D.; Ai, L.; Kim, W.J.; Stanton, V.L.; Reinhard, M.K.; Backman, L.R.F.; Streitfeld, W.S.; Babu, N.R.; Treiber, N.; et al. ATM is required for SOD2 expression and homeostasis within the mammary gland. *Breast Cancer Res. Treat.* **2017**, *166*, 725–741. [CrossRef] [PubMed]
46. Bai, D.; Ueno, L.; Vogt, P.K. Akt-mediated regulation of NFkappaB and the essentialness of NFkappaB for the oncogenicity of PI3K and Akt. *Int. J. Cancer* **2009**, *125*, 2863–2870. [CrossRef] [PubMed]
47. Carloni, S.; Girelli, S.; Scopa, C.; Buonocore, G.; Longini, M.; Balduini, W. Activation of autophagy and Akt/CREB signaling play an equivalent role in the neuroprotective effect of rapamycin in neonatal hypoxia-ischemia. *Autophagy* **2010**, *6*, 366–377. [CrossRef]
48. De Rosa, V.; Iommelli, F.; Monti, M.; Fonti, R.; Votta, G.; Stoppelli, M.P.; Del Vecchio, S. Reversal of Warburg Effect and Reactivation of Oxidative Phosphorylation by Differential Inhibition of EGFR Signaling Pathways in Non-Small Cell Lung Cancer. *Clin. Cancer Res.* **2015**, *21*, 5110–5120. [CrossRef]
49. Xu, Y.; Porntadavity, S.; St Clair, D.K. Transcriptional regulation of the human manganese superoxide dismutase gene: The role of specificity protein 1 (Sp1) and activating protein-2 (AP-2). *Biochem. J.* **2002**, *362 Pt 2*, 401–412. [CrossRef]
50. Gunnell, A.S.; Tran, T.N.; Torrang, A.; Dickman, P.W.; Sparen, P.; Palmgren, J.; Ylitalo, N. Synergy between cigarette smoking and human papillomavirus type 16 in cervical cancer in situ development. *Cancer Epidemiol. Biomark. Prev.* **2006**, *15*, 2141–2147. [CrossRef]
51. Louie, K.S.; Castellsague, X.; de Sanjose, S.; Herrero, R.; Meijer, C.J.; Shah, K.; Munoz, N.; Bosch, F.X. Smoking and passive smoking in cervical cancer risk: Pooled analysis of couples from the IARC multicentric case-control studies. *Cancer Epidemiol. Biomark. Prev.* **2011**, *20*, 1379–1390. [CrossRef]
52. Pena, N.; Carrillo, D.; Munoz, J.P.; Chnaiderman, J.; Urzua, U.; Leon, O.; Tornesello, M.L.; Corvalan, A.H.; Soto-Rifo, R.; Aguayo, F. Tobacco smoke activates human papillomavirus 16 p97 promoter and cooperates with high-risk E6/E7 for oxidative DNA damage in lung cells. *PLoS ONE* **2015**, *10*, e0123029. [CrossRef]
53. Munoz, J.P.; Carrillo-Beltran, D.; Aedo-Aguilera, V.; Calaf, G.M.; Leon, O.; Maldonado, E.; Tapia, J.C.; Boccardo, E.; Ozbun, M.A.; Aguayo, F. Tobacco Exposure Enhances Human Papillomavirus 16 Oncogene Expression via EGFR/PI3K/Akt/c-Jun Signaling Pathway in Cervical Cancer Cells. *Front. Microbiol.* **2018**, *9*, 3022. [CrossRef]
54. Ndisang, D.; Khan, A.; Lorenzato, F.; Sindos, M.; Singer, A.; Latchman, D.S. The cellular transcription factor Brn-3a and the smoking-related substance nicotine interact to regulate the activity of the HPV URR in the cervix. *Oncogene* **2010**, *29*, 2701–2711. [CrossRef]
55. Koshiol, J.; Schroeder, J.; Jamieson, D.J.; Marshall, S.W.; Duerr, A.; Heilig, C.M.; Shah, K.V.; Klein, R.S.; Cu-Uvin, S.; Schuman, P.; et al. Smoking and time to clearance of human papillomavirus infection in HIV-seropositive and HIV-seronegative women. *Am. J. Epidemiol.* **2006**, *164*, 176–183. [CrossRef]
56. Trushin, N.; Alam, S.; El-Bayoumy, K.; Krzeminski, J.; Amin, S.G.; Gullett, J.; Meyers, C.; Prokopczyk, B. Comparative metabolism of benzo[a]pyrene by human keratinocytes infected with high-risk human papillomavirus types 16 and 18 as episomal or integrated genomes. *J. Carcinog.* **2012**, *11*, 1. [CrossRef]

57. Moktar, A.; Ravoori, S.; Vadhanam, M.V.; Gairola, C.G.; Gupta, R.C. Cigarette smoke-induced DNA damage and repair detected by the comet assay in HPV-transformed cervical cells. *Int. J. Oncol.* **2009**, *35*, 1297–1304. [CrossRef] [PubMed]
58. Chen, L.; Wang, H. eIF4E is a critical regulator of human papillomavirus (HPV)-immortalized cervical epithelial (H8) cell growth induced by nicotine. *Toxicology* **2019**, *419*, 1–10. [CrossRef]
59. Ang, K.K.; Harris, J.; Wheeler, R.; Weber, R.; Rosenthal, D.I.; Nguyen-Tan, P.F.; Westra, W.H.; Chung, C.H.; Jordan, R.C.; Lu, C.; et al. Human papillomavirus and survival of patients with oropharyngeal cancer. *N. Engl. J. Med.* **2010**, *363*, 24–35. [CrossRef] [PubMed]
60. Elhalawani, H.; Mohamed, A.S.R.; Elgohari, B.; Lin, T.A.; Sikora, A.G.; Lai, S.Y.; Abusaif, A.; Phan, J.; Morrison, W.H.; Gunn, G.B.; et al. Tobacco exposure as a major modifier of oncologic outcomes in human papillomavirus (HPV) associated oropharyngeal squamous cell carcinoma. *BMC Cancer* **2020**, *20*, 912. [CrossRef] [PubMed]
61. Fakhry, C.; Gillison, M.L.; D'Souza, G. Tobacco use and oral HPV-16 infection. *JAMA* **2014**, *312*, 1465–1467. [CrossRef] [PubMed]
62. Kiessling, S.Y.; Broglie, M.A.; Soltermann, A.; Huber, G.F.; Stoeckli, S.J. Comparison of PI3K Pathway in HPV-Associated Oropharyngeal Cancer with and without Tobacco Exposure. *Laryngoscope Investig. Otolaryngol.* **2018**, *3*, 283–289. [CrossRef] [PubMed]
63. Dikalov, S.; Itani, H.; Richmond, B.; Vergeade, A.; Rahman, S.M.J.; Boutaud, O.; Blackwell, T.; Massion, P.P.; Harrison, D.G.; Dikalova, A. Tobacco smoking induces cardiovascular mitochondrial oxidative stress, promotes endothelial dysfunction, and enhances hypertension. *Am. J. Physiol. Heart Circ. Physiol.* **2019**, *316*, H639–H646. [CrossRef] [PubMed]
64. Dai, D.F.; Rabinovitch, P. Mitochondrial oxidative stress mediates induction of autophagy and hypertrophy in angiotensin-II treated mouse hearts. *Autophagy* **2011**, *7*, 917–918. [CrossRef]
65. Lisanti, M.P.; Martinez-Outschoorn, U.E.; Lin, Z.; Pavlides, S.; Whitaker-Menezes, D.; Pestell, R.G.; Howell, A.; Sotgia, F. Hydrogen peroxide fuels aging, inflammation, cancer metabolism and metastasis: The seed and soil also needs "fertilizer". *Cell Cycle* **2011**, *10*, 2440–2449. [CrossRef]
66. White, J.S.; Weissfeld, J.L.; Ragin, C.C.; Rossie, K.M.; Martin, C.L.; Shuster, M.; Ishwad, C.S.; Law, J.C.; Myers, E.N.; Johnson, J.T.; et al. The influence of clinical and demographic risk factors on the establishment of head and neck squamous cell carcinoma cell lines. *Oral Oncol.* **2007**, *43*, 701–712. [CrossRef]

International Journal of *Molecular Sciences*

MDPI

Article

Cholesterol Is a Regulator of CAV1 Localization and Cell Migration in Oral Squamous Cell Carcinoma

Nyein Nyein Chan [1,2], Manabu Yamazaki [1,*], Satoshi Maruyama [3], Tatsuya Abé [1], Kenta Haga [2], Masami Kawaharada [2], Kenji Izumi [4], Tadaharu Kobayashi [2] and Jun-ichi Tanuma [1,3]

1 Division of Oral Pathology, Department of Tissue Regeneration and Reconstruction, Faculty of Dentistry & Graduate School of Medical and Dental Sciences, Niigata University, Niigata 951-8514, Japan
2 Division of Reconstructive Surgery for Oral and Maxillofacial Region, Faculty of Dentistry & Graduate School of Medical and Dental Sciences, Niigata University, Niigata 951-8514, Japan
3 Oral Pathology Section, Department of Surgical Pathology, Niigata University Hospital, Niigata 951-8520, Japan
4 Division of Biomimetics, Department of Oral Health Science, Faculty of Dentistry & Graduate School of Medical and Dental Sciences, Niigata University, Niigata 951-8514, Japan
* Correspondence: manyamaz@dent.niigata-u.ac.jp; Tel.: +81-25-227-2834; Fax: +81-25-227-0805

Abstract: Cholesterol plays an important role in cancer progression, as it is utilized in membrane biogenesis and cell signaling. Cholesterol-lowering drugs have exhibited tumor-suppressive effects in oral squamous cell carcinoma (OSCC), suggesting that cholesterol is also essential in OSCC pathogenesis. However, the direct effects of cholesterol on OSCC cells remain unclear. Here, we investigated the role of cholesterol in OSCC with respect to caveolin-1 (CAV1), a cholesterol-binding protein involved in intracellular cholesterol transport. Cholesterol levels in OSCC cell lines were depleted using methyl-β-cyclodextrin and increased using the methyl-β-cyclodextrin-cholesterol complex. Functional analysis was performed using timelapse imaging, and CAV1 expression in cholesterol-manipulated cells was investigated using immunofluorescence and immunoblotting assays. CAV1 immunohistochemistry was performed on surgical OSCC samples. We observed that cholesterol addition induced polarized cell morphology, along with CAV1 localization at the trailing edge, and promoted cell migration. Moreover, CAV1 was upregulated in the lipid rafts and formed aggregates in the plasma membrane in cholesterol-added cells. High membranous CAV1 expression in tissue specimens was associated with OSCC recurrence. Therefore, cholesterol promotes the migration of OSCC cells by regulating cell polarity and CAV1 localization to the lipid raft. Furthermore, membranous CAV1 expression is a potential prognostic marker for OSCC patients.

Keywords: caveolin-1; cell polarization; cholesterol; migration; oral squamous cell carcinoma

Citation: Chan, N.N.; Yamazaki, M.; Maruyama, S.; Abé, T.; Haga, K.; Kawaharada, M.; Izumi, K.; Kobayashi, T.; Tanuma, J.-i. Cholesterol Is a Regulator of CAV1 Localization and Cell Migration in Oral Squamous Cell Carcinoma. *Int. J. Mol. Sci.* **2023**, *24*, 6035. https://doi.org/10.3390/ijms24076035

Academic Editors: Marko Tarle and Ivica Lukšić

Received: 3 March 2023
Revised: 20 March 2023
Accepted: 20 March 2023
Published: 23 March 2023

1. Introduction

Cholesterol constitutes 30–40% of the lipid component of the plasma membrane [1]. As cancer cells proliferate rapidly, they require high levels of cholesterol for membrane biogenesis and other cellular functions, such as cell signaling [2]. Therefore, cancer cells reprogram cholesterol metabolism by increasing cholesterol influx via lipid receptors [3] or by upregulating de novo biosynthesis of cholesterol via the mevalonate pathway [4], whereas normal cells strictly regulate the cholesterol content of the plasma membrane [5].

Derangement of cholesterol metabolism and its role in tumor progression have been observed in various types of cancers [2]. Cholesterol supplementation in prostate cancer cells enhances cell survival via the PI3K/Akt pathway, but it has a lower effect on normal prostate epithelial cells [6]. Moreover, cholesterol serves as a mitogen for cell proliferation in intestinal stem cells by increasing cholesterol biosynthesis [7]. Cholesterol reprogramming is also observed in oral squamous cell carcinoma (OSCC), with higher cellular cholesterol levels in OSCC tissues than in normal oral mucosa in the same patient [8]. In addition, one of the lipid receptors, CD36, is overexpressed in OSCC and participates in the proliferation and migration of OSCC cells [9]. However, the serum lipid profile, including cholesterol level, was reported to be lower in OSCC patients than in healthy controls [10,11], suggesting a possibility that cancer cells demand and utilize serum cholesterol and lipids for membrane formation and cancer progression [12,13]. Therefore, cellular cholesterol metabolism is vital for carcinogenesis and cancer progression rather than serum cholesterol level [14]. Moreover, cholesterol-lowering agents, such as statins, can inhibit OSCC progression in several ways. Simvastatin decreases the proliferation of oral cancer cells by inhibiting cell-cycle-regulated protein DNA methyltransferase I [15]. Xu et al. reported that pitavastatin can be used as an anticancer drug, as it downregulates MET signaling in oral and esophageal cancers [16]. Thus, cholesterol is suggested to play an important role in the carcinogenesis and progression of OSCC. However, the direct effect of cellular cholesterol levels on OSCC development and pathogenesis has rarely been reported.

Cellular cholesterol metabolism involves various processes, including cholesterol influx, efflux, esterification, and de novo synthesis, in which the metabolism depends on intracellular cholesterol trafficking [17]. In addition to the endolysosomal pathway, caveolin-1 (CAV1), a major structural protein of caveolae in lipid rafts [18], directly binds to cholesterol and transports it between intracellular organelles and caveolae of the plasma membrane [19–21] through receptor-independent endocytosis [22]. In OSCC, CAV1 is overexpressed [23,24] and is linked to carcinogenesis, tumor progression, lymph node metastasis, chemoresistance, and poor prognosis [25–28]. Although intracellular cholesterol and CAV1 levels are increased in OSCC cells, the role of CAV1 with respect to cellular cholesterol levels in the progression of OSCC remains unclear.

Therefore, we hypothesized that cellular cholesterol levels affect the biological activities of OSCC cells by regulating CAV1 expression. In this study, we investigated the functional changes in OSCC cells with respect to cellular cholesterol levels and the underlying mechanisms involving CAV1 expression. In this study, we found that cholesterol manipulations modified CAV1 localization and cell polarity in OSCC cells. Moreover, membranous CAV1 expression could be a potential prognostic biomarker for patients with OSCC.

2. Results

2.1. Cholesterol Influences the Morphology of OSCC Cells and Promotes Their Migration

To investigate the role of cholesterol in OSCC pathogenesis, we depleted or increased cholesterol levels in cells and observed the viability of cells at different time points. Methyl-β-cyclodextrin (MβCD) is widely used for cholesterol depletion because of its fast extractability, compatibility with live cells, and reversibility [29]. In contrast, the MβCD-cholesterol complex enriches cholesterol in cells [30]. However, the vulnerability of the cells to cholesterol depletion by MβCD depends on its concentration, the incubation duration, and the cell type [30]. In the present study, the viability of treated and untreated cells was comparable up to 8 h, although the HSC-3 cells treated with MβCD for 24 h exhibited a drastic decrease in viability (Figure S1, Supplementary Materials). Thus, we analyzed cellular changes and cell migration after 4 and 8 h of treatment, respectively. Total cholesterol levels were significantly decreased in the MβCD-treated cells ($p < 0.05$ in HSC-2, $p < 0.01$ in HSC-3) and increased in the cells treated with the MβCD–cholesterol complex ($p < 0.05$ in HSC-2, $p < 0.01$ in HSC-3) compared with the control cells (Figure 1A), indicating that cholesterol manipulation was successfully performed. Filipin III signals were detected around the nuclei in the control and cholesterol-depleted (CD) cells, indicating the presence of cholesterol; however, no signals were observed in the plasma membrane (Figure 1B). Meanwhile, in the cholesterol-added (CA) cells, the signals increased in the plasma membrane area in both cell lines (Figure 1B, arrows), suggesting that the cholesterol enrichment procedure used in the present study influenced cholesterol content in the plasma membrane. Moreover, we noticed that increased cellular cholesterol levels changed the shape of the cells. Although most control and CD cells were polygonal in shape, the CA cells were fan-shaped, accompanied by the development of lamellipodia-like structures (Figure 1C, arrowheads). Image analysis revealed that in the case of CA cells, the area was significantly increased ($p < 0.0001$ in both HSC-2 and HSC-3), whereas the circularity index was reduced (Figure 1D), indicating that cholesterol addition promoted cell stretching. Since morphological changes are fundamental processes in cell migration, we tracked the cells using timelapse imaging. Migratory parameters, such as distance and velocity, were significantly increased in CA cells ($p < 0.0001$) and decreased in CD cells ($p < 0.001$ in HSC-2, $p < 0.01$ in HSC-3) in both cell lines (Figure 1E).

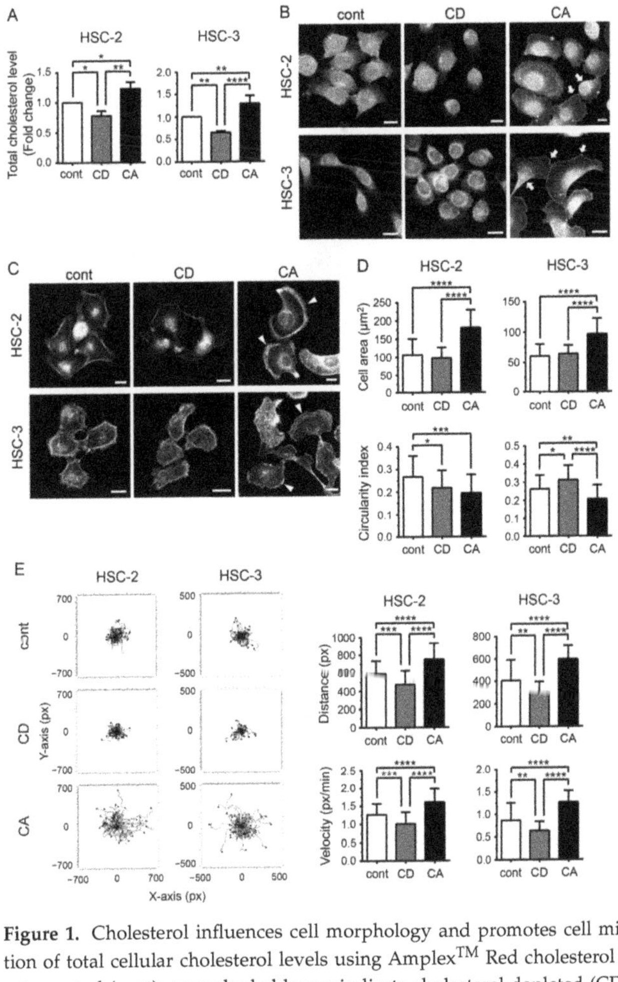

Figure 1. Cholesterol influences cell morphology and promotes cell migration. (**A**) Quantification of total cellular cholesterol levels using Amplex^{TM} Red cholesterol assay. Open boxes indicate control (cont); gray-shaded boxes indicate cholesterol-depleted (CD) cells; solid boxes indicate cholesterol-added (CA) cells. Triplicate results of cholesterol levels represent fold change as mean ± SD (compared to control). * $p < 0.05$, ** $p < 0.01$, and **** $p < 0.0001$. (**B**) Fluorescence staining using a filipin III cholesterol probe. Scale bars, 20 μm. Arrows indicate high filipin III signaling at the periphery of the cells. (**C**) Fluorescence images of F-actin visualized by rhodamine-phalloidin staining to evaluate cellular morphology. Scale bars, 20 μm. Arrowheads indicate the development of a lamellipodia-like structure. (**D**) Bar graphs showing cellular area and circularity index (N ≥ 50) expressed as mean ± SD. * $p < 0.05$, ** $p < 0.01$, *** $p < 0.001$, and **** $p < 0.0001$. (**E**) Cell-tracking plots of timelapse imaging for 8 h (N ≥ 50). Distance and velocity are analyzed using chemotaxis and migration tools (ibidi) and expressed as mean ± SD. ** $p < 0.01$, *** $p < 0.001$, and **** $p < 0.0001$.

2.2. Cholesterol Leads to Cell Polarity by Promoting Asymmetric Membranous Localization of CAV1

To explore the mechanism of cholesterol-regulated cell migration, we focused on the localization of CAV1, a cholesterol-binding protein [20]. In the combined fluorescence images, filipin III and CAV1 signals were similarly distributed in all samples (Figure 2A), suggesting a close relationship between cholesterol and CAV1. In particular, one-sided distribution of both signals was observed in the CA cells, whereas it was attenuated in the CD cells (Figure 2A). Double staining of CAV1 and F-actin revealed that CAV1 localized to the center of the cell in the control and CD cells, whereas CAV1 was asymmetrically localized close to one side of the cell periphery in CA cells (Figure 2B, arrows). Confocal microscopy revealed that CAV1 was primarily localized in the plasma membrane under all three conditions; CAV1 was uniformly distributed in the plasma membrane in the control and CD cells (Figure 2C). In contrast, in the CA cells, CAV1 was asymmetrically distributed in the plasma membrane on the opposite side of lamellipodia (Figure 2C, arrows), and lamellipodia were devoid of CAV1. The asymmetric distribution of CAV1 in the CA cells was also confirmed by the increased distance between the cell centroid and CAV1 centroid (Figure 2D). These data suggest that cholesterol regulates CAV1 distribution.

Since the asymmetric organization of proteins in the plasma membrane is characteristic of cell polarity [31], we investigated CAV1 distribution and cell polarity. As integrins, including ITGB1, translocate to the leading edge [32] and PTEN moves laterally and posteriorly [31] in a migrating cell, ITGB1 and PTEN were used as markers of the leading edge and trailing edge of the polarized cells, respectively. Combined immunofluorescence staining of CAV1 and ITGB1, as well as of CAV1 and PTEN, revealed asymmetric localization of CAV1 on the opposite side of ITGB1 (Figure 3A) and on the same side as PTEN (Figure 3B) in polarized cells. Thus, CAV1 was located at the trailing edge along the plasma membrane in polarized cells. Furthermore, the ratio of polarized cells substantially increased among the CA cells in both cell lines (Figure 3C), indicating that cell migration promoted by cholesterol supplementation was related to front–rear cell polarity.

2.3. Cholesterol Increases the CAV1 Level in Cold Triton X-100 (TX)-Resistant Lipid Raft Region

Next, we assessed whether cholesterol manipulation affected CAV1 expression at the mRNA and protein levels. CAV1 mRNA expression was not altered in the control and cholesterol-manipulated samples (Figure 4A). To determine CAV1 protein levels in the lipid raft, we applied the cold TX pre-extraction method [33], by which detergent-soluble (non-lipid raft) proteins were removed and the detergent-resistant (lipid raft) proteins remained in the cells. We observed that CAV1 signals were markedly decreased in the pre-extracted cells (Figure 4B, lower panels). In the pre-extracted samples, the control and CD cells exhibited a dramatic decrease in CAV1 signals, whereas the CA cells retained high-level asymmetric membranous CAV1 signals (Figure 4B, arrows). These results indicate that cholesterol promotes CAV1 anchoring in the lipid rafts of the plasma membrane. Moreover, the CAV1 level in the detergent-resistant fraction was considerably increased in the CA cells compared to that in the control and CD cells (Figure 4C, Figure S2 in Supplementary Materials). However, significant changes were not observed in the detergent-soluble fraction.

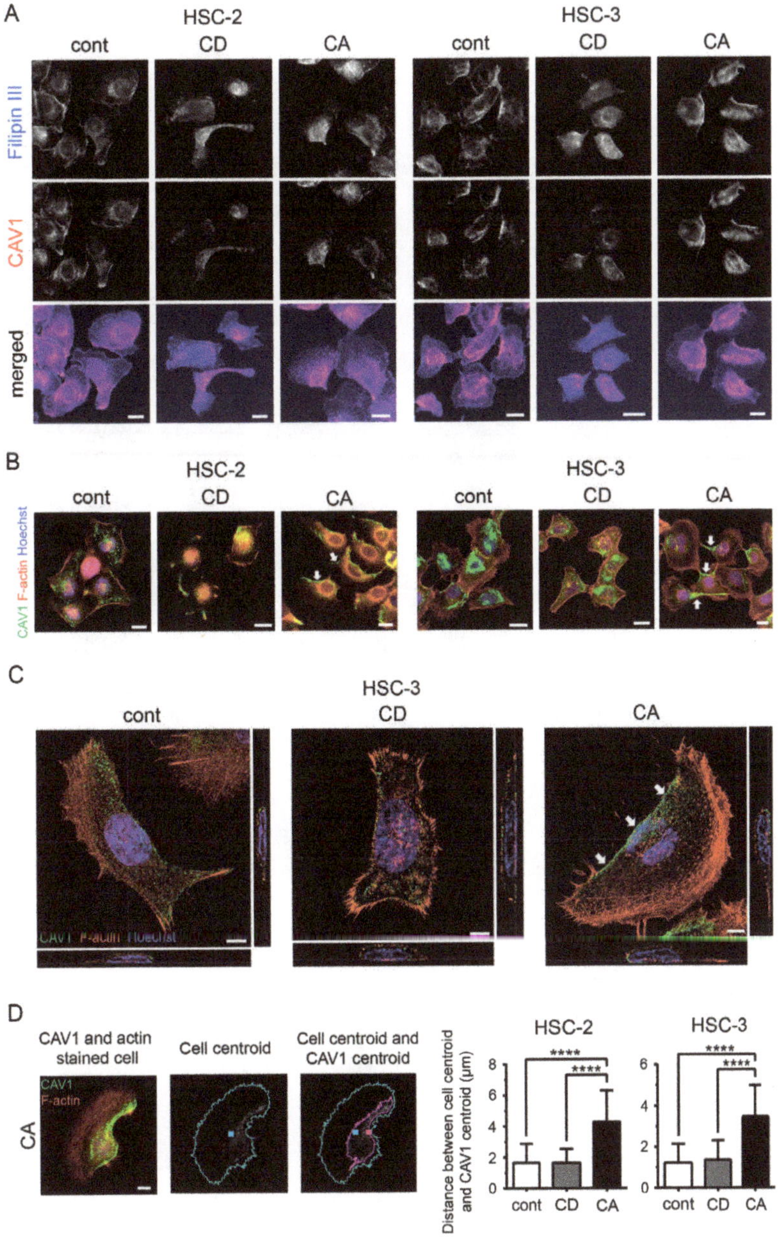

Figure 2. Cholesterol promotes asymmetric membranous localization of CAV1. (**A**) Colocalization of filipin III and CAV1. Blue, filipin III; red, CAV1. Scale bars, 20 μm. (**B**) Fluorescence staining for CAV1 and F-actin. Green, CAV1; red, F-actin; blue, Hoechst. Scale bars, 20 μm. Arrows indicate the asymmetric localization of CAV1. (**C**) CAV1 distribution assessed using confocal microscopy. Green, CAV1; red, F-actin; blue, Hoechst. Scale bars, 5 μm. Arrows indicate the asymmetric localization of CAV1. (**D**) Assessment of CAV1 distribution by centroid position. Cell centroid (blue square) and CAV1 centroid (red square) of CAV1- and actin-stained cells ($N \geq 50$) were determined using ImageJ. The distance between the two points was measured using ImageJ software. Scale bar, 10 μm. Bar graphs represent the distance as mean ± SD. **** $p < 0.0001$.

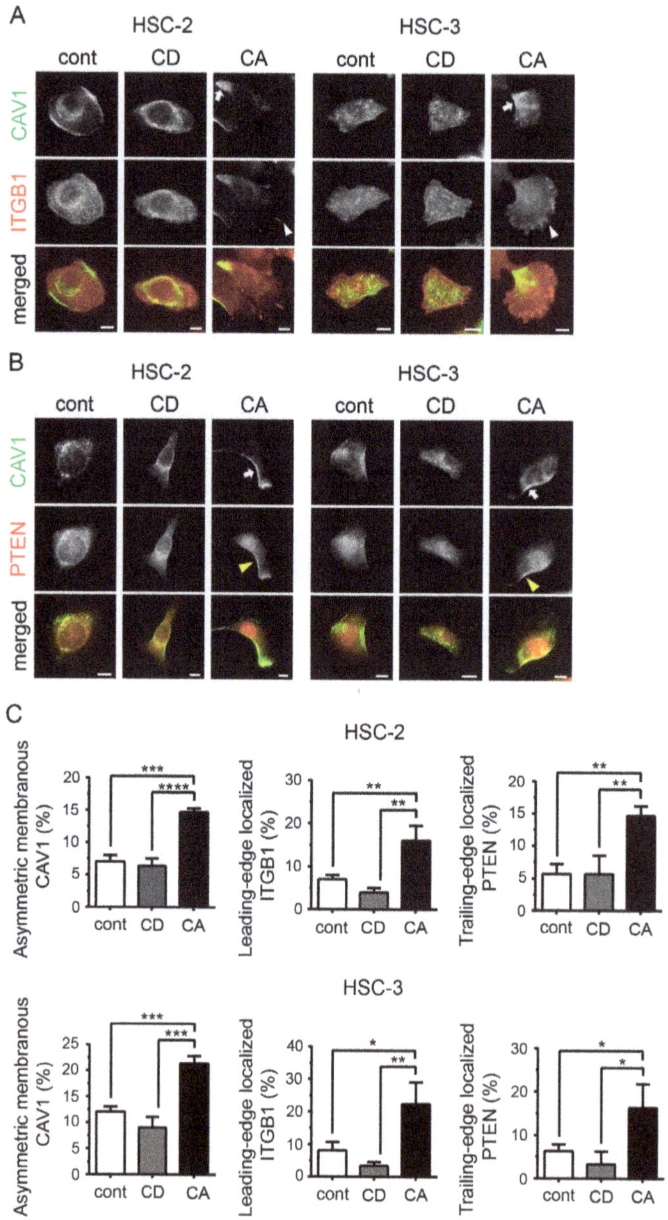

Figure 3. Cholesterol endows cell polarity by asymmetric membranous localization of CAV1. (**A**) Combined immunofluorescence staining of CAV1 and integrin β1 (ITGB1). Green, CAV1; red, ITGB1. Scale bars, 10 μm. White arrows indicate asymmetric membranous localization of CAV1 at the trailing edge of polarized cells; white arrowheads indicate ITGB1 at the cell leading edge in polarized cells. (**B**) Combined immunofluorescence staining of CAV1 and PTEN. Green, CAV1; red, PTEN. Scale bars, 10 μm. White arrow, asymmetric membranous CAV1 at the trailing edge of polarized cells; yellow arrowhead, PTEN at the trailing edge in polarized cells. (**C**) Percentage of polarized cells as per the asymmetric localization of CAV1, ITGB1, and PTEN. Bar graphs show triplicate results of the percentage of polarized cells expressed as mean ± SD. * $p < 0.05$, ** $p < 0.01$, *** $p < 0.001$, and **** $p < 0.0001$.

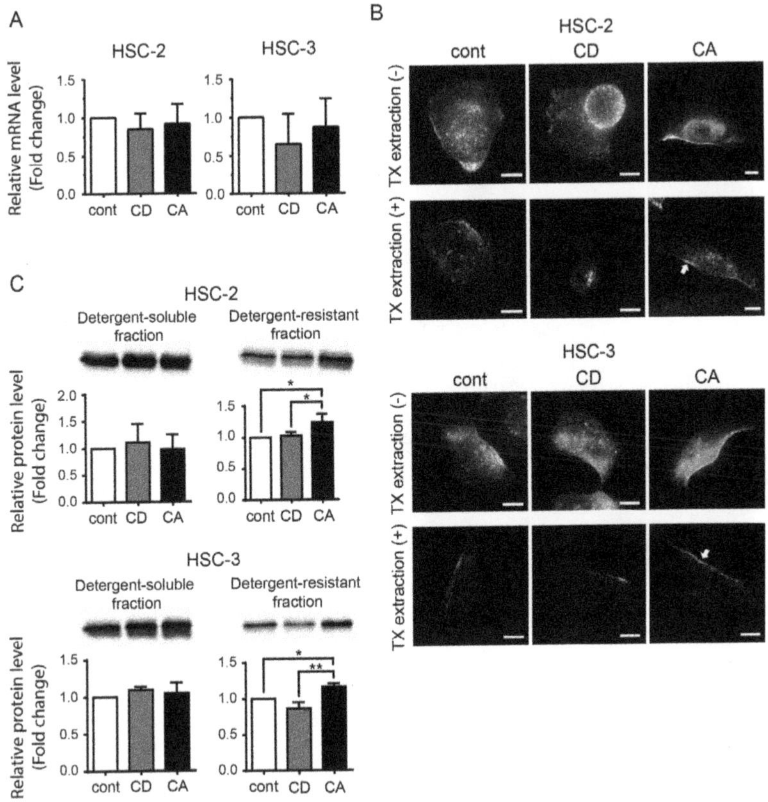

Figure 4. Cholesterol manipulation changes the CAV1 protein level in the cold Triton X-100 (TX)-resistant lipid raft region. (**A**) Quantitative RT-PCR for CAV1. Triplicate results are shown as mean + SD. (**B**) Immunofluorescence staining for CAV1 in cells with or without TX pre-extraction in HSC-2 (upper) and HSC-3 (lower). Scale bars, 10 μm. Arrow indicates asymmetric membranous localization of CAV1 in TX pre-extracted cells. (**C**) CAV1 protein level in detergent-soluble fraction and detergent-resistant fraction in HSC-2 (upper) and HSC-3 (lower). Coomassie blue stain was used as the loading control. Bar graphs show triplicate results of relative protein level expressed as mean ± SD. * $p < 0.05$, ** $p < 0.01$.

2.4. Membranous CAV1 Expression in OSCC Tissue Specimens Is Correlated with the Aggressiveness of the Tumor and Poor Clinical Outcomes

We examined the clinicopathological relationship and prognostic impact of CAV1 expression levels on the survival of OSCC patients. CAV1 positivity was enhanced in OSCC nests compared with that in non-cancerous oral epithelia (Figure 5A–F). In OSCC cells, CAV1 signals were linearly detected in the plasma membrane and granularly in the cytoplasm (Figure 5C,F). Moreover, the staining intensity in the plasma membrane was higher than that in the cytoplasm. However, the degree of CAV1 membrane positivity was heterogeneous across tumors; in some tumors, CAV1 membrane positivity was observed throughout the tumor (Figure 5B–C), whereas in other tumors, it was observed only in limited areas (Figure 5E–F).

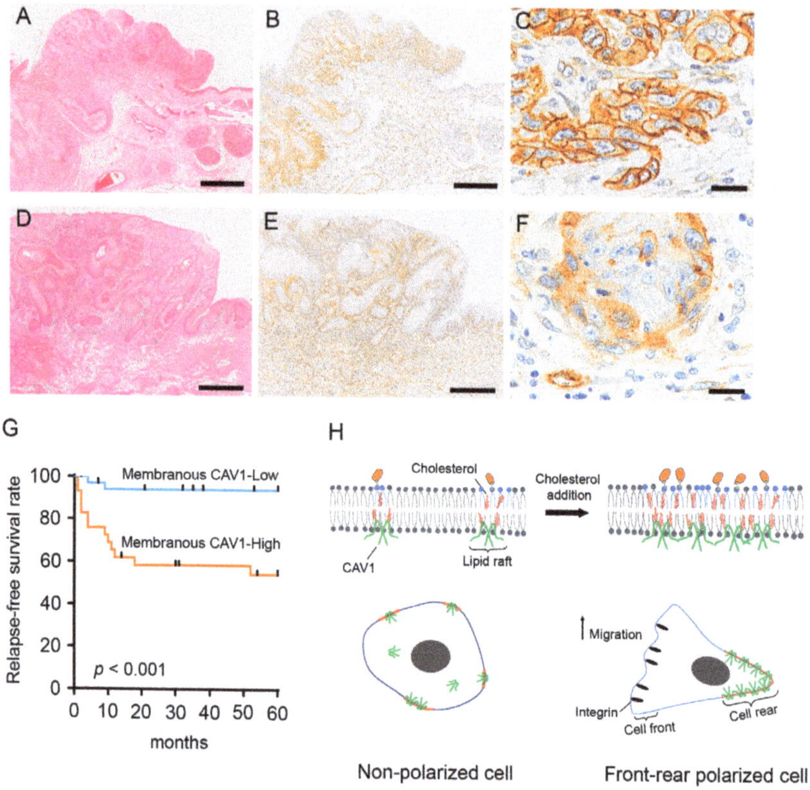

Figure 5. Membranous CAV1 expression in oral squamous cell carcinoma (OSCC) tissue and its correlation with relapse-free survival. (**A–C**) Representative photomicrograph of the tumor with high membranous CAV1 expression (21%). (**D–F**) Representative photomicrograph of the tumor with low membranous CAV1 expression (6%). (**A**,**D**) H&E staining. (**B**,**C**,**E**,**F**) Immunostaining for CAV1. (**C**) and (**F**) are higher-magnification images of (**B**,**E**), respectively. Scale bars, 1 mm (**A**,**B**,**D**,**E**) and 20 μm (**C**,**F**). (**G**) Kaplan–Meier curve showing relapse-free survival of OSCC patients based on membranous CAV1 expression. High membranous CAV1 expression is significantly associated with poor relapse-free survival ($p < 0.001$). (**H**) Schematic diagram showing the conclusions of this study. Cholesterol addition increases the cholesterol level in the plasma membrane and the CAV1 level in the lipid raft. Meanwhile, the cell promotes cell migration by changing its shape from polygonal to fan-shaped; polarized morphology with trailing edge localization of CAV1.

Next, since CAV1 was more intensely distributed in the plasma membrane in the CA cells, as shown in Figure 2B,C, we quantified the area (%) of the OSCC cells with stronger or comparable membranous CAV1 expression compared with that of endothelial cells, and 63 tumors were divided into two groups with a cutoff value of 15% or greater.

Consequently, 29 tumors (46%) were classified into the group with high membranous CAV1 expression, and 34 (54%) were classified into the group with low membranous CAV1 expression. The correlation between membranous CAV1 expression and the clinicopathological parameters is shown in Table 1. High membranous CAV1 expression was significantly associated with age ($p < 0.01$), lymph node metastasis ($p < 0.01$), clinical stage ($p < 0.01$), and regional recurrence ($p < 0.01$). Moreover, OSCC patients with high membrane expression of CAV1 had lower relapse-free survival ($p < 0.001$) (Figure 5G). Next, we performed univariate and multivariate Cox regression analyses of clinicopathological variables, including CAV1 membrane expression, to determine the potential independent prognostic factors for relapse-free survival. The results revealed that the mode of invasion ($p < 0.01$) and membranous CAV1 expression ($p < 0.01$) were significant variables in the univariate and multivariate Cox regression analyses (Table 2).

Table 1. Relationship of clinicopathological factors of the OSCC cases with membranous CAV1 expression.

Characteristic	N	Membranous CAV1 Expression High (≥15%)	Low (<15%)	p-Value
Age				
≤Median (72)	32	9	23	
>Median (72)	31	20	11	<0.01
Gender				
Male	35	14	21	
Female	28	15	13	0.31
T-factor				
T1/T2	54	22	32	
T3/T4	9	7	2	0.07
Primary site				
Tongue	58	28	30	
Buccal mucosa	4	1	3	0.43
Gingiva	1	0	1	
Lymph node metastasis				
Negative	57	23	34	
Positive	6	6	0	<0.01
Clinical stage				
I/II	51	19	32	
III/IV	12	10	2	<0.01
Mode of invasion				
1/2/3	41	15	26	
4C/4D	22	14	8	0.06
Local recurrence				
Negative	61	27	34	0.21
Positive	2	2	0	
Regional recurrence				
Negative	50	18	32	
Positive	13	11	2	<0.01

OSCC, oral squamous cell carcinoma; CAV1, caveolin-1.

Table 2. Univariate and multivariate analyses of clinicopathological parameters and membranous CAV1 expression in relation to relapse-free survival in OSCC.

Variable	Category	N	Univariate Analysis RR	Univariate Analysis p-Value	Multivariate Analysis RR	Multivariate Analysis p-Value
Age	≤72	33	0.59	0.32		
	>72	30	1.68			
Gender	Male	36	0.65	0.41		
	Female	27	1.53			
T-factor	T1/T2	54	0.38	0.13		
	T3/T4	9	2.64			
Lymph node metastasis	Negative	57	0.35	0.15		
	Positive	6	2.86			
Stage	I/II	51	0.4	0.11		
	III/IV	12	2.53			
Mode of invasion	1/2/3	41	0.15	<0.001	0.22	<0.01
	4C/4D	22	6.58		4.51	
Membranous CAV1	High	29	9.16	<0.001	6.47	<0.01
	Low	34	0.1		0.15	

CAV1, caveolin-1; OSCC, oral squamous cell carcinoma; RR, risk ratio.

3. Discussion

The present study demonstrates that cellular cholesterol levels affect the migratory ability of OSCC cells by regulating cell polarity. We revealed that cholesterol-induced cell polarization is characterized by the trailing-edge membranous localization of CAV1, which might be initiated by increased CAV1 in the lipid raft. We also showed that membranous CAV1 expression in OSCC cells is a potential prognostic factor. This study highlights the relationship between cellular cholesterol levels and membranous localization of CAV1, indicating that it potentiates OSCC progression and metastasis.

We showed that cellular cholesterol levels were related to changes in cell morphology and migration. In particular, cholesterol addition resulted in morphological changes in cells, with the development of lamellipodia and an increase in cell size in OSCC cells. Furthermore, cholesterol addition and depletion induced an increase and decrease in OSCC cell migration, respectively. The importance of cholesterol in cell shape and cell migration has been widely studied with respect to membrane cholesterol depletion and replenishment [34,35]. For instance, cholesterol depletion by MβCD induces morphological changes, such as loss of lamellipodia and filopodia, which decrease cell migration [34,35], whereas cholesterol replenishment after depletion restores normal morphological characteristics and cell migration capacity in breast cancer cells [35]. However, the effects of cholesterol supplementation on cellular function have rarely been reported. Qin et al. reported that cholesterol-loaded mouse macrophages exhibit larger cell sizes than control macrophages and develop lamellipodia [36], which is similar to our results. They discovered that cellular cholesterol changes cell shape by increasing pinocytic activity and activating Rac1, the major protein for lamellipodia development; however, cholesterol-loaded macrophages remained polygonal [36]. Nagao et al. reported that cholesterol load suppresses the migration ability of macrophages by interfering with Rho activation [37]. A similar result was reported for tendon-derived stem cells, wherein cholesterol addition disturbed the G0/G1 cell cycle and inhibited directional cell migration [38]. On the contrary, in the present study, cholesterol-added OSCC cells showed fan-shaped morphology with a decreased circularity index, which is interpreted as polarized cells [39] and elevated migration ability. Therefore, we assumed that such cell activation by cholesterol addition may be characteristic of malignant tumor cells.

Our results suggest that CAV1 plays an important role in cholesterol-induced cell polarization. We found that cholesterol addition increased the number of polarized cells exhibiting asymmetric CAV1 distribution at the trailing edge of the plasma membrane. CAV1 localization at the trailing edge of polarized cells has been observed in a variety of cells, such as endothelial cells [40–42], mouse embryonic fibroblasts [43], mouse neuronal cells [44], and prostate cancer cells [45]. CAV1 promotes cell polarization via its inhibitory effects on other proteins [42], such as Rac and Cdc42, which induce cell protrusion [46]. That is, CAV1 localization on one side of the plasma membrane potentially causes an induction in lamellipodia and focal adhesion molecules including ITGB1 on the other side [42]. Beardsley et al. demonstrated the role of CAV1 in cell polarity and migration using CAV1 RNA interference; the suppression of CAV1 attenuates cell polarization and directional migration in endothelial cells [42]. In addition, cholesterol reportedly has a significant influence on the sequestration of integrin $\alpha_V\beta_3$ in a model membrane system [47]. Thus, cholesterol could initiate the segregation of CAV1 and integrins on the plasma membrane, resulting in cell polarization.

Moreover, the increase in CAV1 levels in lipid rafts due to cholesterol addition may be related to CAV1 polarization. We demonstrated that cholesterol addition increased CAV1 protein levels in the detergent-resistant (lipid raft) fraction, whereas the detergent-soluble (non-lipid raft) fraction was less affected; lipid-raft-associated CAV1 was localized at the trailing edge in the CA cells. In the plasma membrane, cholesterol preferentially organizes sphingolipids to form a lipid raft, also called the liquid-ordered domain, in which highly ordered lipid hydrocarbon chains are more tightly packed than the surrounding lipid bilayer [48,49]. Because cholesterol serves as a glue in the tightly organized lipid rafts, the melting temperature of the lipid rafts is higher than that of the non-raft membranes [50]. Therefore, lipid-raft-associated proteins are resistant to TX extraction at low temperatures [48]. CAV1 is a lipid-raft-associated protein [48] that participates in the formation of caveolar lipid rafts [51,52]. Genetic ablation of CAV1 completely eradicates caveolae in mouse embryonic fibroblasts and peritoneal macrophages [52]. Caveolar lipid rafts are considered the major signaling machinery for cell polarity, as their rear-side localization assists directional migration in endothelial [40] and neuronal cells [44]. Moreover, increased CAV1 levels in lipid rafts increase the number of caveolae in the plasma membranes of caveolin cDNA-transfected lymphocytes [53]. Thus, the relationship between cholesterol, CAV1, and caveolae formation is important for cell polarization and migration. Therefore, we assumed that cholesterol initiates cell polarization and promotes migration by upregulating the lipid-raft-associated CAV1 at the trailing edge (Figure 5H), although we could not specify CAV1 localization to caveolae. However, the molecular mechanisms underlying the cell polarity conferred by lipid-raft-associated CAV1 remain unclear, and future studies are warranted.

Apart from cholesterol treatment regulated by MβCD and MβCD–cholesterol complex, other cholesterol-manipulating methods also affect the CAV1 protein level and cell migration. Similar to our findings, high levels of low-density lipoprotein stimulate the development of the actin cytoskeleton in human endothelial cells and raise CAV1 protein levels in lipid rafts without altering overall CAV1 protein levels [54]; however, that study did not examine cell migration. Fluvastatin also affects cytoskeletal organization and inhibits cell migration on fibronectin-coated surfaces in rat vascular smooth muscle cells [55], comparable to our findings. Thus, cellular cholesterol levels may affect CAV1 protein levels in lipid rafts and regulate cell motility without being affected by manipulation techniques. However, activation of cells may vary between cell lines. Contrary to our findings, mevastatin triggers the EGF-Rac1 signaling pathway in primary human keratinocytes by lowering the CAV1 protein level, which promotes cell motility [56].

Membranous expression of CAV1 is a possible predictive marker for worse clinical outcomes in patients with OSCC. In the present study, OSCC with high membranous CAV1 expression exhibited an advanced clinical stage, increased regional metastasis, and shorter relapse-free survival. CAV1 is overexpressed in both the membrane and cytoplasm of OSCC cells [23,24,26,57]. Overexpression of CAV1 is associated with regional metastasis [23,25] and poor survival [25,26], despite different scoring methods for CAV1 immunohistochemistry; however, previous studies have not focused on membranous CAV1 expression. Importantly, membranous CAV1 expression has been recognized as a marker for brain tumors with high-grade malignancies [58]. In astroglial tumors, cytoplasmic dot-like, cytoplasmic and membrane, and intense membrane CAV1 staining are observed in grade II, III, and IV tumors, respectively [58], suggesting that CAV1 membrane expression is an indicator of the aggressiveness of tumors, such as astrocytomas and OSCC. In addition, based on our results, we speculated that membranous CAV1 expression is a surrogate indicator for cellular cholesterol levels. However, tissue-based quantification of cholesterol was not possible because fresh tissue was unavailable in the present study. Further studies are necessary to confirm this hypothesis.

The present study has several limitations. First, we did not investigate whether other cholesterol manipulation methods, such as the use of statins for cholesterol depletion and low-density lipoprotein for cholesterol addition, that have more physio-pharmacological significance would have the same effects. Second, the direct mechanistic relationship and molecular mechanisms between CAV1 and cholesterol-induced cellular changes have not been fully validated. It is also necessary to clarify whether CAV1 reciprocally regulates cellular cholesterol levels. These issues should be addressed in future research. Third, since this work is a preliminary examination of the impact of cellular cholesterol on the activities of OSCC cells, we only evaluated planar cell movement on coverslips. Therefore, planar and vertical migration of cholesterol-manipulated cells will be confirmed in the future using 3D models because OSCC cell migration and invasion also depend on the tumor microenvironment, which can be explored in 3D models [59,60], and are related to the underlying substrates [61].

In conclusion, we found that elevated cellular cholesterol levels in OSCC cells induce an aggressive phenotype by regulating CAV1 in the lipid rafts. Moreover, membranous CAV1 expression in tissue specimens has been suggested to be a reliable marker for the prognosis of OSCC. Further studies determining the correlation between cellular cholesterol levels and CAV1 expression could help in the development of effective treatment strategies for OSCC.

4. Materials and Methods

4.1. Cell Lines

HSC-2, a well-differentiated OSCC cell line, and HSC-3, a poorly differentiated OSCC cell line, developed from the metastatic lymph nodes of the floor of mouth and tongue cancer, respectively, were obtained from the Riken BRC Cell Bank (Tsukuba, Japan). The cells were maintained in minimum essential medium (MEM) (Thermo Fisher Scientific, Waltham, MA, USA) supplemented with 10% fetal bovine serum (FBS) (Thermo Fisher Scientific, Waltham, MA, USA) in a humidified atmosphere with 5% CO_2/95% air at 37 °C.

4.2. Tissue Samples

We included 63 patients who visited the Niigata University Hospital for surgical treatment of primary OSCC between 2006 and 2019. The experimental protocol for analyzing the surgical material was reviewed and approved by the Ethical Board of the Niigata University Graduate School of Medical and Dental Sciences (approval number: 2018-0228). All experiments were conducted in accordance with the guidelines of the Declaration of Helsinki. The median age of the patients was 72 years (range: 29–92 years); 36 patients were male, and 27 were female. Clinical stage was determined according to the Union for International Cancer Control TNM classification system, 8th edition [62]. Serial sections were prepared for hematoxylin and eosin (H&E) and immunohistochemical staining as described in Section 4.12.

4.3. Reagents and Antibodies

MβCD (C4555) and cholesterol (C3045) were purchased from Sigma-Aldrich (St. Louis, MO, USA). Filipin III, a cholesterol probe, was obtained from Cayman Chemical Co. (Ann Arbor, MI, USA). The primary antibodies used for immunofluorescence assay were as follows: anti-CAV1 (1:400; D46G3 rabbit IgG mAb; Cell Signaling Technology, Danvers, MA, USA), anti-PTEN (1:100; clone 17A, mouse IgM mAb, Lab Vision, South San Francisco, CA, USA), and anti-integrin β1 (ITGB1) (1:100; P5D2, mouse IgG mAb, Chemicon International, Temecula, CA, USA). Alexa Fluor™ 488-conjugated goat antibodies against rabbit IgG (1:500), Alexa Fluor™ 488-conjugated goat antibodies against mouse IgG (1:500), Alexa Fluor™ 568-conjugated goat antibodies against rabbit IgG (1:500), and Alexa Fluor™ 555-conjugated goat antibodies against mouse IgM (heavy chain) (1:500) were used as the secondary antibodies and were obtained from Thermo Fisher Scientific (Waltham, MA, USA). Rhodamine-phalloidin conjugate (1:500; Thermo Fisher Scientific, Waltham, MA, USA) was used for F-actin staining, and Hoechst 33342 (1:500; Dojindo Laboratories Co., Ltd., Kumamoto, Japan) was used for nuclear staining.

4.4. Cholesterol Manipulation

For manipulation of cholesterol levels in cells, we depleted the cholesterol levels using MβCD and increased them using the MβCD-cholesterol inclusion complex [30]. We dissolved MβCD powder in distilled water and prepared MβCD stock solution (70 mM), which was stored at 4 °C. For the depletion of cholesterol levels, the cells were grown for 36–48 h and incubated with 1 mM MβCD dissolved in MEM containing 25 mM HEPES in 5% CO_2/95% air at 37 °C. To increase the cholesterol levels, an MβCD-cholesterol complex (8:1 molar ratio) was prepared. First, the cholesterol powder was dissolved in prewarmed

100% ethanol (final concentration: 52 mM). Then, aliquots from the cholesterol–ethanol solution (cholesterol concentration: 10 mM) were prepared, and ethanol was evaporated at 80 °C until only white flakes of cholesterol remained. Subsequently, a solution containing 80 mM MβCD was added to the white flakes of cholesterol, and the mixture was stirred at 80 °C until cholesterol was completely dissolved in MβCD. The stock solution of the MβCD–cholesterol complex was stored at 4 °C. Next, we prepared a cholesterol-supplemented medium by adding MβCD–cholesterol complex (0.125 mM) to 25 mM HEPES containing MEM and incubated the mixture at 37 °C for 1 h in a water bath. Then, the cholesterol-supplemented medium was filtered (pore size, 0.2 μm) and added to the cells and proceeded using the same procedure as cholesterol-depleted cells.

4.5. Cell Viability Assay

The cells (1×10^4) were grown for 36–48 h in 96-well plates, then incubated with 100 μL of FBS-free medium (control) or cholesterol-treated medium in 5% CO_2/95% air at 37 °C for up to 24 h. CellTiter 96® AQueous One reagent (Promega Corporation, Madison, WI, USA) was added, and the absorbance was measured at 490 nm using the GloMax® Discover System (Promega Corporation, Madison, WI, USA). We evaluated cell viability at different time points from 4 to 24 h.

4.6. Quantification of Cellular Cholesterol

An Amplex™ Red cholesterol assay kit (Thermo Fisher Scientific, Waltham, MA, USA) was used for cholesterol quantification. The cells (2×10^5) were grown in a 35 mm dish for 36–48 h; then, cellular cholesterol was manipulated (as mentioned in Section 4.4) for 4 h. After washing with ice-cold phosphate-buffered saline (PBS), 200 μL of 1× reaction buffer was added to the dishes, and they were kept on ice for 25 min. The cells were scraped and centrifuged at 2300× *g* for 5 min at 4 °C. The supernatant was transferred to a tube and divided into 5 μL aliquots for the Bio-Rad protein assay (Bio-Rad Laboratories, Inc., Hercules, CA, USA), and 50 μL/well was added to a 96-well plate for cholesterol quantification. A mixture containing Amplex™ Red reagent, 1× reaction buffer, horseradish peroxidase, cholesterol oxidase, and cholesterol esterase was added to each well of a 96-well plate, and the plate was incubated at 37 °C for 1 h. The fluorescence intensity was measured at 570–590 nm using MikroWin 2000 (Mikrotek Laborsysteme GmbH, Overath, Germany).

4.7. Fluorescence Staining

HSC-2 and HSC-3 cells were seeded on a coverslip in a 35 mm dish at a cell concentration of 0.5×10^5 and grown for 36–48 h. Cellular cholesterol levels were manipulated for 4 h, as mentioned in Section 4.4, and fluorescence staining was performed. Briefly, the cells were fixed using 4% paraformaldehyde in PBS for 15 min and permeabilized using 0.2% TX in PBS at room temperature (RT) for 15 min. To block non-specific binding, the cells were incubated with 2% normal goat serum (Vector Laboratories, Inc., Burlingame, CA, USA) in PBS and reacted with primary antibodies overnight at 4 °C. The cells were then incubated with the respective secondary antibodies and Hoechst 33342 at RT for 1 h. For double staining with F-actin, rhodamine-phalloidin was also added at the time of incubation with secondary antibody. The coverslips were mounted using a mounting medium, and the cells were observed under a conventional fluorescence microscope (Eclipse E600, Nikon Corporation, Tokyo, Japan). In some experiments, a Dragonfly 505 spinning-disk confocal microscope system (Andor Technology, Oxford Instruments plc., Abingdon, UK) with a Zyla 4.2 USB 3.0 detector (Andor Technology, Oxford Instruments plc., Abingdon, UK) and a Ti2-E microscope (Nikon Corporation, Tokyo, Japan) was used to capture confocal images. For filipin III staining, the fixed cells were incubated with filipin III (100 μg/mL in PBS) at RT in the dark for 1 h, and the coverslips were mounted. For filipin III and antibody staining, the fixed cells were incubated with filipin III, then permeabilized using 0.02% TX for 10 min at RT. Afterward, the cells were incubated with primary antibody at 4 °C overnight, then reacted with secondary antibody, and the coverslips were mounted.

To evaluate CAV1 expression in a detergent-resistant membrane, TX pre-extraction of cells was performed as described in a previous study [33]. The cells were washed with ice-cold cytoskeletal-stabilizing buffer [63] and incubated on ice with 1% TX and protease inhibitor cocktail (1:50; Nacalai Tesque, Inc., Kyoto, Japan) for 30 min. Next, the cells were fixed and subjected to immunofluorescent staining without permeabilization.

4.8. Image Analysis

Immunofluorescence images of randomly selected cells (to include at least 50 cells) were captured from triplicate experiments. All cells, excluding those on the margins, were analyzed. Morphology was evaluated by automatic tracing of the area and perimeter of the F-actin-stained cells using ImageJ software (National Institutes of Health, Bethesda, MD, USA), and the circularity index ($4\pi \times \text{Area}/\text{Perimeter}^2$) was calculated. Confocal images were visualized using ImarisViewer 9.9.1 (Oxford Instruments plc., Abingdon, UK). The distribution of CAV1 was assessed by determining the distance between the centroid of the cell and the centroid of CAV1, as per a method reported by Zhang et al. [64]. The cells that exhibited one-sided membranous distribution of CAV1 were manually counted as cells with asymmetric membranous CAV1 using CAV1-specific immunofluorescence analysis. The cells with ITGB1 signals in lamellipodial structures or those with uneven distribution of PTEN were recognized as the cells with ITGB1 on the leading edge or PTEN on the trailing edge, respectively.

4.9. Timelapse Imaging and Cell Tracking Analysis

Both HSC-2 and HSC-3 cells (0.5×10^5) were grown on a coverslip in a 35 mm dish. After aspiration of the old medium, cholesterol-treated medium or control medium was added, and timelapse images were taken by a CytoWatcher instrument (WSL-1800-B, ATTO Corporation, Tokyo, Japan) at 5 min intervals up to 8 h. Then, the images were tracked using NIS-Elements Advanced Research (Nikon, Tokyo, Japan), and the track plots were analyzed using the Chemotaxis and Migration tool 2.0 (ibidi GmbH, Gräfelfing, Germany).

4.10. Quantitative Reverse Transcription-Polymerase Chain Reaction (RT-PCR)

Total RNA was extracted from cultured cells (1×10^6) using Nucleospin (Macherey-Nagel, Düren, Germany) and reverse-transcribed into cDNA using a high-capacity cDNA reverse transcription kit (Thermo Fisher Scientific, Waltham, MA, USA). A polymerase chain reaction (PCR) was performed using a specific primer for CAV1 (qHsaCID0022177, Bio-Rad Laboratories, Inc., Hercules, CA, USA) and SYBR green PCR master mix (Bio-Rad Laboratories, Inc., Hercules, CA, USA) in a QuantStudio 1 RT-PCR system (Thermo Fisher Scientific, Waltham, MA, USA). The expression of the peptidylprolyl isomerase A (PPIA, JBioS, Bio services Co.,LTD, Japan) gene was used to normalize for variance, and 5′-GCA GTA ATG GGT TAC TTC TGA AAC-3′ (forward) and 5′-TGC CTC AGG TAA TAC ATT ACA GAC-3′ (reverse) were used as primers.

4.11. Western Blotting

Cell lysates were prepared using an UltraRIPA kit for lipid rafts (BioDynamics Laboratory Inc., Tokyo, Japan) according to the manufacturer's instructions. In brief, the cells (1×10^6) were seeded in a 60 mm dish and treated with cholesterol for 4 h. Then, the cells were lysed using buffer A on ice for 10 min and centrifuged at $19{,}300\times g$ for 5 min; the supernatant yielded a detergent-soluble fraction, i.e., non-raft proteins. The pellet was washed once with buffer A, incubated with buffer B at RT for 5 min, and centrifuged at $19{,}300\times g$ for 5 min. The B buffer lysate contained the detergent-resistant fraction and lipid raft proteins. A protease inhibitor cocktail (1:50) was added to all buffers. Both detergent-soluble and detergent-resistant lysates (10 μL each) were subjected to a BCA protein assay (Takara Bio Inc., Shiga, Japan). After adjustment for protein concentration, the samples were subjected to sodium dodecyl sulfate-polyacrylamide gel electrophoresis under reducing conditions, and the proteins were transferred to polyvinylidene difluoride membranes (Bio-Rad Laboratories, Inc.). To prevent non-specific protein binding, the membrane was blocked using 0.5% ECL blocking agent (GE Healthcare UK, Little Chalfont, UK) in 50 mM Tris-buffered saline (TBS) (pH 7.4) containing 0.1% Tween-20 (TTBS) for 1 h at RT. Then, the membranes were incubated with anti-CAV1 (1:1000; D46G3 rabbit, Cell Signaling Technology, Danvers, MA, USA) diluted with TTBS at 4 °C overnight. After washing with TTBS, the membranes were incubated with horseradish peroxidase-linked anti-rabbit IgG antibody (7074S, Cell Signaling Technology, Danvers, MA, USA) diluted 1:3000 in TTBS for 1 h at RT. The target protein bands were visualized using ECL Prime Western blotting detection reagents (GE Healthcare UK, Little Chalfont, UK). Coomassie brilliant blue staining was used for protein normalization.

4.12. Immunohistochemistry Staining for CAV1 in Tissue Sections

Immunohistochemistry staining of the paraffin sections was performed using the ChemMate EnVision system (Dako, Glostrup, Denmark). The sections were deparaffinized in xylene and rehydrated in ethanol. Antigens were retrieved by boiling the sections in 0.5 M EDTA (pH 8) using a pressure cooker for 10 min and under high pressure for 3 min. After cooling to RT, endogenous peroxidase was blocked by incubating the sections with 0.3% hydrogen peroxide for 10 min. The sections were incubated with the primary antibody anti-CAV1 (1:400; D46G3 rabbit, Cell Signaling Technology, Danvers, MA, USA) at 4 °C overnight. After washing with TBS, the sections were incubated with EnVision Plus (Dako, Glostrup, Denmark) at RT for 30 min. The signals were developed using 3, 3′-diaminobenzidine (Dako, Glostrup, Denmark), and the sections were counterstained using hematoxylin.

4.13. Immunohistochemistry Analysis

The whole microscope slides were scanned using an Olympus Virtual Transmitted Light Slide Microscope VS120-S5 (Evident, Tokyo, Japan). The images were loaded in QuPath v.0.3.2 software [65] as bright-field images. Since staining of CAV1 was observed in vascular endothelial cells in all sections, the endothelial cells were selected as positive controls. Using a thresholder command in QuPath, we measured the region of tumor cells with membranous CAV1 signals of equal or stronger intensity than those of vascular endothelial cells and calculated the ratio of tumor area with membranous CAV1 and total tumor area on each slide. The tumor cells with CAV1 membrane positivity ≥15% were classified into the high-expression group, and the tumor cells with CAV1 membrane positivity of <15% were classified into the low-expression group.

4.14. Statistical Analysis

Statistical analyses were performed using GraphPad Prism 6 software (GraphPad Software, Inc., La Jolla, CA, USA). Experimental data were analyzed using one-way ANOVA with post hoc Tukey test or Dunn's test. The association between membranous CAV1 expression and patient characteristics was studied using Fisher's exact test or the chi-squared test ($n = 63$). Survival curves were analyzed using the Kaplan–Meier method, and statistical analysis was performed using the log-rank test. Univariate and multivariate Cox regression analyses were performed using JMP 9 software (SAS, Cary, NC, USA). Statistical significance was set at $p < 0.05$.

Supplementary Materials: The following supporting information can be downloaded at: https://www.mdpi.com/article/10.3390/ijms24076035/s1.

Author Contributions: Conceptualization, N.N.C., M.Y., T.K. and J.-i.T.; Methodology, N.N.C., M.Y., T.K. and J.-i.T.; Validation, N.N.C. and M.Y.; Formal analysis, N.N.C., M.Y., S.M., T.A. and J.-i.T.; Investigation, N.N.C., M.Y., S.M., T.A. and J.-i.T.; Resources, N.N.C. and M.Y.; Data curation, M.Y.; Writing–original draft preparation, N.N.C. and M.Y.; Writing–review and editing, N.N.C., M.Y., S.M., T.A., K.H., M.K., K.I., T.K. and J.-i.T.; Visualization, N.N.C. and M.Y.; Supervision, M.Y., T.K. and

J.-i.T.; Project administration, T.K. and J.-i.T.; Funding acquisition, M.Y., T.K. and J.-i.T. All authors have read and agreed to the published version of the manuscript.

Funding: This study was supported by Grants-in-Aid for Scientific Research from the Japan Society for the Promotion of Science (JSPS KAKENHI grant nos. JP18K09533 and JP21K09856 to M.Y.).

Institutional Review Board Statement: This study was conducted in accordance with the Declaration of Helsinki, and ethical approval was obtained from the Ethical Board of the Niigata University Graduate School of Medical and Dental Sciences (approval number 2018-0228).

Informed Consent Statement: Informed consent was obtained in the form of an opt-out on the website. Patients who were rejected were excluded.

Data Availability Statement: The data are available from the corresponding author upon reasonable request.

Conflicts of Interest: The authors declare no conflict of interest.

References

1. Skotland, T.; Kavaliauskiene, S.; Sandvig, K. The Role of Lipid Species in Membranes and Cancer-Related Changes. *Cancer Metastasis Rev.* **2020**, *39*, 343–360. [CrossRef] [PubMed]
2. Huang, B.; Song, B.-L.; Xu, C. Cholesterol Metabolism in Cancer: Mechanisms and Therapeutic Opportunities. *Nat. Metab.* **2020**, *2*, 132–141. [CrossRef] [PubMed]
3. Chang, W.-C.; Huang, S.-F.; Lee, Y.-M.; Lai, H.-C.; Cheng, B.-H.; Cheng, W.-C.; Ho, J.Y.-P.; Jeng, L.-B.; Ma, W.-L. Cholesterol Import and Steroidogenesis Are Biosignatures for Gastric Cancer Patient Survival. *Oncotarget* **2017**, *8*, 692–704. [CrossRef] [PubMed]
4. Oni, T.E.; Biffi, G.; Baker, L.A.; Hao, Y.; Tonelli, C.; Somerville, T.D.D.; Deschênes, A.; Belleau, P.; Hwang, C.; Sánchez-Rivera, F.J.; et al. SOAT1 Promotes Mevalonate Pathway Dependency in Pancreatic Cancer. *J. Exp. Med.* **2020**, *217*, e20192389. [CrossRef] [PubMed]
5. Hryniewicz-Jankowska, A.; Augoff, K.; Sikorski, A.F. Highlight Article: The Role of Cholesterol and Cholesterol-Driven Membrane Raft Domains in Prostate Cancer. *Exp. Biol. Med.* **2019**, *244*, 1053–1061. [CrossRef]
6. Zhuang, L.; Kim, J.; Adam, R.M.; Solomon, K.R.; Freeman, M.R. Cholesterol Targeting Alters Lipid Raft Composition and Cell Survival in Prostate Cancer Cells and Xenografts. *J. Clin. Investig.* **2005**, *115*, 959–968. [CrossRef]
7. Wang, B.; Rong, X.; Palladino, E.N.D.; Wang, J.; Fogelman, A.M.; Martín, M.G.; Alrefai, W.A.; Ford, D.A.; Tontonoz, P. Phospholipid Remodeling and Cholesterol Availability Regulate Intestinal Stemness and Tumorigenesis. *Cell Stem Cell* **2018**, *22*, 206–220. [CrossRef]
8. Dickinson, A.; Saraswat, M.; Joenväärä, S.; Agarwal, R.; Jyllikoski, D.; Wilkman, T.; Mäkitie, A.; Silén, S. Mass Spectrometry–Based Lipidomics of Oral Squamous Cell Carcinoma Tissue Reveals Aberrant Cholesterol and Glycerophospholipid Metabolism—A Pilot Study. *Transl. Oncol.* **2020**, *13*, 100807. [CrossRef]
9. Sakurai, K.; Tomihara, K.; Yamazaki, M.; Heshiki, W.; Moniruzzaman, R.; Sekido, K.; Tachinami, H.; Ikeda, A.; Imaue, S.; Fujiwara, K.; et al. CD36 Expression on Oral Squamous Cell Carcinoma Cells Correlates with Enhanced Proliferation and Migratory Activity. *Oral Dis.* **2020**, *26*, 745–755. [CrossRef]
10. Ganavi, B.S.; Patil, S.; Rao, R.S. Evaluation of Serum Lipids and Lipoproteins as Prognosticators in Leukoplakia. *J. Contemp. Dent. Pract.* **2015**, *15*, 294–299. [CrossRef]
11. Acharya, S.; Rai, P.; Hallikeri, K.; Anehosur, V.; Kale, J. Serum Lipid Profile in Oral Squamous Cell Carcinoma: Alterations and Association with Some Clinicopathological Parameters and Tobacco Use. *Int. J. Oral Maxillofac. Surg.* **2016**, *45*, 713–720. [CrossRef] [PubMed]
12. Bailwad, S.; Singh, N.; Bailwad, S.A.; Jani, D.R.; Patil, P.; Singh, M.; Deep, G.; Singh, S. Alterations in serum lipid profile patterns in oral cancer: Correlation with histological grading and tobacco abuse. *Oral Health Dent. Manag.* **2014**, *13*, 573–579.
13. Kumar, P.; Augustine, J.; Urs, A.B.; Arora, S.; Gupta, S.; Mohanty, V.R. Serum Lipid Profile in Oral Cancer and Leukoplakia: Correlation with Tobacco Abuse and Histological Grading. *J. Cancer Res. Ther.* **2012**, *8*, 384–388. [CrossRef] [PubMed]
14. Codini, M.; Garcia-Gil, M.; Albi, E. Cholesterol and Sphingolipid Enriched Lipid Rafts as Therapeutic Targets in Cancer. *Int. J. Mol. Sci.* **2021**, *22*, 726. [CrossRef]
15. Dongoran, R.A.; Wang, K.H.; Lin, T.J.; Yuan, T.C.; Liu, C.H. Anti-Proliferative Effect of Statins Is Mediated by DNMT1 Inhibition and P21 Expression in OSCC Cells. *Cancers* **2020**, *12*, 2084. [CrossRef]
16. Xu, B.; Muramatsu, T.; Inazawa, J. Suppression of Met Signaling Mediated by Pitavastatin and Capmatinib Inhibits Oral and Esophageal Cancer Cell Growth. *Mol. Cancer Res.* **2021**, *19*, 585–597. [CrossRef]
17. Xu, H.; Zhou, S.; Tang, Q.; Xia, H.; Bi, F. Cholesterol Metabolism: New Functions and Therapeutic Approaches in Cancer. *Biochim. Et Biophys. Acta—Rev. Cancer* **2020**, *1874*, 188394. [CrossRef]
18. Ketteler, J.; Klein, D. Caveolin-1, Cancer and Therapy Resistance. *Int. J. Cancer* **2018**, *14*, 2092–2104. [CrossRef]
19. Liu, P.; Rudick, M.; Anderson, R.G.W. Multiple Functions of Caveolin-1. *J. Biol. Chem.* **2002**, *277*, 41295–41298. [CrossRef]
20. Ikonen, E.; Parton, R.G. Caveolins and Cellular Cholesterol Balance. *Traffic* **2000**, *1*, 212–217. [CrossRef]

21. Simón, L.; Campos, A.; Leyton, L.; Quest, A.F.G. Caveolin-1 Function at the Plasma Membrane and in Intracellular Compartments in Cancer. *Cancer Metastasis Rev.* **2020**, *39*, 435–453. [CrossRef]
22. Surguchov, A. Caveolin: A New Link between Diabetes and AD. *Cell Mol. Neurobiol.* **2020**, *40*, 1059–1066. [CrossRef] [PubMed]
23. Hung, K.F.; Lin, S.C.; Liu, C.J.; Chang, C.S.; Chang, K.W.; Kao, S.Y. The Biphasic Differential Expression of the Cellular Membrane Protein, Caveolin-1, in Oral Carcinogenesis. *J. Oral Pathol. Med.* **2003**, *32*, 461–467. [CrossRef]
24. Xue, J.; Chen, H.; Diao, L.; Chen, X.; Xia, D. Expression of Caveolin-1 in Tongue Squamous Cell Carcinoma by Quantum Dots. *Eur. J. Histochem.* **2010**, *54*, 99–103. [CrossRef]
25. Kato, K.; Miyazawa, H.; Kobayashi, H.; Noguchi, N.; Lambert, D.; Kawashiri, S. Caveolin-1 Expression at Metastatic Lymph Nodes Predicts Unfavorable Outcome in Patients with Oral Squamous Cell Carcinoma. *Pathol. Oncol. Res.* **2020**, *26*, 2105–2113. [CrossRef]
26. Auzair, L.B.M.; Vincent-Chong, V.K.; Ghani, W.M.N.; Kallarakkal, T.G.; Ramanathan, A.; Lee, C.E.; Rahman, Z.A.A.; Ismail, S.M.; Abraham, M.T.; Zain, R.B. Caveolin 1 (Cav-1) and Actin-Related Protein 2/3 Complex, Subunit 1B (ARPC1B) Expressions as Prognostic Indicators for Oral Squamous Cell Carcinoma (OSCC). *Eur. Arch. Otorhinolaryngol.* **2016**, *273*, 1885–1893. [CrossRef]
27. Huang, C.-F.; Yu, G.-T.; Wang, W.-M.; Liu, B.; Sun, Z.-J. Original Article Prognostic and Predictive Values of SPP1, PAI and Caveolin-1 in Patients with Oral Squamous Cell Carcinoma. *Int. J. Clin. Exp. Pathol.* **2014**, *7*, 6032–6039. [PubMed]
28. Nakatani, K.; Wada, T.; Nakamura, M.; Uzawa, K.; Tanzawa, H.; Fujita, S. Expression of Caveolin-1 and Its Correlation with Cisplatin Sensitivity in Oral Squamous Cell Carcinoma. *J. Cancer Res. Clin. Oncol.* **2005**, *131*, 445–452. [CrossRef] [PubMed]
29. Mahammad, S.; Parmryd, I. Cholesterol Depletion Using Methyl-β-Cyclodextrin. *Methods Mol. Biol.* **2015**, *1232*, 91–102. [CrossRef]
30. Zidovetzki, R.; Levitan, I. Use of Cyclodextrins to Manipulate Plasma Membrane Cholesterol Content: Evidence, Misconceptions and Control Strategies. *Biochim. Biophys. Acta* **2007**, *1768*, 1311–1324. [CrossRef]
31. Orlando, K.; Guo, W. Membrane Organization and Dynamics in Cell Polarity. *Cold Spring Harb. Perspect. Biol.* **2009**, *1*, a001321. [CrossRef] [PubMed]
32. Ridley, A.J.; Schwartz, M.A.; Burridge, K.; Firtel, R.A.; Ginsberg, M.H.; Borisy, G.; Parsons, J.T.; Horwitz, A.R. Cell Migration: Integrating Signals from Front to Back. *Science* **2003**, *302*, 1704–1709. [CrossRef]
33. Seveau, S.; Eddy, R.J.; Maxfield, F.R.; Pierini, L.M. Cytoskeleton-Dependent Membrane Domain Segregation during Neutrophil Polarization. *Mol. Biol. Cell.* **2001**, *12*, 3550–3562. [CrossRef] [PubMed]
34. Guerra, F.S.; da Silva Sampaio, L.; Konig, S.; Bonamino, M.; Rossi, M.I.D.; Costa, M.L.; Fernandes, P.; Mermelstein, C. Membrane Cholesterol Depletion Reduces Breast Tumor Cell Migration by a Mechanism That Involves Non-Canonical Wnt Signaling and IL-10 Secretion. *Transl. Med. Commun.* **2016**, *1*, 3. [CrossRef]
35. Kumar, M.; Irungbam, K.; Kataria, M. Depletion of Membrane Cholesterol Compromised Caspase-8 Imparts in Autophagy Induction and Inhibition of Cell Migration in Cancer Cells. *Cancer Cell Int.* **2018**, *18*, 23. [CrossRef] [PubMed]
36. Qin, C.; Nagao, T.; Grosheva, I.; Maxfield, F.R.; Pierini, L.M. Elevated Plasma Membrane Cholesterol Content Alters Macrophage Signaling and Function. *Arterioscler. Thromb. Vasc. Biol.* **2006**, *26*, 372–378. [CrossRef]
37. Nagao, T.; Qin, C.; Grosheva, I.; Maxfield, F.R.; Pierini, L.M. Elevated Cholesterol Levels in the Plasma Membranes of Macrophages Inhibit Migration by Disrupting Rhoa Regulation. *Arterioscler. Thromb. Vasc. Biol.* **2007**, *27*, 1596–1602. [CrossRef]
38. Li, K.; Deng, Y.; Deng, G.; Chen, P.; Wang, Y.; Wu, H.; Ji, Z.; Yao, Z.; Zhang, X.; Yu, B.; et al. High Cholesterol Induces Apoptosis and Autophagy through the ROS-Activated AKT/FOXO1 Pathway in Tendon-Derived Stem Cells. *Stem. Cell Res. Ther.* **2020**, *11*, 131. [CrossRef]
39. Lomakin, A.J.; Lee, K.C.; Han, S.J.; Bui, D.A.; Davidson, M.; Mogilner, A.; Danuser, G. Competition for Actin between Two Distinct F-Actin Networks Defines a Bistable Switch for Cell Polarization. *Nat. Cell Biol.* **2015**, *17*, 1435–1445. [CrossRef]
40. Isshiki, M.; Ando, J.; Yamamoto, K.; Fujita, T.; Ying, Y.; Anderson, R.G.W. Sites of Ca^{2+} wave initiation move with caveolae to the trailing edge of migrating cells. *J. Cell. Sci.* **2001**, *115*, 475–484. [CrossRef]
41. Parat, M.O.; Anand-Apte, B.; Fox, P.L. Differential Caveolin-1 Polarization in Endothelial Cells during Migration in Two and Three Dimensions. *Mol. Biol. Cell* **2003**, *14*, 3156–3168. [CrossRef] [PubMed]
42. Beardsley, A.; Fang, K.; Mertz, H.; Castranova, V.; Friend, S.; Liu, J. Loss of Caveolin-1 Polarity Impedes Endothelial Cell Polarization and Directional Movement. *J. Biol. Chem.* **2005**, *280*, 3541–3547. [CrossRef]
43. Sun, X.H.; Flynn, D.C.; Castranova, V.; Millecchia, L.L.; Beardsley, A.R.; Liu, J. Identification of a Novel Domain at the N Terminus of Caveolin-1 That Controls Rear Polarization of the Protein and Caveolae Formation. *J. Biol. Chem.* **2007**, *282*, 7232–7241. [CrossRef] [PubMed]
44. Lentini, D.; Guzzi, F.; Pimpinelli, F.; Zaninetti, R.; Cassetti, A.; Coco, S.; Maggi, R.; Parenti, M. Polarization of Caveolins and Caveolae during Migration of Immortalized Neurons. *J. Neurochem.* **2008**, *104*, 514–523. [CrossRef] [PubMed]
45. Hill, M.M.; Daud, N.H.; Aung, C.S.; Loo, D.; Martin, S.; Murphy, S.; Black, D.M.; Barry, R.; Simpson, F.; Liu, L.; et al. Co-Regulation of Cell Polarization and Migration by Caveolar Proteins PTRF/Cavin-1 and Caveolin-1. *PLoS ONE* **2012**, *7*, e43041. [CrossRef]
46. Grande-García, A.; Echarri, A.; de Rooij, J.; Alderson, N.B.; Waterman-Storer, C.M.; Valdivielso, J.M.; del Pozo, M.A. Caveolin-1 Regulates Cell Polarization and Directional Migration through Src Kinase and Rho GTPases. *J. Cell Biol.* **2007**, *177*, 683–694. [CrossRef]
47. Ge, Y.; Gao, J.; Jordan, R.; Naumann, C.A. Changes in Cholesterol Level Alter Integrin Sequestration in Raft-Mimicking Lipid Mixtures. *Biophys. J.* **2018**, *114*, 158–167. [CrossRef]
48. Simons, K.; Ehehalt, R. Cholesterol, Lipid Rafts, and Disease. *J. Clin. Investig.* **2002**, *110*, 597–603. [CrossRef]

49. Schmidt, M.L.; Davis, J.H. Liquid Disordered-Liquid Ordered Phase Coexistence in Lipid/Cholesterol Mixtures: A Deuterium 2D NMR Exchange Study. *Langmuir* **2017**, *33*, 1881–1890. [CrossRef]
50. London, E.; Brown, D.A. Insolubility of Lipids in Triton X-100: Physical Origin and Relationship to Sphingolipid/Cholesterol Membrane Domains (Rafts). *Biochim. Biophys. Acta* **2000**, *1508*, 182–195. [CrossRef]
51. Fra, A.M.; Williamson, E.; Simons, K.; Parton, R.G. De Novo Formation of Caveolae in Lymphocytes by Expression of VIP21-Caveolin. *Proc. Natl. Acad. Sci. USA* **1995**, *92*, 8655–8659. [CrossRef]
52. Frank, P.G.; W-C Cheung, M.; Pavlides, S.; Llaverias, G.; Park, D.S.; Lisanti, M.P.; Pav-lides, S. Caveolin-1 and Regulation of Cellular Cholesterol Homeostasis. *Am. J. Physiol. Heart Circ. Physiol.* **2006**, *291*, 677–686. [CrossRef]
53. Smart, E.J.; Ying, Y.S.; Donzell, W.C.; Anderson, R.G.W. A Role for Caveolin in Transport of Cholesterol from Endoplasmic Reticulum to Plasma Membrane. *J. Biol. Chem.* **1996**, *271*, 29427–29435. [CrossRef]
54. Zhu, Y.; Liao, H.L.; Niu, X.L.; Yuan, Y.; Lin, T.; Verna, L.; Stemerman, M.B. Low Density Lipoprotein Induces eNOS Translocation to Membrane Caveolae: The Role of RhoA Activation and Stress Fiber Formation. *Biochim. Biophys. Acta* **2003**, *1635*, 117–126. [CrossRef]
55. Sanyour, H.J.; Li, N.; Rickel, A.P.; Torres, H.M.; Anderson, R.H.; Miles, M.R.; Childs, J.D.; Francis, K.R.; Tao, J.; Hong, Z. Statin-Mediated Cholesterol Depletion Exerts Coordinated Effects on the Alterations in Rat Vas-cular Smooth Muscle Cell Biomechanics and Migration. *J. Physiol.* **2020**, *598*, 1505–1522. [CrossRef] [PubMed]
56. Sawaya, A.P.; Jozic, I.; Stone, R.C.; Pastar, I.; Egger, A.N.; Stojadinovic, O.; Glinos, G.D.; Kirsner, R.S.; Tom-ic-Canic, M. Mevastatin Promotes Healing by Targeting Caveolin-1 to Restore EGFR Signaling. *JCI Insight* **2019**, 4. [CrossRef] [PubMed]
57. Jaafari-Ashkavandi, Z.; Aslani, E. Caveolin-1 Expression in Oral Lichen Planus, Dysplastic Lesions and Squamous Cell Carcinoma. *Pathol. Res. Pract.* **2017**, *213*, 809–814. [CrossRef] [PubMed]
58. Cassoni, P.; Senetta, R.; Castellano, I.; Ortolan, E.; Bosco, M.; Magnani, I.; Ducati, A. Caveolin-1 Expression Is Variably Displayed in Astroglial-Derived Tumors and Absent in Oligodendrogliomas: Concrete Premises for a New Reliable Diagnostic Marker in Gliomas. *Am. J. Surg. Pathol.* **2007**, *31*, 760–769. [CrossRef]
59. Hoque Apu, E.; Akram, S.U.; Rissanen, J.; Wan, H.; Salo, T. Desmoglein 3—Influence on Oral Carcinoma Cell Migration and Invasion. *Exp. Cell Res.* **2018**, *370*, 353–364. [CrossRef]
60. Haga, K.; Yamazaki, M.; Maruyama, S.; Kawaharada, M.; Suzuki, A.; Hoshikawa, E.; Chan, N.N.; Funayama, A.; Mi-kami, T.; Kobayashi, T.; et al. Crosstalk between Oral Squamous Cell Carcinoma Cells and Can-cer-Associated Fibroblasts via the TGF-β/SOX9 Axis in Cancer Progression. *Transl. Oncol.* **2021**, *14*. [CrossRef]
61. Salo, T.; Sutinen, M.; Hoque Apu, E.; Sundquist, E.; Cervigne, N.K.; de Oliveira, C.E.; Akram, S.U.; Ohlmeier, S.; Suomi, F.; Eklund, L.; et al. A Novel Human Leiomyoma Tissue Derived Matrix for Cell Culture Studies. *BMC Cancer* **2015**, *15*, 981. [CrossRef] [PubMed]
62. Brierley, J.D.; Gospodarowicz, M.K.; Wittekind, C. *TNM Classification of Malignant Tumors*, 8th ed.; John Wiley & Sons: Oxford, UK, 2017; pp. 17–21.
63. Conrad, P.A.; Nederlof, M.A.; Herman, I.M.; Lansing Taylor, D. Correlated Distribution of Actin, Myosin, and Microtubules at the Leading Edge of Migrating Swiss 3T3 Fibroblasts. *Cell Motil. Cytoskeleton.* **1989**, *14*, 527–543. [CrossRef] [PubMed]
64. Zhang, X.; Hu, Z.; Guo, Y.; Shan, X.; Li, X.; Lin, J. High-Efficiency Procedure to Characterize, Segment, and Quantify Complex Multicellularity in Raw Micrographs in Plants. *Plant Methods* **2020**, *16*, 100. [CrossRef] [PubMed]
65. Bankhead, P.; Loughrey, M.B.; Fernández, J.A.; Dombrowski, Y.; McArt, D.G.; Dunne, P.D.; McQuaid, S.; Gray, R.T.; Murray, L.J.; Coleman, H.G.; et al. QuPath: Open Source Software for Digital Pathology Image Analysis. *Sci. Rep.* **2017**, *7*, 16878. [CrossRef] [PubMed]

International Journal of *Molecular Sciences*

MDPI

Communication

Positive Linear Relationship between Nucleophosmin Protein Expression and the Viral Load in HPV-Associated Oropharyngeal Squamous Cell Carcinoma: A Possible Tool for Stratification of Patients

Marco D'Agostino [1], Marco Di Cecco [1], Carla Marani [2], Maurizio Giovanni Vigili [3], Sara Sileno [4], Chiara Costanza Volpi [5], Annunziata Gloghini [5], Daniele Avitabile [6], Alessandra Magenta [4,*,†] and Siavash Rahimi [7,*,†]

1 Experimental Immunology Laboratory, Istituto Dermopatico dell'Immacolata, IDI-IRCCS, 00167 Rome, Italy
2 Division of Histopathology, Ospedale San Carlo di Nancy, 00165 Rome, Italy
3 Head and Neck Surgery Departments, Istituto Dermopatico dell'Immacolata, IDI-IRCCS, 00167 Rome, Italy
4 Institute of Translational Pharmacology IFT, National Research Council of Italy (CNR), 00133 Rome, Italy
5 Diagnostic Pathology and Laboratory Medicine Department, Fondazione IRCCS Istituto Nazionale Tumori, 20133 Milan, Italy
6 Idi Farmaceutici S.R.L., Pomezia, 00071 Rome, Italy
7 Anatomic Pathology Department, Istituto Dermopatico dell'Immacolata IDI-IRCCS, 00167 Rome, Italy
* Correspondence: ale.magenta@gmail.com (A.M.); s.rahimi@idi.it (S.R.)
† These authors contributed equally to this work.

Citation: D'Agostino, M.; Di Cecco, M.; Marani, C.; Vigili, M.G.; Sileno, S.; Volpi, C.C.; Gloghini, A.; Avitabile, D.; Magenta, A.; Rahimi, S. Positive Linear Relationship between Nucleophosmin Protein Expression and the Viral Load in HPV-Associated Oropharyngeal Squamous Cell Carcinoma: A Possible Tool for Stratification of Patients. *Int. J. Mol. Sci.* **2023**, *24*, 3482. https://doi.org/10.3390/ijms24043482

Academic Editors: Marko Tarle and Ivica Lukšić

Received: 12 January 2023
Revised: 2 February 2023
Accepted: 6 February 2023
Published: 9 February 2023

Abstract: Most oropharyngeal squamous cell carcinomas (OPSCCs) are human papillomavirus (HPV)-associated, high-risk (HR) cancers that show a better response to chemoradiotherapy and are associated with improved survival. Nucleophosmin (NPM, also called NPM1/B23) is a nucleolar phosphoprotein that plays different roles within the cell, such as ribosomal synthesis, cell cycle regulation, DNA damage repair and centrosome duplication. NPM is also known as an activator of inflammatory pathways. An increase in NPM expression has been observed in vitro in E6/E7 overexpressing cells and is involved in HPV assembly. In this retrospective study, we investigated the relationship between the immunohistochemical (IHC) expression of NPM and HR-HPV viral load, assayed by RNAScope in situ hybridization (ISH), in ten patients with histologically confirmed p16-positive OPSCC. Our findings show that there is a positive correlation between NPM expression and HR-HPV mRNA ($Rs = 0.70$, $p = 0.03$), and a linear regression ($r^2 = 0.55$; $p = 0.01$). These data support the hypothesis that NPM IHC, together with HPV RNAScope, could be used as a predictor of transcriptionally active HPV presence and tumor progression, which is useful for therapy decisions. This study includes a small cohort of patients and, cannot report conclusive findings. Further studies with large series of patients are needed to support our hypothesis.

Keywords: oropharyngeal squamous cell carcinoma; HPV; nucleophosmin; inflammation

1. Introduction

Oral squamous cell carcinoma (OSCC) and oropharyngeal squamous cell carcinoma (OPSCC) are the most common types of HNSCC [1–3]. It is well known that tobacco smoking and alcohol consumption are the main causes of HNSCC [4,5], and despite the reduction in these risk factors, the incidence of HNSCC has increased [6]. Most OPSCCs are high-risk (HR) human papillomavirus (HPV)-related [7–9], with HPV16, the most common genotype involved, representing 86.7% of all HPV-positive OSCCs, followed by HPV18 and HPV33 [10].

Patients with HPV-induced OPSCC have been shown to be younger and are less likely to have a history of tobacco or alcohol use than patients with HPV-negative OPSCCs. A superior socioeconomic status and sexual behaviors have also been associated with the development of HPV-positive OPSCC [11]. Patients with HPV-associated OPSCC showed a better clinical outcome compared to those with HPV-negative tumors, with a good response to chemoradiotherapy. Hence, HPV status is included as a stratification factor for clinical trials using patients with OPSCC [12,13].

The HPV genome consists of a small double-stranded DNA and includes three major regions. The early genes (E1-E7) are expressed early in the viral infectious cycle for the regulation of transcription, plasmid replication and transformation. They encode the E6 and E7 oncoproteins, which are responsible for tumorigenesis [6]. The late genes code for the major (L1) and minor (L2) capsid proteins involved in the packaging of the viral genome and virus release. The long control region (LCR) contains the regulatory elements for transcription and replication. E6 protein binds the tumor suppressor p53 that is involved in apoptosis and cellular senescence, promoting its degradation [14]. Moreover, the E7 protein interacts and inactivates the retinoblastoma (Rb) tumor suppressor, which plays an important role in the regulation of the cell cycle. The inactivation of p53 and pRb causes uncontrolled cell proliferation and apoptosis inhibition, resulting in cellular transformation and genomic instability [15]. E6 and E7 expression inhibition in oropharyngeal cancer cells is associated with the restoration of p53 and Rb pathways and increased apoptosis [16].

The nucleolus is known to have a central role in the interaction between the virus and the infected cell. Indeed, several viruses, including HPV, have evolved molecular strategies to take control of nucleolar functions, ultimately favoring viral replication and maturation, such as ribosomal biogenesis, cell cycle progression and apoptosis [17].

The E7 protein has been colocalized with pRB in the nucleolus [18]. It interacts with p14arf and the Upstream Binding Factor 1 (UBF1), a key factor in the activation of RNA polymerase I machinery, thus favoring rDNA transcription [19]. The expression and/or localization of other nucleolar proteins, such as PICT-1 [20] and nucleolin [21], has been shown to correlate with HPV18-dependent carcinogenesis [21].

In keeping with the nucleolar role of HPV infection, changes in numbers or in morphometric parameters of silver-stained nucleolar organizer regions (AgNORs) have been previously proposed as useful predictors of worse prognosis in different forms of HPV-infected squamous cell carcinomas [22–25]. Recently, the presence of hyperchromasia, thickening of nuclear contour, and prominent nucleoli on Pap smear have been proposed as strong indicators of the presence of intraepithelial neoplasia grade 1 (CIN1) or greater CIN 2-3 [26]. Indeed, AgNOR areas greater than 3.3 μm^2 with concomitant expression of p16INK4a have been shown to be useful in the identification of high-risk human papillomaviruses (HR-HPV) for the development of cervical cancer [27].

Nucleophosmin (NPM, also called NPM1/B23) is a nucleolar phosphoprotein that plays different roles within the cell, such as ribosomal synthesis, cell cycle regulation, repair of DNA damage and centrosome duplication [28].

NPM interacts with different proteins from RNA and DNA viruses, including HIV, HCV, HBV and HPV, and affects the infection process [29]. In fact, NPM is implicated in different steps of the viral replicative cycle, including cytoplasmic nuclear traffic and the final assembly of viral particles, thus impacting the viral replication efficiency [29]. It has been shown that NPM levels increased in human foreskin keratinocytes (HFK) overexpressing E7, following differentiation induced by methylcellulose. Furthermore, in cultured cells and organotypic structures overexpressing E7 and E6/E7, an NPM protein level upregulation was found [30]. In addition, NPM downregulation in E6/E7 overexpressing cells provoked induction of p53 and pRb levels, causing replicative capacity reduction and an increase in the differentiation marker, Keratin 1, in HFKs [30].

Therefore, NPM is required for proliferation and inhibition of differentiation in primary keratinocyte cells expressing HPV's E6 and E7 [30]. The host nucleolar protein NPM is also required during HPV16 pseudovirus (PsV) assembly since it interacts with L2 minor capsid protein, playing an important role in establishing the correct interactions between L2 and L1 during the assembly of the HPV capsid [31].

Given the importance of the nucleolus in HPV infection and the pivotal role of the nucleolar protein NPM in the replicative capacity of HPV-infected cells, the aim of this study is to elucidate the relationship between NPM and the HR-HPV viral load, assessed by RNAScope, in p16-positive HPV-associated OPSCC.

2. Results

All cases show non-keratinized ("basaloid") and mixed-type ("keratinized" and "basaloid") SCC morphology [32] and positive p16 immunohistochemical staining according to the Lewis et al., criteria (Figure 1b) [33].

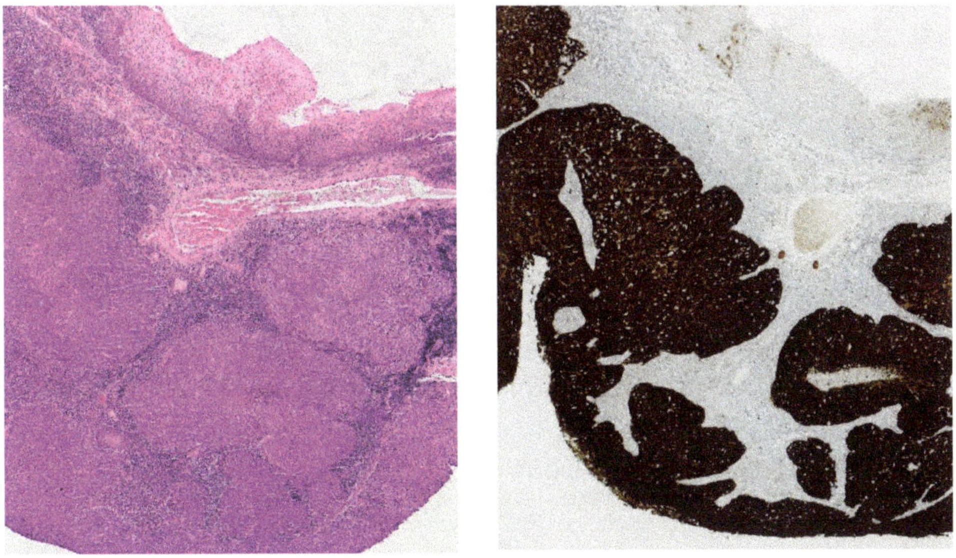

(a) (b)

Figure 1. HPV-OPSCC: morphology and immunohistochemistry (**a**) H&E image of "basaloid" invasive squamous cell carcinoma; (**b**) Intense and diffuse positive IHC staining with anti-p16 antibody.

RNAScope-ISH revealed positive staining for E6/E7 mRNA HR-HPV (Figure 2a,c). There was a different degree of intensity of staining among the cases. In some cases, the strong signals formed clusters, indicating a high viral load. The staining was specific and limited only to the neoplastic cells and dysplastic epithelium. The lymphoid stroma and normal squamous epithelium were negative.

In a similar way, we found that NPM IHC positivity was also variable in FFPE tissue. Some cases had low IHC positive staining, whereas others showed intense areas of positive staining (Figure 2b,d).

Interestingly, NPM IHC intensity positively correlated with high-risk HPV mRNA-IHS in OPSCC (Rs = 0.70, $p = 0.03$) (Figure 3). Moreover, a linear relationship was found between NPM IHC and HR-HPV mRNA, detected by RNAScope (Figure 3). Our data indicate that NPM is a positively signed direct regressor for HR-HPV mRNA expression. Thus, NPM expression level could be a predictor of HR-HPV mRNA levels with an average increase of 1.15 units for each 1-unit increase in NPM expression level. The "true" mean increase could plausibly be expected to lie between 0.30 and 2.00 (95% confidence interval). The r^2 suggests that about 55% of the variability in the HR-HPV mRNA can be explained by its relationship with NPM expression. The results show that NPM and E6/E7 mRNA HR-HPV positivity were very similar in patients' categorization.

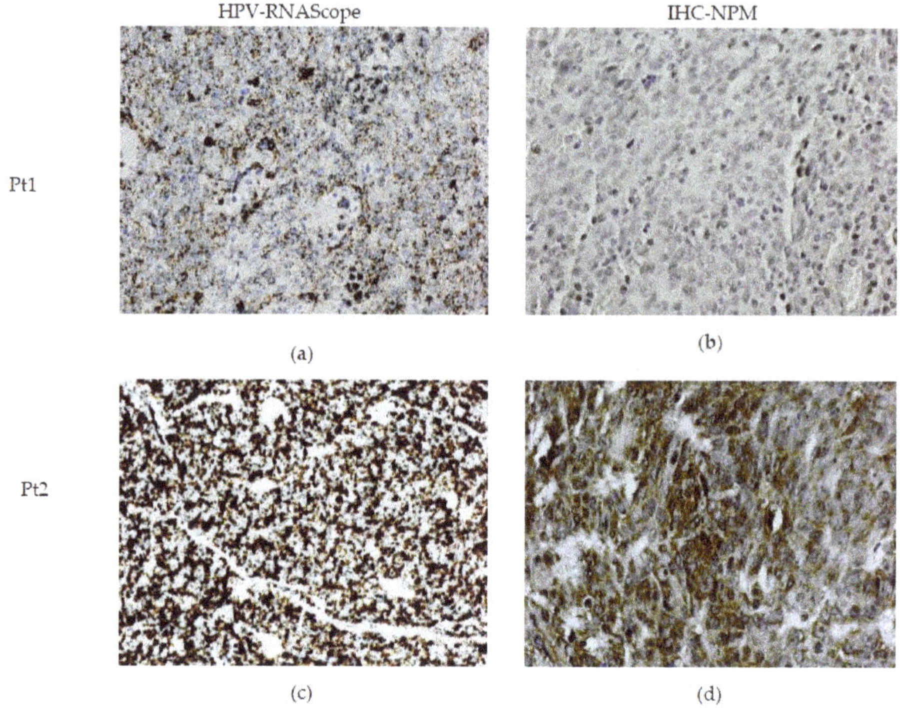

Figure 2. HR-HPV ISH and IHC of NPM protein in OPSCC (**a**,**c**) RNAScope ISH showing mild/moderate and large amounts of E6/E7 mRNA HR-HPV, respectively, (**b**,**d**) representative images of NPM IHC staining of same patients (Pt1, Pt2) depicted in (**a**,**c**). Weak and intense staining correlates with the amount of E6/E7 mRNA.

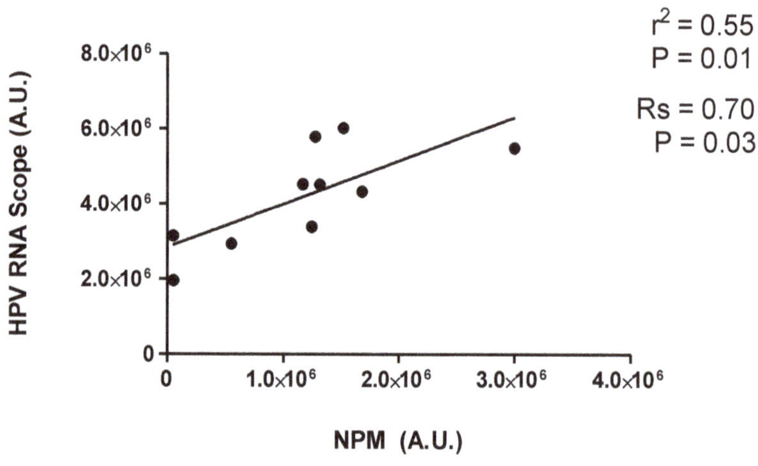

Figure 3. Correlation analysis and linear regression between NPM levels and mRNA HR-HPV expression in OPCCS. Spearman correlation analysis (Rs) and linear regression (r^2) between NPM IHC positivity and mRNA HR-HPV ISH levels. IHC quantification of NPM and E6/E7 mRNA HR-HPV ISH were quantified by Image J color deconvolution of three adjacent fields for each section and transformed in arbitrary units (A.U.) of positivity for each patient.

3. Discussion

The majority of the OPSCCs are HR-HPV-dependent and present a good clinical outcome in terms of chemoradiotherapy sensitivity compared with HPV-negative HNSCC [34]. p16 is a tumor suppressor protein and belongs to the family of INK4 cyclin-dependent-kinase inhibitors. Immunohistochemistry with p16 is an excellent surrogate of high-risk HPV infection [35,36].

However, approximately 20% of p16-positive OPSCC patients may lack transcriptionally-active HR-HPV [37–40].

In addition, a positive immunohistochemical reaction with p16 shows the presence or absence of HR-HPV infection and does not assess the amount of the viral load. Assuming that the amount of HPV viral load does establish the progression of the disease, then the p16 immunohistochemical test could not define the aggressiveness of the disease. RNAScope complementary to HPV E6/E7 mRNA is a molecular technique, which allows visualizing viral transcripts in FFPE tissue. HPV-RNAScope demonstrates high sensitivity and specificity for detection of HPV infection and has been proposed as the clinical standard for assigning a diagnosis of HPV-positive OPSCC [41–44].

Viral proteins often target the nucleolus, nucleolar proteins are released into the nucleoplasm and cytoplasm, and in most cases, viral nucleic acids are localized in the nucleolus. On the other hand, cellular proteins can be relocated to the nucleolus and participate in the infectious process [17]. Nucleolar proteins, in association with viral proteins, participate in replicating viruses in the capsid assembly and are often implicated in the transport of viral particles in the nucleoplasm and cytoplasm. Indeed, several viruses, including HPV, take advantage of nucleolar functions in order to increase viral replication and maturation, controlling ribosomal biogenesis, cell cycle progression and apoptosis [17].

The expression of different biomarkers has been linked to HPV carcinogenesis. Given the importance of the nucleolus, different nucleolar proteins have been used to determine the progression of HPV infection. For example, PITC1 [20] and nucleolin [21] are two nucleolar proteins whose expression has been linked to uterine cervical cancer aggressivity. Additionally, the expression of another cellular protein, proliferating cell nuclear antigen (PCNA), a protein essential for DNA replication, has been used for this aim [24]. PCNA expression was associated with high-risk HPV and the progression of cervical intraepithelial neoplasia (CIN).

In keeping with the nucleolar role of HPV infection, the numbers and the morphometric parameters of AgNORs have been proposed as useful predictors of worse prognosis in different forms of HPV-infected squamous cell carcinomas [22–25].

Further, hyperchromasia, thickening of nuclear contour, and prominent nucleoli on Pap smear have been used as indicators of intraepithelial neoplasia grade 1 (CIN1) or greater CIN 2–3 [26]. Moreover, AgNOR areas and p16INK4a positivity have been associated with HR-HPV for the development of cervical cancer [27].

Since NPM is a nucleolar protein that is frequently overexpressed in different types of tumours [45], we investigated the possible correlation between NPM and HR-HPV viral load in a small cohort of HPV-related OPSCC, using immunohistochemistry and RNAScope, respectively.

Our results showed a positive correlation and a linear relationship between the expression of NPM and HPV E6/E7 mRNA. These data support the hypothesis that NPM could be used as a predictor of transcriptionally active HPV presence and possibly tumor progression.

NPM up-regulation is required for the inhibition of differentiation and promotion of proliferation in differentiating cells, which express E6–E7 [30]. In addition, NPM has a role in establishing the correct interactions between L2 and L1 during HPV capsid assembly [31].

We previously showed that NPM intracellular protein level is increased by inflammatory cytokines and is released into the extracellular space by fibroblasts and primary keratinocytes upon cytokine stimulation associated with psoriasis [46].

Interestingly, circulating NPM is upregulated in the plasma of psoriatic patients and positively correlated with the severity of the disease and some determinants of cardiovascular risk [46].

Moreover, we demonstrated that NPM acts as an alarmin after genotoxic stress treatment and, when it is secreted in the extracellular space, induces inflammation by binding the Toll-Like Receptor 4 (TLR4) receptor. This interaction activates a signaling pathway that leads to the translocation of NF-kB in the nucleus with consequent induction of inflammatory genes, such as interleukin 6 (IL-6) and cyclooxygenase 2 (COX-2) [47].

We know that an increased level of reactive oxygen and nitrogen species (ROS and RNS), produced during chronic inflammation, play a pivotal role in tumor progression, and it is established that NPM is a modulator of the cellular oxidative stress response and an activator of inflammation pathway. Given the fact that inflammation-mediated DNA damage provides a potential mechanism of HPV integration and that an excessive amount of ROS and RNS promote DNA damage [48], it would be reasonable to speculate that NPM could potentially contribute to HPV integration and the promotion of tumor progression.

Targeting a single host protein to simultaneously impact different steps of viral replication is an appealing solution. Since NPM induction increases viral replication and also cell cycle progression, targeting NPM might simultaneously impact on viral replication and on the neoplastic state that emerges from it [29].

Different groups are currently studying the development and preclinical/clinical evaluation of NPM inhibitors. Among these, only two have been evaluated in Phase I/II cancer clinical trials, the CIGB-300 peptide in HPV-positive cervical cancers [49] and the synthetic pseudopeptide N6L (NCT01711398) in all solid tumors. CIGB-300 has also been tested in an HIV infection model with success [50].

Moreover, in cervical cancers treatment, 75% of the patients showed tumor reduction at colposcopy and 19% exhibited full histological regression. In addition, HPV DNA was negative in 48% of the previously positive patients. Long-term follow-up did not show adverse events or recurrences [49].

Since we demonstrated in previous papers that NPM could be considered an extracellular alarmin, the circulating expression of NPM could also be exploited in future applications as a predictor of HPV viral load by salivary or blood test screening in OPSCC.

In conclusion, our results show that a combination of tests, immunohistochemistry of NPM and HR-HPV RNAScope-ISH could be used in routine practice to stratify patients with HPV-positive OPSCC into a group with relatively stable disease and a group with the progression of malignancy. This finding potentially could have clinical implications because NPM inhibition could offer therapeutic benefits to these patients.

This study includes a small cohort of patients and, by definition, cannot be regarded as yielding conclusive findings. Further studies with a larger cohort of patients are needed to support this hypothesis.

4. Materials and Methods

4.1. Patients

Ten cases of OPSCC were retrieved from archives of Histopathology Division of San Carlo di Nancy Hospital and Istituto Dermopatico dell'Immacolata (IDI-IRCCS), Rome-Italy. Haematoxylin and eosin (H&E) stained slides obtained from formalin-fixed paraffin-embedded (FFPE) lesion tissue were examined.

4.2. Immunohistochemistry (IHC)

Leica Stainer Immunohistochemistry System was used for the p16 antibody (BD Biosciences, purified mouse anti-human p16, product number 550834, concentration 31.25 μg/mL, dilution 1:10). Appropriate positive and negative control tissue was used.

NPM IHC was performed on FFPE tissue as previously described [46]. Briefly, sections were incubated with the anti-human NPM rabbit polyclonal antibody (ab15440; dilution 1:200). Rabbit IgG isotype control (Santa Cruz Biotechnology, Dallas, TX, USA) was used at the same concentration of primary antibody. Polyclonal biotinylated secondary Abs and staining kits were obtained from Vector Laboratories. Immunoreactivity was visualized using the peroxidase reaction with 3-amino-9-ethylcarbazole (AEC, Vector Laboratories, Burlingame, CA, USA) in H_2O_2 as a substrate and samples were counterstained with hematoxylin. As a negative control, primary Abs were omitted. Stained sections were analyzed with the AxioCam digital camera coupled to the Axioplan 2 microscope (Carl Zeiss AG, Oberkochen, Germany). NPM staining intensity was evaluated by quantitative analysis (Image J color deconvolution) in three adjacent fields of each section by two independent observers, not aware of the status of the specimens. The mean values for each patient's section expressed as arbitrary units (A.U.) of NPM IHC positivity area were used for correlation and regression analyses.

4.3. RNAscope-In Situ Hybridization (ISH)

RNAscope-ISH was carried out on sections obtained from FFPE tissue. Bond III Automated. ISH for HR-HPV E6/E7 mRNA was performed using the RNAscope 2.5 VS HPV HR18 probe (cat. #312599; Advanced Cell Diagnostics, Inc., Newark, CA, USA), which recognizes HPV 16, 18, 26, 31, 33, 35, 39, 45, 51, 52, 53, 56, 58, 59, 66, 68, 73 and 82, genotypes. ISH was performed on an automated platform (Discovery Ultra, Ventana, Roche, Basel, Switzerland) by using the RNAscope VS Universal HRP assay (Advanced Cell Diagnostics, Inc.), according to the manufacturer's instructions. Positive staining has been identified as brown, punctate dots present in the nucleus and/or cytoplasm. Control probes for the bacterial gene 4-hydroxy-tetrahydrodipicolinate reductase (DapB), negative control, and for the housekeeping gene ubiquitin C (UbC), positive control for the evidence of preserved RNA, have also been included for each case.

4.4. Statistical Analysis

Because of the novelty of the study, whose primary objectives are mainly descriptive and exploratory, the minimum sample size has not been pre-determined.

Spearman correlation analysis and linear regression analysis were carried out using GraphPad Prism (version 5.0., GraphPad Software San Diego, CA, USA). A $p < 0.05$ was considered statistically significant.

Author Contributions: Conceptualization, A.M. and S.R.; data curation, M.D.; formal analysis, A.M.; funding acquisition, M.D., C.C.V., A.G., A.M. and S.R.; investigation, M.D., M.G.V., S.S., C.C.V. and A.G.; methodology, M.D., M.D.C., C.M., M.G.V., S.S., C.C.V. and A.G.; writing—original draft, M.D.; writing—review and editing, A.M., D.A. and S.R. All authors have read and agreed to the published version of the manuscript.

Funding: This study was supported by Italian Ministry of Health: RF-02362708 granted to A.M.; SG-12358253 granted to M.D.; RC-2022 granted to S.R.; and Lega Italiana per la Lotta ai Tumori: LILT-5X1000-2018 granted to C.C.V.; A.G.

Institutional Review Board Statement: The study was conducted according to the guidelines of the Declaration of Helsinki and approved by the Ethics Committee of IDI-IRCCS, Rome, Italy (Prot. n. 29 CE/2022 N° Registro Pareri: 698/1-2022).

Informed Consent Statement: Informed consent was obtained from all subjects involved in the study.

Data Availability Statement: The datasets generated during and/or analyzed during the current study are available from the corresponding author upon reasonable request.

Conflicts of Interest: The authors declare no conflict of interest.

References

1. Jemal, A.; Bray, F.; Center, M.M.; Ferlay, J.; Ward, E.; Forman, D. Global Cancer Statistics. *CA. Cancer J. Clin.* **2011**, *61*, 69–90. [CrossRef] [PubMed]
2. Patil, S.; Habib Awan, K.; Arakeri, G.; Jayampath Seneviratne, C.; Muddur, N.; Malik, S.; Ferrari, M.; Rahimi, S.; Brennan, P.A. Machine Learning and Its Potential Applications to the Genomic Study of Head and Neck Cancer—A Systematic Review. *J. Oral Pathol. Med.* **2019**, *48*, 773–779. [CrossRef]
3. Green, B.; Elhamshary, A.; Gomez, R.; Rahimi, S.; Brennan, P.A. An Update on the Current Management of Head and Neck Mucosal Melanoma. *J. Oral Pathol. Med.* **2017**, *46*, 475–479. [CrossRef]
4. Sturgis, E.M.; Cinciripini, P.M. Trends in Head and Neck Cancer Incidence in Relation to Smoking Prevalence: An Emerging Epidemic of Human Papillomavirus-Associated Cancers? *Cancer* **2007**, *110*, 1429–1435. [CrossRef] [PubMed]
5. Hashibe, M.; Brennan, P.; Benhamou, S.; Castellsague, X.; Chen, C.; Curado, M.P.; Dal Maso, L.; Daudt, A.W.; Fabianova, E.; Fernandez, L.; et al. Alcohol Drinking in Never Users of Tobacco, Cigarette Smoking in Never Drinkers, and the Risk of Head and Neck Cancer: Pooled Analysis in the International Head and Neck Cancer Epidemiology Consortium. *J. Natl. Cancer Inst.* **2007**, *99*, 777–789. [CrossRef]
6. Chai, R.C.; Lambie, D.; Verma, M.; Punyadeera, C. Current Trends in the Etiology and Diagnosis of HPV-Related Head and Neck Cancers. *Cancer Med.* **2015**, *4*, 596–607. [CrossRef]
7. Chaturvedi, A.K.; Engels, E.A.; Pfeiffer, R.M.; Hernandez, B.Y.; Xiao, W.; Kim, E.; Jiang, B.; Goodman, M.T.; Sibug-Saber, M.; Cozen, W.; et al. Human Papillomavirus and Rising Oropharyngeal Cancer Incidence in the United States. *J. Clin. Oncol.* **2011**, *29*, 4294–4301. [CrossRef]
8. Marur, S.; D'Souza, G.; Westra, W.H.; Forastiere, A.A. HPV-Associated Head and Neck Cancer: A Virus-Related Cancer Epidemic. *Lancet. Oncol.* **2010**, *11*, 781–789. [CrossRef]
9. de Martel, C.; Plummer, M.; Vignat, J.; Franceschi, S. Worldwide Burden of Cancer Attributable to HPV by Site, Country and HPV Type. *Int. J. Cancer* **2017**, *141*, 664–670. [CrossRef]
10. Kreimer, A.R.; Clifford, G.M.; Boyle, P.; Franceschi, S. Human Papillomavirus Types in Head and Neck Squamous Cell Carcinomas Worldwide: A Systematic Review. *Cancer Epidemiol. Biomark. Prev.* **2005**, *14*, 467–475. [CrossRef]
11. Castle, P.E.; Shields, T.; Kirnbauer, R.; Manos, M.M.; Burk, R.D.; Glass, A.G.; Scott, D.R.; Sherman, M.E.; Schiffman, M. Sexual Behavior, Human Papillomavirus Type 16 (HPV 16) Infection, and HPV 16 Seropositivity. *Sex. Transm. Dis.* **2002**, *29*, 182–187. [CrossRef]
12. Fakhry, C.; Westra, W.H.; Li, S.; Cmelak, A.; Ridge, J.A.; Pinto, H.; Forastiere, A.; Gillison, M.L. Improved Survival of Patients with Human Papillomavirus-Positive Head and Neck Squamous Cell Carcinoma in a Prospective Clinical Trial. *J. Natl. Cancer Inst.* **2008**, *100*, 261–269. [CrossRef]
13. Albers, A.E.; Qian, X.; Kaufmann, A.M.; Coordes, A. Meta Analysis: HPV and P16 Pattern Determines Survival in Patients with HNSCC and Identifies Potential New Biologic Subtype. *Sci. Rep.* **2017**, *7*, 16715. [CrossRef]
14. Scheffner, M.; Werness, B.A.; Huibregtse, J.M.; Levine, A.J.; Howley, P.M. The E6 Oncoprotein Encoded by Human Papillomavirus Types 16 and 18 Promotes the Degradation of P53. *Cell* **1990**, *63*, 1129–1136. [CrossRef]
15. Ramón, A.C.; Basukala, O.; Massimi, P.; Thomas, M.; Perera, Y.; Banks, L.; Perea, S.E. CIGB-300 Peptide Targets the CK2 Phospho-Acceptor Domain on Human Papillomavirus E7 and Disrupts the Retinoblastoma (RB) Complex in Cervical Cancer Cells. *Viruses* **2022**, *14*, 1681. [CrossRef]
16. Rampias, T.; Sasaki, C.; Weinberger, P.; Psyrri, A. E6 and E7 Gene Silencing and Transformed Phenotype of Human Papillomavirus 16-Positive Oropharyngeal Cancer Cells. *J. Natl. Cancer Inst.* **2009**, *101*, 412–423. [CrossRef]
17. Iarovaia, O.V.; Ioudinkova, E.S.; Velichko, A.K.; Razin, S. V Manipulation of Cellular Processes via Nucleolus Hijaking in the Course of Viral Infection in Mammals. *Cells* **2021**, *10*, 1597. [CrossRef]
18. Zatsepina, O.; Braspenning, J.; Robberson, D.; Hajibagheri, M.A.; Blight, K.J.; Ely, S.; Hibma, M.; Spitkovsky, D.; Trendelenburg, M.; Crawford, L.; et al. The Human Papillomavirus Type 16 E7 Protein Is Associated with the Nucleolus in Mammalian and Yeast Cells. *Oncogene* **1997**, *14*, 1137–1145. [CrossRef]
19. Dichamp, I.; Séité, P.; Agius, G.; Barbarin, A.; Beby-Defaux, A. Human Papillomavirus 16 Oncoprotein E7 Stimulates UBF1-Mediated RDNA Gene Transcription, Inhibiting a P53-Independent Activity of P14ARF. *PLoS ONE* **2014**, *9*, e96136. [CrossRef]
20. Yoshimoto, M.; Tokuda, A.; Nishiwaki, K.; Sengoku, K.; Yaginuma, Y. The Protein Interacting with Carboxyl Terminus-1 Codon 389 Polymorphism Impairs Protein Interacting with Carboxyl Terminus-1 Function and Is a Risk Factor for Uterine Cervical Cancer. *Mol. Carcinog.* **2017**, *56*, 1484–1492. [CrossRef]
21. Grinstein, E.; Wernet, P.; Snijders, P.J.F.; Rösl, F.; Weinert, I.; Jia, W.; Kraft, R.; Schewe, C.; Schwabe, M.; Hauptmann, S.; et al. Nucleolin as Activator of Human Papillomavirus Type 18 Oncogene Transcription in Cervical Cancer. *J. Exp. Med.* **2002**, *196*, 1067–1078. [CrossRef]
22. Tosi, P.; Cintorino, M.; Santopietro, R.; Lio, R.; Barbini, P.; Ji, H.; Chang, F.; Kataja, V.; Syrjänen, S.; Syrjänen, K. Prognostic Factors in Invasive Cervical Carcinomas Associated with Human Papillomavirus (HPV). Quantitative Data and Cytokeratin Expression. *Pathol. Res. Pract.* **1992**, *188*, 866–873. [CrossRef]
23. Del Carmen Alarcón-Romero, L.; Illades-Aguiar, B.; Flores-Alfaro, E.; Terán-Porcayo, M.A.; Antonio-Véjar, V.; Reyes-Maldonado, E. AgNOR Polymorphism Association with Squamous Intraepithelial Lesions and Invasive Carcinoma with HPV Infection. *Salud Publica Mex.* **2009**, *51*, 134–140. [CrossRef]

24. Donofrio, V.; Lo Muzio, L.; Mignogna, M.D.; Troncone, G.; Staibano, S.; Boscaino, A.; De Rosa, G. Prognostic Evaluation of HPV-Associated Precancerous and Microinvasive Carcinoma of the Oral Cavity: Combined Use of Nucleolar Organiser Regions (AgNOR) and Proliferating Cell Nuclear Antigen (PCNA). *Eur. J. Cancer. B. Oral Oncol.* **1995**, *31*, 174–180. [CrossRef]
25. Lo Muzio, L.; Mignogna, M.D.; Staibano, S.; de Vico, G.; Salvatore, G.; Damiano, S.; Bucci, E.; Procaccini, M.; Mezza, E.; De Rosa, G. Morphometric Study of Nucleolar Organiser Regions (AgNOR) in HPV-Associated Precancerous Lesions and Microinvasive Carcinoma of the Oral Cavity. *Oral Oncol.* **1997**, *33*, 247–259. [CrossRef]
26. Hata, H.; Okayama, K.; Iijima, J.; Teruya, K.; Shiina, N.; Caniz, T.; Ishii, Y.; Fujii, M.; Oda, M.; Okodo, M. A Comparison of Cytomorphological Features of ASC-H Cells Based on Histopathological Results Obtained from a Colposcopic Target Biopsy Immediately after Pap Smear Sampling. *Asian Pac. J. Cancer Prev.* **2019**, *20*, 2139–2143. [CrossRef]
27. Hidalgo, J.V.; Rocher, A.E.; López, J.L.; Gamboni, M.; Vighi, S.; Canessa, O.E.; Peressini, S.; Guerra, F.; di Carlo, M.B.; Palaoro, L.A.; et al. AgNOR, P16 and Human Papillomavirus in Low-Grade Squamous Intra-Epithelial Lesions of the Uterine Cervix. Preliminary Report. *Biotech. Histochem.* **2012**, *87*, 257–264. [CrossRef]
28. Box, J.K.; Paquet, N.; Adams, M.N.; Boucher, D.; Bolderson, E.; O'Byrne, K.J.; Richard, D.J. Nucleophosmin: From Structure and Function to Disease Development. *BMC Mol. Biol.* **2016**, *17*, 19. [CrossRef]
29. Lobaina, Y.; Perera, Y. Implication of B23/NPM1 in Viral Infections, Potential Uses of B23/NPM1 Inhibitors as Antiviral Therapy. *Infect. Disord. Drug Targets* **2019**, *19*, 2–16. [CrossRef]
30. McCloskey, R.; Menges, C.; Friedman, A.; Patel, D.; McCance, D.J. Human Papillomavirus Type 16 E6/E7 Upregulation of Nucleophosmin Is Important for Proliferation and Inhibition of Differentiation. *J. Virol.* **2010**, *84*, 5131–5139. [CrossRef]
31. Day, P.M.; Thompson, C.D.; Pang, Y.Y.; Lowy, D.R.; Schiller, J.T. Involvement of Nucleophosmin (NPM1/B23) in Assembly of Infectious HPV16 Capsids. *Papillomavirus Res.* **2015**, *1*, 74–89. [CrossRef] [PubMed]
32. Rahimi, S.; Akaev, I.; Brennan, P.A.; Virgo, A.; Marani, C.; Gomez, R.S.; Yeoh, C.C. A Proposal for Classification of Oropharyngeal Squamous Cell Carcinoma: Morphology and Status of HPV by Immunohistochemistry and Molecular Biology. *J. Oral Pathol. Med.* **2020**, *49*, 110–116. [CrossRef]
33. Lewis, J.S.; Chernock, R.D.; Ma, X.-J.; Flanagan, J.J.; Luo, Y.; Gao, G.; Wang, X.; El-Mofty, S.K. Partial P16 Staining in Oropharyngeal Squamous Cell Carcinoma: Extent and Pattern Correlate with Human Papillomavirus RNA Status. *Mod. Pathol.* **2012**, *25*, 1212–1220. [CrossRef] [PubMed]
34. Rahimi, S. HPV-Related Squamous Cell Carcinoma of Oropharynx: A Review. *J. Clin. Pathol.* **2020**, *73*, 624–629. [CrossRef] [PubMed]
35. Lewis, J.S.; Beadle, B.; Bishop, J.A.; Chernock, R.D.; Colasacco, C.; Lacchetti, C.; Moncur, J.T.; Rocco, J.W.; Schwartz, M.R.; Seethala, R.R.; et al. Human Papillomavirus Testing in Head and Neck Carcinomas: Guideline from the College of American Pathologists. *Arch. Pathol. Lab. Med.* **2018**, *142*, 559–597. [CrossRef] [PubMed]
36. Lydiatt, W.M.; Patel, S.G.; O'Sullivan, B.; Brandwein, M.S.; Ridge, J.A.; Migliacci, J.C.; Loomis, A.M.; Shah, J.P. Head and Neck Cancers-Major Changes in the American Joint Committee on Cancer Eighth Edition Cancer Staging Manual. CA. *Cancer J. Clin.* **2017**, *67*, 122–137. [CrossRef]
37. Ndiaye, C.; Mena, M.; Alemany, L.; Arbyn, M.; Castellsagué, X.; Laporte, L.; Bosch, F.X.; de Sanjosé, S.; Trottier, H. HPV DNA, E6/E7 MRNA, and P16INK4a Detection in Head and Neck Cancers: A Systematic Review and Meta-Analysis. *Lancet. Oncol.* **2014**, *15*, 1319–1331. [CrossRef]
38. Mirghani, H.; Casiraghi, O.; Guerlain, J.; Amen, F.; He, M.-X.; Ma, X.-J.; Luo, Y.; Mourareau, C.; Drusch, F.; Lakdhar, A.B.; et al. Diagnosis of HPV Driven Oropharyngeal Cancers: Comparing P16 Based Algorithms with the RNAscope HPV Test. *Oral Oncol.* **2016**, *62*, 101–108. [CrossRef]
39. Smith, E.M.; Wang, D.; Kim, Y.; Rubenstein, L.M.; Lee, J.H.; Haugen, T.H.; Turek, L.P. P16INK4a Expression, Human Papillomavirus, and Survival in Head and Neck Cancer. *Oral Oncol.* **2008**, *44*, 133–142. [CrossRef]
40. Rietbergen, M.M.; Brakenhoff, R.H.; Bloemena, E.; Witte, B.I.; Snijders, P.J.F.; Heideman, D.A.M.; Boon, D.; Koljenovic, S.; Baatenburg-de Jong, R.J.; Leemans, C.R. Human Papillomavirus Detection and Comorbidity: Critical Issues in Selection of Patients with Oropharyngeal Cancer for Treatment De-Escalation Trials. *Ann. Oncol.* **2013**, *24*, 2740–2745. [CrossRef]
41. Schache, A.G.; Liloglou, T.; Risk, J.M.; Jones, T.M.; Ma, X.-J.; Wang, H.; Bui, S.; Luo, Y.; Sloan, P.; Shaw, R.J.; et al. Validation of a Novel Diagnostic Standard in HPV-Positive Oropharyngeal Squamous Cell Carcinoma. *Br. J. Cancer* **2013**, *108*, 1332–1339. [CrossRef] [PubMed]
42. Ukpo, O.C.; Flanagan, J.J.; Ma, X.-J.; Luo, Y.; Thorstad, W.L.; Lewis, J.S. High-Risk Human Papillomavirus E6/E7 MRNA Detection by a Novel in Situ Hybridization Assay Strongly Correlates with P16 Expression and Patient Outcomes in Oropharyngeal Squamous Cell Carcinoma. *Am. J. Surg. Pathol.* **2011**, *35*, 1343–1350. [CrossRef] [PubMed]
43. Lewis, J.S.; Ukpo, O.C.; Ma, X.-J.; Flanagan, J.J.; Luo, Y.; Thorstad, W.L.; Chernock, R.D. Transcriptionally-Active High-Risk Human Papillomavirus Is Rare in Oral Cavity and Laryngeal/Hypopharyngeal Squamous Cell Carcinomas—A Tissue Microarray Study Utilizing E6/E7 MRNA in Situ Hybridization. *Histopathology* **2012**, *60*, 982–991. [CrossRef]
44. Wang, F.; Flanagan, J.; Su, N.; Wang, L.-C.; Bui, S.; Nielson, A.; Wu, X.; Vo, H.-T.; Ma, X.-J.; Luo, Y. RNAscope: A Novel in Situ RNA Analysis Platform for Formalin-Fixed, Paraffin-Embedded Tissues. *J. Mol. Diagn.* **2012**, *14*, 22–29. [CrossRef] [PubMed]
45. Lim, M.J.; Wang, X.W. Nucleophosmin and Human Cancer. *Cancer Detect. Prev.* **2006**, *30*, 481–490. [CrossRef] [PubMed]

46. D'Agostino, M.; Beji, S.; Sileno, S.; Lulli, D.; Mercurio, L.; Madonna, S.; Cirielli, C.; Pallotta, S.; Albanesi, C.; Capogrossi, M.C.; et al. Extracellular Nucleophosmin Is Increased in Psoriasis and Correlates with the Determinants of Cardiovascular Diseases. *Front. Cardiovasc. Med.* **2022**, *9*, 867813. [CrossRef]
47. Beji, S.; D'Agostino, M.; Gambini, E.; Sileno, S.; Scopece, A.; Vinci, M.C.; Milano, G.; Melillo, G.; Napolitano, M.; Pompilio, G.; et al. Doxorubicin Induces an Alarmin-like TLR4-Dependent Autocrine/Paracrine Action of Nucleophosmin in Human Cardiac Mesenchymal Progenitor Cells. *BMC Biol.* **2021**, *19*, 124. [CrossRef]
48. Williams, V.M.; Filippova, M.; Soto, U.; Duerksen-Hughes, P.J. HPV-DNA Integration and Carcinogenesis: Putative Roles for Inflammation and Oxidative Stress. *Future Virol.* **2011**, *6*, 45–57. [CrossRef]
49. Solares, A.M.; Santana, A.; Baladrón, I.; Valenzuela, C.; González, C.A.; Díaz, A.; Castillo, D.; Ramos, T.; Gómez, R.; Alonso, D.F.; et al. Safety and Preliminary Efficacy Data of a Novel Casein Kinase 2 (CK2) Peptide Inhibitor Administered Intralesionally at Four Dose Levels in Patients with Cervical Malignancies. *BMC Cancer* **2009**, *9*, 146. [CrossRef]
50. Nouri, K.; Moll, J.M.; Milroy, L.-G.; Hain, A.; Dvorsky, R.; Amin, E.; Lenders, M.; Nagel-Steger, L.; Howe, S.; Smits, S.H.J.; et al. Biophysical Characterization of Nucleophosmin Interactions with Human Immunodeficiency Virus Rev and Herpes Simplex Virus US11. *PLoS ONE* **2015**, *10*, e0143634. [CrossRef]

International Journal of
Molecular Sciences

MDPI

Article

Potential of uPAR, αvβ6 Integrin, and Tissue Factor as Targets for Molecular Imaging of Oral Squamous Cell Carcinoma: Evaluation of Nine Targets in Primary Tumors and Metastases by Immunohistochemistry

Mads Lawaetz [1,2,*], Anders Christensen [1,2], Karina Juhl [2], Kirstine Karnov [1,2,†], Giedrius Lelkaitis [3], Anne-Marie Kanstrup Fiehn [3,4], Andreas Kjaer [2] and Christian von Buchwald [1]

1 Department of Otolaryngology, Head and Neck Surgery and Audiology, Rigshospitalet, Copenhagen University Hospital, 2100 Copenhagen, Denmark
2 Department of Clinical Physiology, Nuclear Medicine and PET and Cluster for Molecular Imaging, Copenhagen University Hospital-Rigshospitalet & Department of Biomedical Sciences, University of Copenhagen, 2100 Copenhagen, Denmark
3 Department of Pathology, Rigshospitalet, Copenhagen University Hospital, 2100 Copenhagen, Denmark
4 Department of Clinical Medicine, University of Copenhagen, 2200 Copenhagen, Denmark
* Correspondence: mads.lawaetz@regionh.dk
† Before this article was published, Kirstine Kim Schmidt Karnov sadly passed away. Our thoughts are with her family.

Abstract: No clinically approved tumor-specific imaging agents for head and neck cancer are currently available. The identification of biomarkers with a high and homogenous expression in tumor tissue and minimal expression in normal tissue is essential for the development of new molecular imaging targets in head and neck cancer. We investigated the expression of nine imaging targets in both primary tumor and matched metastatic tissue of 41 patients with oral squamous cell carcinoma (OSCC) to assess their potential as targets for molecular imaging. The intensity, proportion, and homogeneity in the tumor and the reaction in neighboring non-cancerous tissue was scored. The intensity and proportion were multiplied to obtain a total immunohistochemical (IHC) score ranging from 0–12. The mean intensity in the tumor tissue and normal epithelium were compared. The expression rate was high for the urokinase-type plasminogen activator receptor (uPAR) (97%), integrin αvβ6 (97%), and tissue factor (86%) with a median total immunostaining score (interquartile range) for primary tumors of 6 (6–9), 12 (12–12), and 6 (2.5–7.5), respectively. For the uPAR and tissue factor, the mean staining intensity score was significantly higher in tumors compared to normal epithelium. The uPAR, integrin αvβ6, and tissue factor are promising imaging targets for OSCC primary tumors, lymph node metastases, and recurrences.

Keywords: oral squamous cell carcinoma; lymph node metastases; molecular imaging; immunohistochemistry; urokinase-type plasminogen activator receptor; tissue factor; integrin αvβ6

Citation: Lawaetz, M.; Christensen, A.; Juhl, K.; Karnov, K.; Lelkaitis, G.; Kanstrup Fiehn, A.-M.; Kjaer, A.; von Buchwald, C. Potential of uPAR, αvβ6 Integrin, and Tissue Factor as Targets for Molecular Imaging of Oral Squamous Cell Carcinoma: Evaluation of Nine Targets in Primary Tumors and Metastases by Immunohistochemistry. *Int. J. Mol. Sci.* **2023**, *24*, 3853. https://doi.org/10.3390/ijms24043853

Academic Editors: Marko Tarle and Ivica Lukšić

Received: 22 December 2022
Revised: 7 February 2023
Accepted: 12 February 2023
Published: 14 February 2023

1. Introduction

Despite advances in diagnostic techniques and postoperative treatment, poor survival and high recurrence rate remain for patients with oral squamous cell carcinoma (OSCC) [1]. The primary curative treatment is surgery, where the adequate resection margins (>5 mm) are one of the most important prognosticators [2,3]. Achieving radical resection margins is challenging when the tumor is surrounded by multiple functionally and aesthetically critical structures and the border between the tumor and normal tissue is not clearly delineated. This is reflected in a positive margin rate of 12–30% for OSCC, one of the highest rates among all solid tumors [2,4,5]. Additionally, the detection and removal of regional lymph

Table 2. Median and interquartile ranges of intensity, proportion, and total immune staining scores for each target in primary tumor, lymph node metastases, and tissue from local recurrence.

Target	Primary Tumor				Lymph Node Metastases				Local Recurrence				Normal Epithelium	
	n	Intensity score (IQR)	Proportion (IQR)	TIS-score (IQR)	n	Intensity score (IQR)	Proportion (IQR)	TIS-score (IQR)	n	Intensity score (IQR)	Proportion (IQR)	TIS-score (IQR)	n	Intensity score (IQR)
Integrin αvβ6	40	3(3-3)	4(4-4)	12(12-12)	28	3(3-3)	4(4-4)	12(9.75-12)	8	3(3-3)	4(4-4)	12(12-12)	47	3(3-3)
Tissue factor	41	3(2-3)	2(1-3)	6(2.5-7.5)	28	2(1-3)	1(1-2)	2(1-5.5)	8	2.5(0-3)	1.5(0-2)	4(0-6)	47	1(1-1)
PARP1	35	2(2-3)	3(3-4)	6(4-9)	24	2(2-3)	3(3-3)	6(6-9)	7	2(2-2)	3(3-4)	6(4-8)	39	2(1-2)
uPAR	34	3(2.75-3)	2(2-3)	6(6-9)	23	3(2-3)	2(2-3)	6(4-6)	6	3(2.75-3)	2.5(2-3.25)	6(6-9.75)	37	0(0-0)
VEGFR1	35	2(2-2)	4(3-4)	8(6-8)	24	2(2-2)	4(3.25-4)	8(6.5-8)	7	2(1-2)	4(3-4)	8(3-8)	40	1.5(1-2)
EpCAM	34	0.5(0-2)	0.5(0-2)	0.5(0-2.5)	24	1.5(0-3)	1(0-1)	1.5(0-3)	7	1(0-3)	1(0-2)	1(0-6)	34	0(0-0)
VEGFR2	35	1(1-2)	1(1-2)	2(1-4)	24	1(1-2)	2(1-2)	2(1-4)	7	1(0-1)	2(0-2)	2(0-2)	39	0(0-1)
Cathepsin E	35	0(0-0)	0(0-0)	0(0-0)	23	0(0-0)	0(0-0)	0(0-0)	7	0(0-0)	0(0-0)	0(0-0)	40	0(0-0.5)
Integrin αvβ3	36	0(0-0)	0(0-0)	0(0-0)	27	0(0-0)	0(0-0)	0(0-0)	8	0(0-0)	0(0-0)	0(0-0)	44	0(0-0)

Table 3. Overview of the expression pattern for all nine included targets.

Target	Tumor-Specific	Homogenous Expression in Tumor Compartment	Expression Rate Primary Tumor	Expression Rate Lymph Node Metastasis	Superficial Margin Contrast Tumor vs. Epithelium	Profound Margin Contrast Tumor vs. Normal Cells
Integrin αvβ6	Partly	80%	95%	100%	No	Yes
Tissue factor	Yes	3%	93%	80%	Yes	Yes
PARP1	No	0%	94%	100%	Yes	No
uPAR	Yes	51%	97%	96%	Yes	Yes
VEGFR1	No	5%	100%	100%	Yes	No
EpCAM	No	3%	50%	66%	No	No
VEGFR2	No	0%	80%	81%	Yes	No
Cathepsin E	NA	0%	3%	13%	NA	NA
Integrin αvβ3	NA	NA	NA	NA	NA	NA

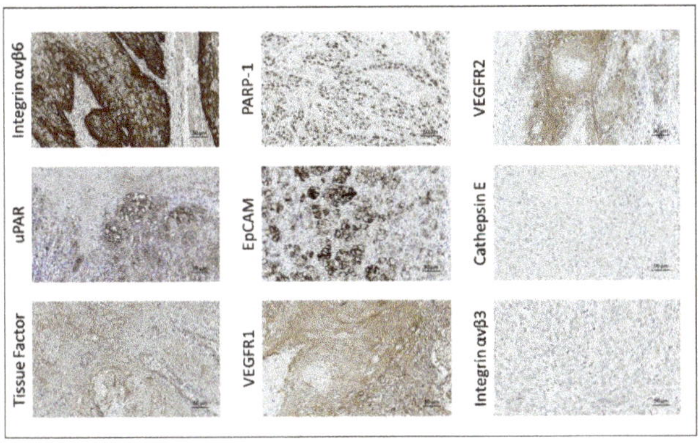

Figure 1. Expression of integrin αvβ6, tissue factor, PARP-1, uPAR, VEGFR1, EpCAM, VEGFR2, Cathepsin E and integrin αvβ3 in primary tumor tissue of OSCC.

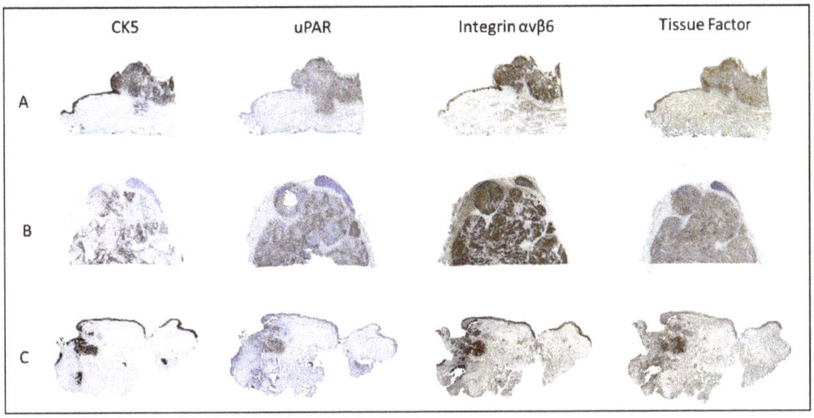

Figure 2. Expression of CK5 (for visualization of tumor localization), uPAR, integrin αvβ6 and tissue factor in (**A**) primary tumor, (**B**) lymph node metastases, and (**C**) local recurrence.

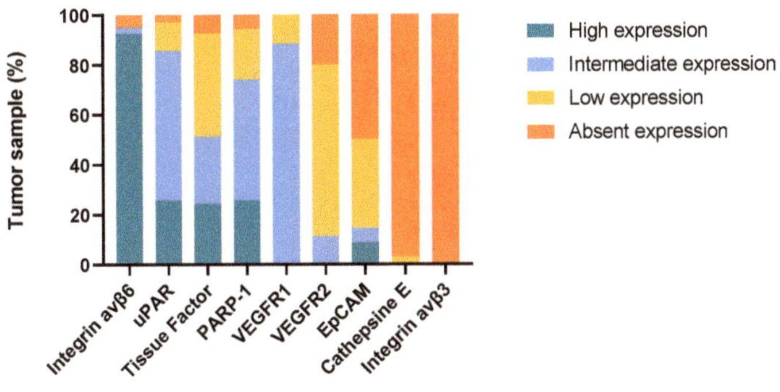

Figure 3. Expression of imaging targets in OSCC primary tumors.

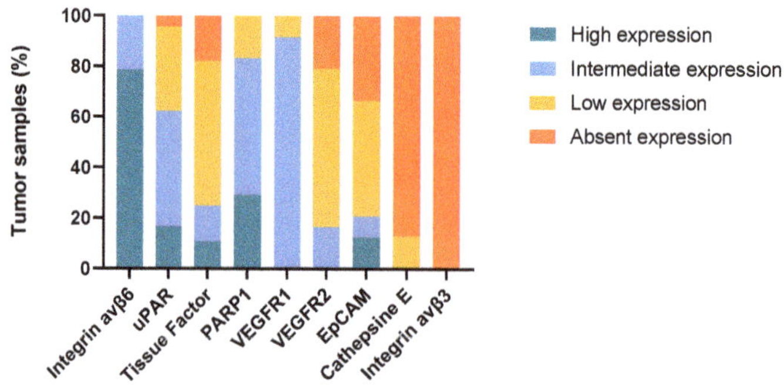

Figure 4. Expression of imaging targets in OSCC lymph node metastases.

2.2.2. uPAR

The overall expression rate was 97% with highly tumor-specific staining, which was rated as homogeneous in 51% of the samples. uPAR was expressed in 23/24 metastases (96%). Both membrane and cytoplasmic staining were found in tumor cells. The total immune staining scores for primary tumor cells, lymph node metastases, and local tumor recurrence tissue were 6 (6–9), 6 (4–8), and 6 (6–9.75), respectively. Normal epithelium exhibited no staining, except for in four cases where weak epithelial staining was seen. In one case, moderate staining of a lichen planus lesion was observed in the periphery of the tumor. There was a clear contrast between tumor and surrounding tissue at the deep tumor margin. Weak to moderate staining was observed in granulocytes.

2.2.3. Tissue Factor

The overall expression rate of tissue factor in tumor tissue was high (86%), but only with a homogenous pattern in 3% of tumor samples. In half of the primary tumor samples, tissue factor showed moderate to intense expression. In lymph node metastases, expression was mainly weak and moderate. Staining scores for primary tumor cells, lymph node metastases, and local recurrence tumor tissue were 6 (2.5–7.5), 2 (1–5.5), and 4 (0–6), respectively. Normal epithelium expressed tissue factor in approximately 80% of the samples, although the staining in this compartment was mostly weak. Salivary duct and acini cells also showed a weak expression of tissue factor.

2.2.4. PARP-1

A high overall expression rate was seen for PARP-1 (97%), with positive staining of tumor nuclei, albeit heterogeneously. For primary tumor cells, lymph node metastases, and local recurrence tumor tissue, the staining scores were 6 (4–9), 6 (6–9), and 6 (4–8), respectively. Nevertheless, the staining was not very tumor-specific, as several normal cells were also stained. Lymphocytes, endothelium, muscle tissues, nerve fibers, salivary gland tissues, plasma cells, and normal epithelium exhibited variable nuclei staining.

2.2.5. VEGFR1

All tumors were positive for VEGFR1, but the staining was not tumor-specific and contrasted poorly with the normal stroma and epithelium. The VEGFR1 staining scores for primary tumor, lymph node metastases, and recurrent tumor tissue were 8 (6–8), 8 (6.5–8), and 8 (3–6), respectively. Macrophages, plasma cells, nerve fibers, endothelium, muscle tissues, and salivary gland tissues had expression of VEGFR.

2.2.6. EpCAM

EpCAM was expressed in 57% of all tumor samples, but only 3% exhibited a homogenous pattern. In tumor cells, membrane and cytoplasmic stains were seen. The intensity of EpCAM positive tumors varied but was generally weak to moderate. Total IHC scores were 0.5 (0–2.5), 1.5 (0–3), and 1 (0–6) for primary tumor cells, lymph node metastases, and local recurrence tumor tissue, respectively. Rarely were EpCAM-positive macrophages and plasma cells observed. Normal epithelium exhibited no staining.

2.2.7. VEGFR2

The overall expression rate of VEGFR2 was 79%, with no tumors displaying homogenous expression pattern. The VEGFR2 antibody staining was present in the cytoplasm of the tumor cells, although it was mainly weak. The staining scores for primary tumor tissue, lymph node metastases, and local recurrence were 2 (1–4), 2 (1–4), and 2 (0–2), respectively. Moderate to weak expression was also seen in normal oral squamous epithelium in 29% of samples. No expression was seen in the stroma surrounding tumor.

2.2.8. Cathepsin E and Integrin αvβ3

Only one primary tumor and three lymph node metastases showed Cathepsin E expression. No expression of integrin αvβ3 was observed in primary tumors, metastases, or tissue from local recurrence. The staining scores for both biomarkers for primary tumor cells, lymph node metastases, and local recurrence tumor tissue were 0 (0–0), 0 (0–0), and 0 (0–0).

2.3. *Intensity of Staining in Normal Oral Mucosal Epithelium vs. Tumor Tissue*

The mean staining intensity score between normal epithelium and tumor tissue was compared for all samples where both components were present. The staining intensity was significantly higher in tumors compared to normal epithelium in uPAR ($p < 0.001$, n = 37), VEGFR2 ($p = 0.002$, n = 41), VEGFR1 ($p = 0.001$, n = 41), PARP-1 ($p = 0.003$, n = 40), and tissue factor ($p < 0.001$, n = 47). No difference in staining intensity between tumor tissue and normal epithelium was seen for integrin αvβ6 ($p = 0.380$, n = 47) or EPCAM ($p = 0.130$, n = 39).

2.4. *Biomarker Expression in Primary Tumor Compared to Lymph Node Metastases and Tissue from Local Recurrence (T-Site)*

We examined the correlation between total immune staining scores in primary tumors and lymph node metastases for each target in cases where tissue from both locations were available. We identified 28 primary cancers with accessible tissue from lymph node metastasis. All targets with tumor staining exhibited a positive Spearman rank correlation value. However, only uPAR (spearman correlation = 0.554, $p = 0.014$), tissue factor (spearman correlation = 0.615, $p = 0.001$), and VEGFR2 (Spearman correlation = 0.765, $p < 0.001$) had a significant positive correlation between total immune staining scores in primary tumor and lymph node metastases. Due to small numbers of cases with recurrence, no significant correlation was found between the total immune staining scores in primary tumors and tumor tissue from local recurrence, but a tendency toward positive correlation was seen for uPAR (spearman correlation = 0.395; $p = 0.510$), EpCAM (spearman correlation = 0.111, $p = 0.834$), and PARP-1 (spearman correlation = 0.064, $p = 0.905$)

3. Discussion

In this study, we have evaluated nine potential molecular imaging targets from 41 OSCC patients with tissue samples from the primary tumor, lymph node metastases, and local recurrence. This is, to the best of our knowledge, the first study to investigate and compare multiple potential targets in both primary OSCC tumors and their metastases. Based on immunohistochemical expression levels and expression patterns in the tumor, normal epithelium, and surrounding tissue, it was revealed that the uPAR, integrin αvβ6, and tissue factor represent attractive molecular imaging targets in OSCC due to a high overall expression rate of 97%, 97%, and 86%, respectively. The high expression rates of uPAR (96%) and integrin αvβ6 (100%) in lymph node metastases indicate a potential in FGS for detecting lymph node metastases during sentinel lymph node biopsy or neck dissection, which could potentially spare healthy nodes.

We found a highly tumor-specific uPAR expression in most tumor samples (97%), with a moderate to intense staining in both primary tumors and metastases. Our results are in accordance with previous immunohistochemical studies that have also found a high tumor-specific expression of uPAR in OSCC, with an absence of staining in the surrounding normal squamous epithelium and weak expression in tumor-associated inflammatory cells (macrophages, neutrophils, and fibroblasts), with a sharp demarcation at the deep tumor margin [37–39]. Interestingly, our current study demonstrated uPAR expression in 96% of metastasis, which indicates that combined targeted strategies against the tumor as well as metastatic disease seem possible. Different molecular imaging modalities have been explored for uPAR. In clinical trials, uPAR-targeted PET imaging using a peptide-based tracer has been studied for several cancers including OSCC, where a prognostic value was demonstrated [40–43]. No studies have yet investigated the diagnostic potential of uPAR-targeted PET imaging in OSCC, but a Phase II clinical trial is currently underway (NCT02960724). Few clinical studies have been conducted on FGS using uPAR-directed probes. In a cell-line-based xenograph proof-of-concept study conducted at our institution, it was shown that uPAR-targeted optical near-infrared fluorescence imaging using ICG conjugated to AE-105 can be used to identify small lymph node metastases during surgery [44]. Boonstra et al. also investigated uPAR-targeted FGS in cell-line-based xenograph models with an antibody-based tracer (hybrid ATN 658) conjugated to a fluorophore (ZW800-1), and showed that this modality could also identify primary tumors and lymph node metastases [45]. Clinical trials investigating uPAR-targeted FGS are ongoing in patients with oral cancer, lung cancer, and glioblastoma (EudraCT no. 2022-001361-12, 2021-004389-37 and 2020-003089-38).

The tissue factor also demonstrated a tumor-specific expression, but at a lower rate (86%) and with a more heterogeneous pattern than uPAR. The expression of the tissue factor in lymph node metastases was less compared to the primary tumor tissue. These results are consistent with similar immunohistochemistry studies on primary tumor tissue from oral and oropharyngeal squamous cell carcinoma, which found tissue factor expression rates of 58% and 76%, respectively [37,46]. As, an imaging target tissue factor has been poorly investigated in OSCC, but the potential in several other cancers has been explored. In preclinical studies, the tissue factor has been investigated as a target for FGS, SPECT, and PET using tissue factor-specific monoclonal antibodies in both anaplastic thyroid cancer, glioblastoma, and pancreatic cancer xenografts with promising effect [47–50]. In 2021, an antibody drug (tisotumab vedotin)-targeting tissue factor was approved by FDA for treatment of metastatic cervical cancer [51]. Subsequently the tissue factor-targeted PET-imaging with a protein (FVIIa) labeled with ^{18}F was successfully tested first in a human study and proposed as a future diagnostic tool prior to tissue factor-targeted treatment [52]. The high expression of the tissue factor in OSCC and the recent development of tissue factor-targeted tracers in other solid cancers makes it a promising imaging agent in OSCC.

Integrin $\alpha v\beta 6$ was also highly expressed in our study, with a clear contrast at the deep tumor margin. However, a high integrin $\alpha v\beta 6$ expression was also seen in normal squamous cell epithelium without a significant difference in the intensity score between a tumor and normal epithelium. Our findings suggest that molecular imaging drugs targeting integrin $\alpha v\beta 6$ may provide a distinct contrast at the deep margin but less at the superficial margins. These results are in line with those obtained by Baart et al., who investigated the immunohistochemical expression of integrin $\alpha v\beta 6$ in both OSCC and cutaneous squamous cell carcinoma of the head and neck [38]. They also proposed integrin $\alpha v\beta 6$ as a target for FGS in OSCC, especially due to the clear discrimination at the deep margin and compared to EGFR, they found less staining of the normal epithelium. Integrin $\alpha v\beta 6$ has been studied as a PET-imaging target in different cancers. In 2019, Hausner et al. successfully performed a first in human studies by exploring PET/CT with a radiolabeled integrin $\alpha v\beta 6$-binding peptide in patients with metastatic colon, breast, and pancreas cancer [18]. Later, Quigley et al. tested a Ga-68-labeled peptide (Ga-68-Trivehexin) for human PET/CT imaging of head, neck, and pancreatic cancer, with results showing a high tumor-specific uptake and no uptake in tumor-associated inflammation [19]. Integrin $\alpha v\beta 6$ has, to our knowledge, not been tested as a target for fluorescent imaging in OSCC patients. However, Ilyia et al. showed imaging potential in in vitro head and neck cancer models with quantum dots conjugated to an integrin $\alpha v\beta 6$-specific peptide [53]. A human trial by de Valk et al. has studied integrin $\alpha v\beta 6$-targeted near-infrared fluorescent peptides (cRGD-ZW800-1) in 12 patients with colon carcinoma and was able to show cancer-specific imaging in both open and laparoscopic surgery [54]. Studies investigating integrin $\alpha v\beta 6$ as a target for fluorescent imaging in OSCC have not yet been published, but a clinical trial with cRGD-ZW800-1 (NCT 04191460) is planned to investigate whether this modality can improve the rate of adequate surgical resection margins in OSCC.

PARP-1 showed mostly moderate and moderate to high expression levels in the tumor nuclei, but it appears less suitable as an imaging target compared to uPAR, $\alpha v\beta 6$, and tissue factor, owing to the non-specific staining of several different cell-types in the lamina propria and submucosa as well as the staining of normal squamous epithelium. Even though some expressions of PARP-1 are present in normal tissues, this biomarker might not be excluded as a target for molecular imaging, because the density of the nuclei in tumor cells are higher compared to normal tissues [28]. Kossatz et al. recently investigated a topically applied PARP-1-specific fluorescence agent for the use of early diagnosis of OSCC in a Phase 1 study with 12 patients, where the fluorescence signal showed a tumor to normal ratio > 3 [30]. However, the topical approach is probably confined to early stage disease or screening of mucosal lesions, as the penetration depth is limited (300 μm in the trial by Kossatz et al.). VEGFR1 and VEGFR2 did not appear promising for imaging purposes in our study, as their expression was limited, and the tumor specificity was low. No studies have yet examined the molecular imaging of these targets in OSCC, but different angiogenesis inhibitors for the treatment of head and neck squamous cell carcinoma have been thoroughly investigated, with bevacizumab being the most promising [55].

This study has some limitations. First, a biomarkers appropriateness as an imaging target is determined by several factors in addition to its overexpression. The target selection criteria system has been suggested as a tool to identify potential imaging targets and consists of seven different criterions. However, several of these are either difficult to measure (tumor to normal ratio greater than 10) or questionable (internalization of the tracer) [56]. Second, immunohistochemistry has several inherited limitations, including the selection of an antibody clone, which can affect the intensity and proportion of the stained tumor tissue substantially. In addition, both a manual and semi-quantitative scoring method were used, and several different scoring systems exists. This is a subjective estimate and interobserver variability is unavoidable. Third, the small sample size of tissues from lymph node metastases and tissues from local tumor recurrence compared to primary tumors limits the interpretation of the results. This study does not provide new diagnostic methods in pathology to diagnose OSCC earlier than with current methods, but rather focuses on the potential future targets for molecular imaging.

4. Materials and Methods

4.1. Patient and Tissue Selection

From an existing, well-defined database consisting of patients diagnosed with OSCC between 2000–2011 and surgically treated at the department of Otolaryngology, Head and Neck Surgery and Audiology at Rigshospitalet (Copenhagen, Denmark), we randomly selected 41 patients. Microscopy slides were retrieved from the archives of the Department of Pathology and one FFPE tissue block containing both tumor tissue and normal epithelium were selected from each patient for following IHC staining. Of the 41 patients, 28 patients also had available tissue from lymph node metastases and 8 patients from recurrent disease. Clinicopathological data were obtained from medical and pathology reports. The 7th edition of the TNM Union for International Cancer Control (UICC) staging system was used.

4.2. Selection of Imaging Targets

Through literature search, we identified nine targets with previously described overexpression in several cancers, including head and neck, and for which there is a potential for rapid translation into clinical settings due to earlier research/probe development. The following biomarkers were selected: integrin αvβ6, tissue factor, poly(ADP-ribose) polymerase 1 (PARP-1), urokinase plasminogen activator receptor (uPAR), vascular endothelial growth factor receptor 1 (VEGFR1), epithelial cell adhesion molecule (EpCAM), vascular endothelial growth factor receptor 2 (VEGFR2), Cathepsin E, and integrin αvβ3. Immunohistochemical staining for cytokeratin 5 (CK5) was used to visualize tumor location. Despite its great imaging potential, epidermal growth factor receptor (EGFR) was not included as it is very well characterized in OSCC and clinical trials with targeted tracers are currently being performed (NCT03134846 and NCT03733210).

4.3. Immunohistochemistry

The expression of all targets was determined for both the primary tumor, metastasis, and tissue from local recurrence. Tumor tissue had been fixated in 10% formalin solution at room temperature for 24 h and then embedded in paraffin at the time of collection. FFPE blocks were stored at room temperature. Tissue sections of 4 µm were cut and IHC staining with integrin αvβ3, integrin αvβ6, tissue factor, and EPCAM were performed using a semi-automated autostainer, Ventana Benchmark Ultra (Roche Diagnostics). Manual staining was performed for the following biomarkers: Cathepsin E, PARP-1, uPAR, VEGFR1, and VEGFR2. Antibodies, reagents, and methods used for IHC analysis are listed in Appendix A. Briefly, the slides were incubated at 60 °C for 60 min before being deparaffinized in HistoClear solution, rehydrated in graded ethanol, and submerged in water. Different antigen retrieval methods were used depending on the target. All antibodies were used at optimal dilutions, which were determined using positive and negative control staining (data not shown). Secondary staining with HRP-conjugated antibody was performed by incubation for 30–40 min. The reaction was visualized with Envision DAB+ for the manual staining and with DAB+ chromogen solution for the autostainer. Digital pictures for Figure 4 were obtained using Zeiss Axioscan with 10 × zoom.

4.4. Assessment of Immunohistochemical Staining

Two specialized head and neck pathologists (GL and AF) reviewed and scored all samples blinded to clinical data. In the event of a disagreement, individual slides were examined together to obtain a consensus score. Each sample was assessed according to highest staining intensity in tumor compartment, proportion of stained malignant tumor tissue in the total tumor area, expression pattern in tumor tissue (homogenous or heterogeneous), and intensity in normal epithelium. Proportion and intensity scores were generated using a point system: 0% (0), 1–10% (1), 11–50% (2), 51–75% (3), and 76–100% (4), and none (0), weak (1), medium (2), and strong (3), respectively. The staining intensity of normal epithelium around the tumor tissue was scored in the same way. The proportion and intensity scores for tumor tissue were multiplied to provide a single combined score and a total immune staining score (TIS), which is similar to previous studies [38,57–59]. This resulted in a score ranging from 0 to 12, which was divided into four final expression categories: 0 = absent; 1–5 = low; 6–8 = intermediate; and 9–12 = high expression. For each target, the proportion of patients categorized as low, intermediate, and high expression was calculated. The expression rate was calculated as the proportion of samples with low, intermediate, and high expression.

4.5. Statistical Analysis

Statistical analysis was performed using IBM SPSS statistics 25.0. The median and interquartile range of the staining score were calculated for primary tumor, lymph node metastases, and recurrence. Wilcoxon signed-rank test was used to compare the intensity of immunohistochemistry staining of tumor to normal oral mucosal epithelium. Correlation between total immune staining scores in primary tumor and in lymph node metastases was tested using Spearman's correlation test. Results were considered statistically significant at the level of $p < 0.05$.

Bar charts were made using GraphPad Prism version 9.3 for PC, GraphPad Software, La Jolla, California, USA.

5. Conclusions

In conclusion, the uPAR, integrin $\alpha v\beta 6$, and tissue factor are promising imaging targets for OSCC. Molecular imaging based on a single target that could be used for both pre- and intraoperative imaging of a primary tumor, lymph node metastases, and in cases, of recurrence would be a powerful tool for the diagnosis and treatment of OSCC.

Author Contributions: Conceptualization, M.L., A.C., K.J., A.K., K.K. and C.v.B.; data curation, M.L. and K.J.; formal analysis, M.L., K.J., G.L., K.K. and A.-M.K.F.; funding acquisition, C.v.B.; methodology, M.L., A.C., K.J., A.-M.K.F., A.K., K.K. and C.v.B.; software, M.L.; supervision, A.C., G.L., A.-M.K.F., A.K. and C.v.B.; writing—original draft, M.L.; writing—review and editing, M.L., A.C., K.J., G.L., A.-M.K.F. and C.v.B. All authors have read and agreed to the published version of the manuscript.

Funding: This research was funded by the Candys Foundation, grant number no. 2015-138.

Institutional Review Board Statement: The study was conducted in accordance with the Declaration of Helsinki and was approved by the Danish National Committee on Health and Research Ethics (H-2-2012-050). Data were handled according to the rules of the Danish Data Protection Agency.

Informed Consent Statement: Not applicable.

Data Availability Statement: The data reported in this study are available from the corresponding authors upon reasonable request.

Conflicts of Interest: The authors declare no conflict of interest.

Appendix A

Table A1. Primary antibodies used for immunohistochemistry.

Target	Source	Catalog Number	Species	Monoclonal/ Polyclonal	Dilution	Staining Method
Cytokeratin 5	Novocastra	CK5-L-CE	Mouse	Monoclonal	No dilution	Automatic, VENTANA BenchMark IHC
Integrin $\alpha v\beta 3$	R&D Systems	MAB3050	Mouse	Monoclonal	1:500	Automatic, VENTANA BenchMark IHC
Integrin $\alpha v\beta 6$	ABCAM	ab181551	Mouse	Monoclonal	1:500	Automatic, VENTANA BenchMark IHC
Tissue Factor	Sekisui	4509	Mouse	Monoclonal	1:50	Automatic, VENTANA BenchMark IHC
EPCAM	Cell Marque	5435676001	Mouse	Monoclonal	No dilution	Automatic, VENTANA BenchMark IHC
Cathepsin E	Abcam	Ab36996	Rabbit	Polyclonal	1:2000	Manual
PARP1	Abcam	Ab32138	Rabbit	Monoclonal	1:25	Manual
uPAR	Genetex	GTX100467	Mouse	Monoclonal	1:500	Manual
VEGFR1	Abcam	Ab32152	Rabbit	Monoclonal	1:75	Manual
VEGFR2	Cell Signaling	55B11	Rabbit	Monoclonal	1:300	Manual

References

1. Leoncini, E.; Vukovic, V.; Cadoni, G.; Giraldi, L.; Pastorino, R.; Arzani, D.; Petrelli, L.; Wünsch-Filho, V.; Toporcov, T.N.; Moyses, R.A.; et al. Tumour Stage and Gender Predict Recurrence and Second Primary Malignancies in Head and Neck Cancer: A Multicentre Study within the INHANCE Consortium. *Eur. J. Epidemiol.* **2018**, *33*, 1205. [CrossRef] [PubMed]
2. Orosco, R.K.; Tapia, V.J.; Califano, J.A.; Clary, B.; Cohen, E.E.W.; Kane, C.; Lippman, S.M.; Messer, K.; Molinolo, A.; Murphy, J.D.; et al. Positive Surgical Margins in the 10 Most Common Solid Cancers. *Sci. Rep.* **2018**, *8*, 5686. [CrossRef] [PubMed]

3. Eldeeb, H.; Macmillan, C.; Elwell, C.; Hammod, A. The Effect of the Surgical Margins on the Outcome of Patients with Head and Neck Squamous Cell Carcinoma: Single Institution Experience. *Cancer Biol. Med.* **2012**, *9*, 29–33. [CrossRef]
4. Binahmed, A.; Nason, R.W.; Abdoh, A.A. The Clinical Significance of the Positive Surgical Margin in Oral Cancer. *Oral Oncol.* **2007**, *43*, 780–784. [CrossRef] [PubMed]
5. Mcmahon, J.; O'brien, C.J.; Pathak, I.; Hamill, R.; Mcneil, E.; Hammersley, N.; Gardiner, S.; Junor, E. Influence of Condition of Surgical Margins on Local Recurrence and Disease-Specific Survival in Oral and Oropharyngeal Cancer. *Br. J. Oral Maxillofac. Surg.* **2003**, *41*, 224–231. [CrossRef]
6. Ahmed, M.U.; Khawar, A.; Ahmed, J.; Ajmal, M.; Bangash, W.K.; Akhter, M.R. Occult Metastasis in Carcinoma of Oral Cavity. *J. Coll. Physicians Surg. Pak.* **2007**, *17*, 313–315.
7. Du, E.; Ow, T.J.; Lo, Y.T.; Gersten, A.; Schiff, B.A.; Tassler, A.B.; Smith, R.V. Refining the Utility and Role of Frozen Section in Head and Neck Squamous Cell Carcinoma Resection. *Laryngoscope* **2016**, *126*, 1768–1775. [CrossRef]
8. Wu, J.; Yuan, Y.; Tao, X.F.; Lyu, P. Targeted Molecular Imaging of Head and Neck Squamous Cell Carcinoma: A Window into Precision Medicine. *Chin. Med. J.* **2020**, *133*, 1325. [CrossRef]
9. Zhang, R.R.; Schroeder, A.B.; Grudzinski, J.J.; Rosenthal, E.L.; Warram, J.M.; Pinchuk, A.N.; Eliceiri, K.W.; Kuo, J.S.; Weichert, J.P. Beyond the Margins: Real-Time Detection of Cancer Using Targeted Fluorophores. *Nat. Rev. Clin. Oncol.* **2017**, *14*, 347. [CrossRef]
10. Van Schaik, J.E.; Halmos, G.B.; Witjes, M.J.H.; Plaat, B.E.C. An Overview of the Current Clinical Status of Optical Imaging in Head and Neck Cancer with a Focus on Narrow Band Imaging and Fluorescence Optical Imaging. *Oral Oncol.* **2021**, *121*, 105504. [CrossRef]
11. Crawford, K.L.; Pacheco, F.V.; Lee, Y.J.; Hom, M.; Rosenthal, E.L.; Nguyen, Q.T.; Orosco, R.K. A Scoping Review of Ongoing Fluorescence-Guided Surgery Clinical Trials in Otolaryngology. *Laryngoscope* **2022**, *132*, 36–44. [CrossRef] [PubMed]
12. Johnstone, S.; Logan, R.M. The Role of Vascular Endothelial Growth Factor (VEGF) in Oral Dysplasia and Oral Squamous Cell Carcinoma. *Oral Oncol.* **2006**, *42*, 337–342. [CrossRef] [PubMed]
13. Stîngă, A.C.; Mărgăritescu, O.; Stîngă, A.S.; Pirici, D.; Ciurea, R.; Bunget, A.; Cruce, M. VEGFR1 and VEGFR2 Immunohistochemical Expression in Oral Squamous Cell Carcinoma: A Morphometric Study. *Rom. J. Morphol. Embryol.* **2011**, *52*, 1269–1275. [PubMed]
14. Masłowska, K.; Halik, P.K.; Tymecka, D.; Misicka, A.; Gniazdowska, E. The Role of VEGF Receptors as Molecular Target in Nuclear Medicine for Cancer Diagnosis and Combination Therapy. *Cancers* **2021**, *13*, 1072. [CrossRef]
15. Brooks, P.C.; Clark, R.A.F.; Cheresh, D.A. Requirement of Vascular Integrin Avβ3 for Angiogenesis. *Science* **1994**, *264*, 569–571. [CrossRef] [PubMed]
16. Beer, A.J.; Schwaiger, M. Imaging of Integrin Avβ3 Expression. *Cancer Metastasis Rev.* **2008**, *27*, 631–644. [CrossRef] [PubMed]
17. Niu, J.; Li, Z. The Roles of Integrin Avβ6 in Cancer. *Cancer Lett.* **2017**, *403*, 128–137. [CrossRef] [PubMed]
18. Hausner, S.H.; Bold, R.J.; Cheuy, L.Y.; Chew, H.K.; Daly, M.E.; Davis, R.A.; Foster, C.C.; Kim, E.J.; Sutcliffe, J.L. Preclinical Development and First-in-Human Imaging of the Integrin a v b 6 with [18 F]a v b 6 -Binding Peptide in Metastatic Carcinoma. *Clin. Cancer Res.* **2019**, *25*, 1206–1215. [CrossRef] [PubMed]
19. Quigley, N.G.; Steiger, K.; Hoberück, S.; Czech, N.; Zierke, M.A.; Kossatz, S.; Pretze, M.; Richter, F.; Weichert, W.; Pox, C.; et al. PET/CT Imaging of Head-and-Neck and Pancreatic Cancer in Humans by Targeting the "Cancer Integrin" Avβ6 with Ga-68-Trivehexin. *Eur. J. Nucl. Med. Mol. Imaging* **2022**, *49*, 1136–1147. [CrossRef]
20. Li, H.X.; Zheng, J.H.; Fan, H.X.; Li, H.P.; Gao, Z.X.; Chen, D. Expression of Avβ6 Integrin and Collagen Fibre in Oral Squamous Cell Carcinoma: Association with Clinical Outcomes and Prognostic Implications. *J. Oral Pathol. Med.* **2013**, *42*, 547–556. [CrossRef] [PubMed]
21. Ramos, D.M.; Dang, D.; Sadler, S. The Role of the Integrin Avβ6 in Regulating the Epithelial to Mesenchymal Transition in Oral Cancer. *Anticancer Res.* **2009**, *29*, 125–130.
22. Ramos, D.M.; But, M.; Regezi, J.; Schmidt, B.L.; Atakilit, A.; Dang, D.; Ellis, D.; Jordan, R.; Li, X. Expression of Integrin Β6 Enhances Invasive Behavior in Oral Squamous Cell Carcinoma. *Matrix Biol.* **2002**, *21*, 297–307. [CrossRef]
23. Winter, M.J.; Nagtegaal, I.D.; Van Krieken, J.H.J.M.; Litvinov, S.V. The Epithelial Cell Adhesion Molecule (Ep-CAM) as a Morphoregulatory Molecule Is a Tool in Surgical Pathology. *Am. J. Pathol.* **2003**, *163*, 2139. [CrossRef] [PubMed]
24. van Driel, P.B.A.A.; Boonstra, M.C.; Prevoo, H.A.J.M.; van de Giessen, M.; Snoeks, T.J.A.; Tummers, Q.R.J.G.; Keereweer, S.; Cordfunke, R.A.; Fish, A.; van Eendenburg, J.D.H.; et al. EpCAM as Multi-Tumour Target for near-Infrared Fluorescence Guided Surgery. *BMC Cancer* **2016**, *16*, 884. [CrossRef] [PubMed]
25. Boogerd, L.S.F.; Boonstra, M.C.; Prevoo, H.A.J.M.; Handgraaf, H.J.M.; Kuppen, P.J.K.; Van De Velde, J.H.; Fish, A.; Cordfunke, R.A.; Rob, A.; Valentijn, P.M.; et al. Fluorescence-Guided Tumor Detection with a Novel Anti-EpCAM Targeted Antibody Fragment: Preclinical Validation. *Surg. Oncol.* **2019**, *28*, 1–8. [CrossRef] [PubMed]
26. Pontious, C.; Kaul, S.; Hong, M.; Hart, P.A.; Krishna, S.G.; Lara, L.F.; Conwell, D.L.; Cruz-Monserrate, Z. Cathepsin E Expression and Activity: Role in the Detection and Treatment of Pancreatic Cancer. *Pancreatology* **2019**, *19*, 951. [CrossRef] [PubMed]
27. Wang, L.; Liang, C.; Li, F.; Guan, D.; Wu, X.; Fu, X.; Lu, A.; Zhang, G. PARP1 in Carcinomas and PARP1 Inhibitors as Antineoplastic Drugs. *Int. J. Mol. Sci.* **2017**, *18*, 2111. [CrossRef]
28. Kossatz, S.; Brand, C.; Gutiontov, S.; Liu, J.T.C.; Lee, N.Y.; Gonen, M.; Weber, W.A.; Reiner, T. Detection and Delineation of Oral Cancer with a PARP1 Targeted Optical Imaging Agent. *Sci. Rep.* **2016**, *6*, 21371. [CrossRef]

29. Sankaranarayanan, R.A.; Kossatz, S.; Weber, W.; Beheshti, M.; Morgenroth, A.; Mottaghy, F.M. Advancements in PARP1 Targeted Nuclear Imaging and Theranostic Probes. *J. Clin. Med.* **2020**, *9*, 2130. [CrossRef]
30. Demétrio de Souza França, P.; Kossatz, S.; Brand, C.; Karassawa Zanoni, D.; Roberts, S.; Guru, N.; Adilbay, D.; Mauguen, A.; Valero Mayor, C.; Weber, W.A.; et al. A Phase I Study of a PARP1-Targeted Topical Fluorophore for the Detection of Oral Cancer. *Eur. J. Nucl. Med. Mol. Imaging* **2021**, *48*, 3618–3630. [CrossRef]
31. Abd-Elgaliel, W.R.; Cruz-Monserrate, Z.; Logsdon, C.D.; Tung, C.H. Molecular Imaging of Cathepsin E-Positive Tumors in Mice Using a Novel Protease-Activatable Fluorescent Probe. *Mol. Biosyst.* **2011**, *7*, 3207. [CrossRef]
32. Noh, H.; Hong, S.; Huang, S. Role of Urokinase Receptor in Tumor Progression and Development. *Theranostics* **2013**, *3*, 487–495. [CrossRef]
33. Lv, T.; Zhao, Y.; Jiang, X.; Yuan, H.; Wang, H.; Cui, X.; Xu, J.; Zhao, J.; Wang, J. UPAR: An Essential Factor for Tumor Development. *J. Cancer* **2021**, *12*, 7026. [CrossRef]
34. Van Den Berg, Y.W.; Osanto, S.; Reitsma, P.H.; Versteeg, H.H. The Relationship between Tissue Factor and Cancer Progression: Insights from Bench and Bedside. *Blood* **2012**, *119*, 924–932. [CrossRef] [PubMed]
35. Seto, S.; Onodera, H.; Kaido, T.; Yoshikawa, A.; Ishigami, S.; Arii, S.; Imamura, M. Tissue Factor Expression in Human Colorectal Carcinoma Correlation with Hepatic Metastasis and Impact on Prognosis. *Cancer* **2000**, *88*, 295–301. [CrossRef]
36. Akashi, T.; Furuya, Y.; Ohta, S.; Fuse, H. Tissue Factor Expression and Prognosis in Patients with Metastatic Prostate Cancer. *Urology* **2003**, *62*, 1078–1082. [CrossRef]
37. Christensen, A.; Grønhøj, C.; Jensen, J.S.; Lelkaitis, G.; Kiss, K.; Juhl, K.; Charabi, B.W.; Mortensen, J.; Kjær, A.; Buchwald, C. von Expression Patterns of UPAR, TF and EGFR and Their Potential as Targets for Molecular Imaging in Oropharyngeal Squamous Cell Carcinoma. *Oncol. Rep.* **2022**, *48*, 147. [CrossRef]
38. Baart, V.M.; van Duijn, C.; van Egmond, S.L.; Dijckmeester, W.A.; Jansen, J.C.; Vahrmeijer, A.L.; Sier, C.F.M.; Cohen, D. Egfr and Avβ6 as Promising Targets for Molecular Imaging of Cutaneous and Mucosal Squamous Cell Carcinoma of the Head and Neck Region. *Cancers* **2020**, *12*, 1474. [CrossRef] [PubMed]
39. Serpa, M.S.; Mafra, R.P.; Queiroz, S.I.M.L.; da Silva, L.P.; de Souza, L.B.; Pinto, L.P. Expression of Urokinase-Type Plasminogen Activator and Its Receptorin Squamous Cell Carcinoma of the Oral Tongue. *Braz. Oral Res.* **2018**, *32*. [CrossRef]
40. Carlsen, E.A.; Loft, M.; Loft, A.; Berthelsen, A.K.; Langer, S.W.; Knigge, U.; Kjaer, A. Prospective Phase II Trial of Prognostication by 68 Ga-NOTA-AE105 UPAR PET in Patients with Neuroendocrine Neoplasms: Implications for UPAR Targeted Therapy. *J. Nucl. Med.* **2022**, *63*, 1371–1377. [CrossRef]
41. Fosbøl, M.Ø.; Kurbegovic, S.; Johannesen, H.H.; Røder, M.A.; Hansen, A.E.; Mortensen, J.; Loft, A.; Petersen, P.M.; Madsen, J.; Brasso, K.; et al. Urokinase-Type Plasminogen Activator Receptor (UPAR) PET/MRI of Prostate Cancer for Noninvasive Evaluation of Aggressiveness: Comparison with Gleason Score in a Prospective Phase 2 Clinical Trial. *J. Nucl. Med.* **2021**, *62*, 354–359. [CrossRef]
42. Persson, M.; Skovgaard, D.; Brandt-Larsen, M.; Christensen, C.; Madsen, J.; Nielsen, C.H.; Thurison, T.; Klausen, T.L.; Holm, S.; Loft, A.; et al. First-in-Human UPAR PET: Imaging of Cancer Aggressiveness. *Theranostics* **2015**, *5*, 1303–1316. [CrossRef]
43. Risoer, L.M.; Clausen, M.M.; Ujmajuridze, Z.; Farhadi, M.; Andersen, K.F.; Loft, A.; Kjaer, A. Prognostic Value of Urokinase-Type Plasminogen Activator Receptor (UPAR)-PET/CT in Head and Neck Squamous Cell Carcinomas and Comparison with 18 F-FDG-PET/CT: A Single-Center Prospective Study. *J. Nucl. Med.* **2021**, *63*, 1169–1176. [CrossRef] [PubMed]
44. Christensen, A.; Juhl, K.; Persson, M.; Charabi, B.W.; Mortensen, J.; Kiss, K.; Lelkaitis, G.; Rubek, N.; von Buchwald, C.; Kjær, A. UPAR-Targeted Optical near-Infrared (NIR) Fluorescence Imaging and PET for Image-Guided Surgery in Head and Neck Cancer: Proof-of-Concept in Orthotopic Xenograft Model. *Oncotarget* **2017**, *8*, 15407–15419. [CrossRef]
45. Boonstra, M.C.; Van Driel, P.B.A.A.; Keereweer, S.; Prevoo, H.A.J.M.; Stammes, M.A.; Baart, V.M.; Löwik, C.W.G.M.; Mazar, A.P.; van de Velde, C.J.H.; Vahrmeijer, A.L.; et al. Preclinical UPAR-Targeted Multimodal Imaging of Locoregional Oral Cancer. *Oral Oncol.* **2017**, *66*, 1–8. [CrossRef]
46. Christensen, A.; Kiss, K.; Lelkaitis, G.; Juhl, K.; Persson, M.; Charabi, B.W.; Mortensen, J.; Forman, J.L.; Sørensen, A.L.; Jensen, D.H.; et al. Urokinase-Type Plasminogen Activator Receptor (UPAR), Tissue Factor (TF) and Epidermal Growth Factor Receptor (EGFR): Tumor Expression Patterns and Prognostic Value in Oral Cancer. *BMC Cancer* **2017**, *17*, 572. [CrossRef] [PubMed]
47. Wei, W.; Liu, Q.; Jiang, D.; Zhao, H.; Kutyreff, C.J.; Engle, J.W.; Liu, J.; Cai, W. Tissue Factor-Targeted ImmunoPET Imaging and Radioimmunotherapy of Anaplastic Thyroid Cancer. *Adv. Sci.* **2020**, *7*, 1903595. [CrossRef]
48. Nielsen, C.H.; Erlandsson, M.; Jeppesen, T.E.; Jensen, M.M.; Kristensen, L.K.; Madsen, J.; Petersen, L.C.; Kjaer, A. Quantitative PET Imaging of Tissue Factor Expression Using 18F-Labeled Active Site–Inhibited Factor VII. *J. Nucl. Med.* **2016**, *57*, 89–95. [CrossRef] [PubMed]
49. Takashima, H.; Tsuji, A.B.; Saga, T.; Yasunaga, M.; Koga, Y.; Kuroda, J.I.; Yano, S.; Kuratsu, J.I.; Matsumura, Y. Molecular Imaging Using an Anti-Human Tissue Factor Monoclonal Antibody in an Orthotopic Glioma Xenograft Model. *Sci. Rep.* **2017**, *71*, 12341. [CrossRef] [PubMed]
50. Sugyo, A.; Aung, W.; Tsuji, A.B.; Sudo, H.; Takashima, H.; Yasunaga, M.; Matsumura, Y.; Saga, T.; Higashi, T. Anti-tissue Factor Antibody-mediated Immuno-SPECT Imaging of Tissue Factor Expression in Mouse Models of Pancreatic Cancer. *Oncol. Rep.* **2019**, *41*, 2371–2378. [CrossRef]

51. Food and Drug Administration FDA Grants Accelerated Approval to Tisotumab Vedotin-Tftv for Recurrent or Metastatic Cervical Cancer. Available online: https://www.fda.gov/drugs/resources-information-approved-drugs/fda-grants-accelerated-approval-tisotumab-vedotin-tftv-recurrent-or-metastatic-cervical-cancer (accessed on 19 September 2022).
52. Loft, M.; Christensen, C.; Clausen, M.M.; Carlsen, E.A.; Hansen, C.P.; Kroman, N.; Langer, S.W.; Høgdall, C.; Madsen, J.; Gillings, N.; et al. First-in-Human PET Imaging of Tissue Factor in Patients with Primary and Metastatic Cancers Using 18F-Labeled Active-Site Inhibited Factor VII (18F-ASIS): Potential as Companion Diagnostic. *J. Nucl. Med.* **2022**, *63*, 1871–1879. [CrossRef]
53. Yakavets, I.; Francois, A.; Guiot, M.; Lequeux, N.; Fragola, A.; Pons, T.; Bezdetnaya, L.; Marchal, F. NIR Imaging of the Integrin-Rich Head and Neck Squamous Cell Carcinoma Using Ternary Copper Indium Selenide/Zinc Sulfide-Based Quantum Dots. *Cancers* **2020**, *12*, 3727. [CrossRef]
54. de Valk, K.S.; Deken, M.M.; Handgraaf, H.J.M.; Bhairosingh, S.S.; Bijlstra, O.D.; van Esdonk, M.J.; Terwisscha van Scheltinga, A.G.T.; Valentijn, A.R.P.M.; March, T.L.; Vuijk, J.; et al. First-in-Human Assessment of CRGD-ZW800-1, a Zwitterionic, Integrin-Targeted, Near-Infrared Fluorescent Peptide in Colon Carcinoma. *Clin. Cancer Res.* **2020**, *26*, 3990–3998. [CrossRef] [PubMed]
55. Hyytiäinen, A.; Wahbi, W.; Väyrynen, O.; Saarilahti, K.; Karihtala, P.; Salo, T.; Al-Samadi, A. Angiogenesis Inhibitors for Head and Neck Squamous Cell Carcinoma Treatment: Is There Still Hope? *Front. Oncol.* **2021**, *11*, 2123. [CrossRef] [PubMed]
56. Van Oosten, M.; Crane, L.M.A.; Bart, J.; Van Leeuwen, F.W.; Van Dam, G.M. Selecting Potential Targetable Biomarkers for Imaging Purposes in Colorectal Cancer Using TArget Selection Criteria (TASC): A Novel Target Identification Tool. *Transl. Oncol.* **2011**, *4*, 71–82. [CrossRef]
57. van der Fels, C.A.M.; Palthe, S.; Buikema, H.; van den Heuvel, M.C.; Leliveld, A.; de Jong, I.J. Potential Receptors for Targeted Imaging of Lymph Node Metastases in Penile Cancer. *Diagnostics* **2020**, *10*, 694. [CrossRef] [PubMed]
58. de Gooyer, J.M.; Versleijen-Jonkers, Y.M.H.; Hillebrandt-Roeffen, M.H.S.; Frielink, C.; Desar, I.M.E.; de Wilt, J.H.W.; Flucke, U.; Rijpkema, M. Immunohistochemical Selection of Biomarkers for Tumor-Targeted Image-Guided Surgery of Myxofibrosarcoma. *Sci. Rep.* **2020**, *10*, 2915. [CrossRef] [PubMed]
59. Linders, D.; Deken, M.; van der Valk, M.; Tummers, W.; Bhairosingh, S.; Schaap, D.; van Lijnschoten, G.; Zonoobi, E.; Kuppen, P.; van de Velde, C.; et al. CEA, EpCAM, Avβ6 and UPAR Expression in Rectal Cancer Patients with a Pathological Complete Response after Neoadjuvant Therapy. *Diagnostics* **2021**, *11*, 516. [CrossRef]

International Journal of *Molecular Sciences*

Communication

Is CCL2 an Important Mediator of Mast Cell–Tumor Cell Interactions in Oral Squamous Cell Carcinoma?

Bernhard Hemmerlein [1], Luisa Reinhardt [2], Bernhard Wiechens [3], Tatjana Khromov [4], Henning Schliephake [2] and Phillipp Brockmeyer [2,*]

1 Institute of Pathology, Helios Klinikum Krefeld, 47805 Krefeld, Germany
2 Department of Oral and Maxillofacial Surgery, University Medical Center Goettingen, 37075 Goettingen, Germany
3 Department of Orthodontics, University Medical Center Goettingen, 37075 Goettingen, Germany
4 Institute for Clinical Chemistry, University Medical Center Goettingen, 37075 Goettingen, Germany
* Correspondence: ph.brockmeyer@gmail.com

Abstract: In this study, we aimed to evaluate the influence of interactions between mast cells (MCs) and oral squamous cell carcinoma (OSCC) tumor cells on tumor proliferation and invasion rates and identify soluble factors mediating this crosstalk. To this end, MC/OSCC interactions were characterized using the human MC cell line LUVA and the human OSCC cell line PCI-13. The influence of an MC-conditioned (MCM) medium and MC/OSCC co-cultures on the proliferative and invasive properties of the tumor cells was investigated, and the most interesting soluble factors were identified by multiplex ELISA analysis. LUVA/PCI-13 co-cultures increased tumor cell proliferation significantly ($p = 0.0164$). MCM reduced PCI-13 cell invasion significantly ($p = 0.0010$). CC chemokine ligand 2 (CCL2) secretion could be detected in PCI-13 monocultures and be significantly ($p = 0.0161$) increased by LUVA/PCI-13 co-cultures. In summary, the MC/OSCC interaction influences tumor cell characteristics, and CCL2 could be identified as a possible mediator.

Keywords: mast cells; MCs; oral squamous cell carcinoma; OSCC; soluble factors; CC chemokine ligand 2; CCL2; MCP-1

Citation: Hemmerlein, B.; Reinhardt, L.; Wiechens, B.; Khromov, T.; Schliephake, H.; Brockmeyer, P. Is CCL2 an Important Mediator of Mast Cell–Tumor Cell Interactions in Oral Squamous Cell Carcinoma? *Int. J. Mol. Sci.* **2023**, *24*, 3641. https://doi.org/10.3390/ijms24043641

Academic Editors: Marko Tarle and Ivica Lukšić

Received: 24 January 2023
Revised: 8 February 2023
Accepted: 9 February 2023
Published: 11 February 2023

1. Introduction

Mast cells (MCs) are potent effector cells of the immune system involved in numerous physiological and pathological conditions, such as angiogenesis, tissue remodeling, wound healing, IgE-dependent allergic disease, infection-induced immune responses, and autoimmune inflammatory disease [1].

Depending on the tumor entity and MC localization (intratumoral vs. tumor stroma), tumor-promoting and tumor-inhibiting effects have been described. Evidence also suggests that MCs are involved in the progression of various malignomas. Thus, MCs in the stroma of malignant melanoma, pancreatic carcinoma, or gastrointestinal adenocarcinoma are associated with poor patient prognosis [2]. In contrast, a tumor-suppressive effect has been demonstrated for intratumoral MCs in prostate carcinoma [3].

During tumor progression, MCs accumulate near blood vessels located around the tumor, secreting several mediators promoting angiogenesis and suppressing the immune response, including vascular endothelial growth factor (VEGF), histamine, tumor necrosis factors (TNF-α), and interleukin 18 (IL-18) [4]. Similarly, MC-specific proteases such as chymase and tryptase (MCT) are crucial for degrading the extracellular matrix (ECM) and inducing angiogenesis, thereby promoting tumor progression [4]. Stem cell factor (SCF) is critical in the MC/tumor cell interaction. Therefore, SCF expressed by tumor cells promotes MC migration and activation, leading to an increased release of more SCF molecules by tumor cells in a positive feedback loop [5].

In addition to their importance in local tumor progression, MCs are involved in lymph node metastasis (LNM) [6]. Hence, it has been demonstrated that the number of MCT-positive (MCT^+) intratumoral MCs positively correlates with the number of emerging LNMs in gastrointestinal malignancies. These properties additionally attribute a special role to MCs as biomarkers for prognosis assessment and as potential targets for future tumor therapies [4,6].

In addition to their effect on tumor progression and metastasis, MCs seem relevant in drug-based tumor therapy. Immune checkpoint inhibitors (ICIs) may experience reduced efficacy due to the presence of MCs. In a mouse model, a high intratumoral MC density was associated with a lower efficacy of immunotherapies targeting programmed cell death protein 1 (PD-1) inhibitors in melanoma cells [7]. Combining tyrosine kinase inhibitors, such as sunitinib or imatinib, which target MCs, substantially increases the response to therapy with PD-1 inhibitors in mice [7]. High MC density has also been associated with increased resistance to therapy in other malignancies, such as breast or prostate tumors [3,8].

In the oral cavity, a high MC density mainly aids inflammatory processes in diseases such as gingivitis or periodontitis [9]. The relevance of tumor-associated MCs in oral squamous cell carcinoma (OSCC) progression has been controversially described [9]. Angiogenesis plays a crucial role in OSCC progression and promotes local spread and metastasis [10]. It has been shown that more blood vessels and MCs are found in the environment of OSCC compared to healthy oral mucosa, supporting the hypothesis that MCs have a tumor-promoting effect in OSCC by inducing angiogenesis [10]. In contrast, MC density has recently been shown to decrease from oral potentially malignant disorders (OPMD) to OSCC [11], and increased vascularity in OSCC appears to be inversely related to MC density [12,13]. These findings suggest a protective role of MCs in OSCC. Increased MC density has also been described in oral leukoplakia, which may be associated with the progression toward invasive carcinoma [14]. Various studies have shown a tumor-promoting effect through the induction of angiogenesis and degradation of the ECM. MC density has been associated with increased tumor progression in lip carcinoma [15] and with a poorer prognosis in tongue malignancies [16]. However, a low MC density in the stroma of OSCC was associated with poorer prognoses for patients compared to those with a high MC density [17]. In line with these results, we recently showed in many patient tissue samples that a high MC density in the tumor-associated stroma of OSCC is positively correlated with longer overall survival (OS) and reduced MC degranulation [18].

Although the influence of MCs on OSCC progression is already known, it is still unclear which molecules mediate MC/OSCC interactions. In this study, we investigated MC/OSCC interactions, considering the influence on tumor cell proliferation and invasion and identified CC chemokine ligand 2 (CCL2) as a potential interaction mediator.

2. Results

2.1. Influence of the MC/OSCC Interaction on Tumor Cell Proliferation

To investigate the influence of the MC/OSCC interaction on tumor cell proliferative behavior, OSCC cell line PCI-13 was cultured in LUVA (MC)-conditioned medium (MCM), and LUVA/PCI-13 co-cultures were performed. Proliferation was measured using a BrdU uptake assay. Untreated PCI-13 cells served as controls. Data show that PCI-13 cell proliferation increased when treated with MCM compared with untreated controls. A significant ($p = 0.0164$) increase in PCI-13 cell proliferation was demonstrated for LUVA/PCI-13 co-cultivation compared to the untreated controls (Figure 1A).

In summary, a significant effect of direct MC/OSCC interactions on PCI-13 cell proliferation was observed ($p = 0.0164$).

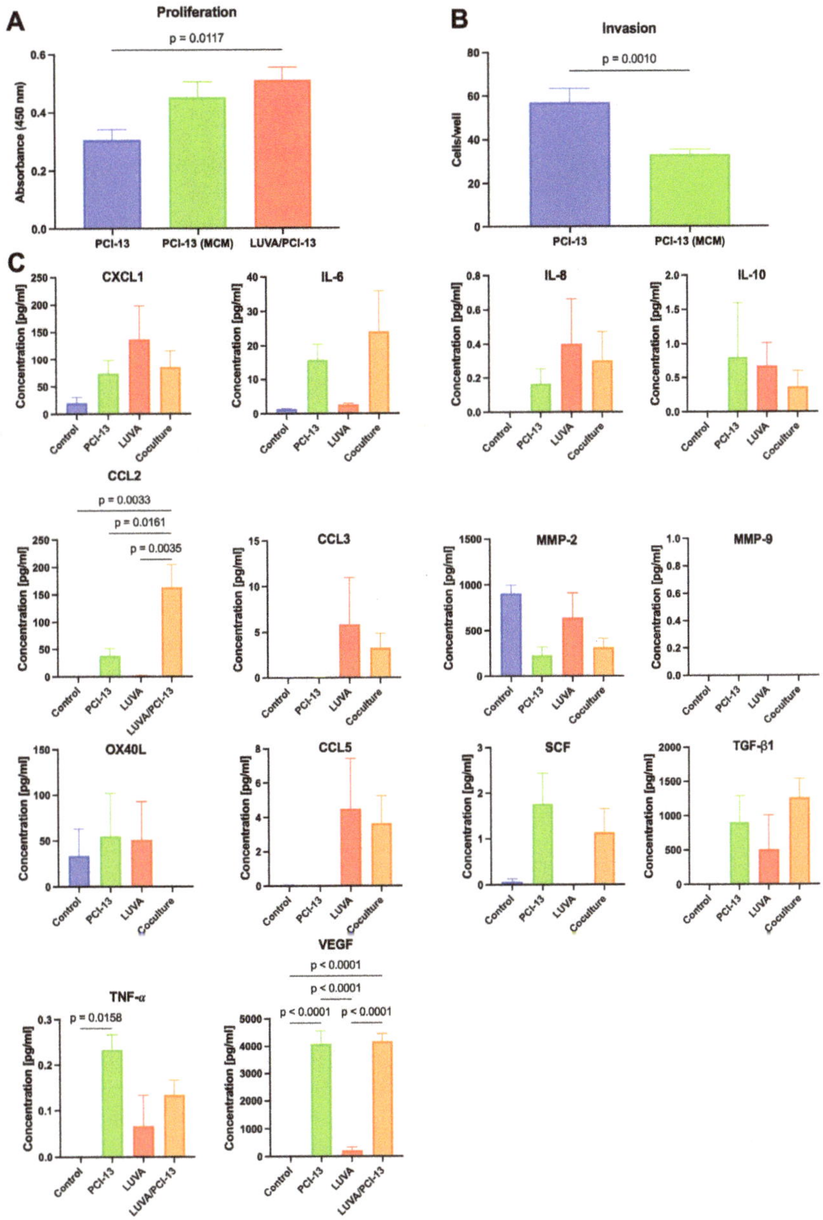

Figure 1. In vitro analysis of MC/OSCC interactions: (**A**) Influence on OSCC cell proliferation. PCI-13 cells cultured in unconditioned medium (PCI-13), PCI-13 cultured in MC-conditioned medium (MCM), and LUVA/PCI-13 co-cultures, based on 5×10^3 OSCC cells, respectively. (**B**) Influence on OSCC cell invasion. PCI-13 cells cultured in unconditioned medium (PCI-13) and PCI-13 cells cultured in MCM. (**C**) Multiplex ELISA analysis of known MC/tumor cell interaction partners: CXCL1, IL-6, IL-8, IL-10, CCL2, CCL3, MMP-2, MMP-9, OX40L, CCL5, SCF, TGF-β1, TNF-α, and VEGF. Cell medium alone as control (control), PCI-13 conditioned medium (PCI-13), LUVA conditioned medium (LUVA), and medium from LUVA/PCI-13 co-cultures (LUVA/OCI-13).

2.2. Influence of the MC/OSCC Interaction on Tumor Cell Invasion

PCI-13 cells were cultured in MCM, and tumor cell invasion assays were performed to investigate the effects of the MC/OSCC interaction on tumor cell invasive behavior. PCI-13 cells cultured in an untreated medium served as controls. The invasion analysis data revealed a significant ($p = 0.0010$) reduction in PCI-13 tumor cell invasion compared to untreated controls (Figure 1B).

In conclusion, a significant effect of the indirect OSCC cell stimulation on PCI-13 tumor cell invasion was observed ($p = 0.0010$).

2.3. Identification of Known MC/Tumor Cell Mediators

An individual multiplex ELISA assay was performed with MC/tumor cell interaction partners already known from the literature [19] to identify potent factors in the conditioned media mediating the MC/OSCC interaction: chemokine (C-X-C motif) ligand 1 (CXCL1), interleukin 6 (IL-6), interleukin 8 (IL-8), interleukin 10 (IL-10), chemokine (C-C motif) ligand 3 (CCL3), matrix metalloproteinase 2 (MMP-2), matrix metalloproteinase 9 (MMP-9), OX40 ligand (OX40L), CC chemokine ligand 5 (CCL5), stem cell factor (SCF), transforming growth factor beta 1 (TGF-β1), tumor necrosis factor alpha (TNF-α), vascular endothelial growth factor (VEGF), and CC chemokine ligand 2 (CCL2). Conditioned media of PCI-13 and LUVA monocultures and LUVA/PCI-13 co-cultures were compared accordingly. Unconditioned cell culture media was the control.

Of the soluble factors mentioned above, significant release differences could only be detected for CCL2, TNF-α, and VEGF, shown in Figure 1C (all p-values < 0.05). CCL2 was not detectable in the control media and was only detected to a minor extent in the PCI-13- and LUVA-conditioned media. However, a significant increase in CCL2 release was detected in the co-cultures, compared with the PCI-13- and LUVA-conditioned media ($p = 0.0161$ and $p = 0.0035$, respectively; Figure 1C). While TNF-α was undetectable in the control media, the high release could be detected in PCI-13-conditioned media and a low release in LUVA-conditioned media. However, co-culturing did not significantly increase or decrease TNF-α release in either cell line (Figure 1C). VEGF could not be detected in the control media, but a strong release was detectable in the tumor cell-conditioned media and a low release in the MC-conditioned media. However, no significant increase or decrease in VEGF release could be detected in the co-cultures compared with the tumor cell-only-conditioned media (Figure 1C).

In conclusion, a significant increase in CCL2 release could be detected by MC/OSCC co-culturing (all p-values < 0.05), suggesting that this factor may be a mediator in the MC/OSCC interaction.

3. Discussion

Despite advances in diagnostic and therapeutic options, the prognosis of patients with high OSCC stages has hardly improved over the past decades [20]. MC density in the tumor microenvironment (TME) of OSCC influences the OS and thus could be an interesting approach for targeted tumor therapy [18]. However, the factors mediating MC/OSCC interactions are far from known. In this study, we investigated the effect of direct and indirect MC stimulation on the proliferative and invasive behavior of OSCC tumor cells in vitro. We identified CCL2 as a potential mediator in OSCC for the first time.

The TME, with its numerous tumor-infiltrating host cells, is critical for disease progression and metastasis [21]. Mast cells comprise a large proportion of immune cells in the TME [22]. However, in several studies, precise MC localization has already been defined as a critical factor for the effect of MCs on tumor cells and patient survival. Therefore, high MC density in TME leads to a more prognostically favorable outcome because MCs inhibit tumor expansion and invasion [2]. In OSCC, different effects have been described for the same MC localization patterns, ranging from antitumor to tumor-promoting [15,17,23]. Iamaroon and colleagues analyzed the association between MCs and angiogenesis in OSCC and premalignant dysplasia by immunohistochemistry [23]. The authors demonstrated an association between high MC density and OSCC progression and invasion, which were also positively correlated with increased vascular sprouting in tumor tissue [23]. Rojas et al. described a tumor-promoting MC effect in lip carcinoma [15]. Moreover, healthy and premalignant altered lip tissue was analyzed for MC density by immunohistochemistry. The analysis confirmed increased immune cells and blood vessel density in carcinomas compared to healthy lip tissue [12]. In contrast, Attramadal et al. demonstrated that low MC density was associated with decreased OS in OSCC patients [17]. An immunohistochemical analysis was performed on 62 tissue samples from patients with T stages 1 and 2 OSCC. The MC number in the immediate tumor-surrounding stroma indicated a tumor-suppressive effect of MC in OSCC [17].

MCs have the ability to promote tumor proliferation and invasion both by direct stimulation and indirectly by modulating the TME [24]. The mitogenic activity of tumor cells is partially dependent on the secretion of MC proteases, such as tryptase and chymase [24]. In this study, we confirmed this direct effect through MC/OSCC co-cultivation. However, our studies of indirect MC stimulation of OSCC invasion suggest a reciprocal effect. Thus, different effects appear to occur in the interaction between MCs and OSCC, highlighting the opposing roles of MCs in tumor progression and complicating our current understanding.

It has been described that CCL2 is able to trigger tumor inflammation. TME is a major cause of immunosuppression, while CCL2 is the most potent chemoattractant in macrophage recruitment and a potent trigger of chronic inflammation [21]. Hence, various proinflammatory, stimulatory and signaling molecules, such as TNF-α, can transcriptionally activate CCL2, and oncogenes such as p53 and RB directly regulate CCL2 expression [21]. Moreover, tumor cells can actively secrete CCL2. This CCL2 is responsible for recruiting various immune effector cells, such as macrophages, myeloid-derived suppressor cells (MDSCs), mesenchymal stem cells (MSCs), and regulatory T cells (Tregs) [21]. A mouse model study demonstrated that the CCL2/CCR2 axis is involved in MC recruitment during the inflammatory response [25]. MC attraction via CCL2 has also been demonstrated for pancreatic tumors [26].

In OSCC, we demonstrated for the first time a possible link between MCs and tumor cells via CCL2 as a mediator, consistent with these results. The CCL2 increase by co-cultivation seems parallel to the increase in tumor cell proliferation, suggesting a possible autocrine tumor cell activation. Indirect MC stimulation resulted in a reduction in tumor cell invasiveness. Therefore, as mentioned, MC localization (in direct tumor cell contact vs. more distant in the TME) exerts a differential influence in OSCC. In our opinion, CCL2 may be involved in MC recruitment and could be an interesting starting point for targeted antitumor therapy. However, further studies are needed to understand the exact functional relationships better.

4. Materials and Methods

All further described measurements were performed in triplicate in three independent experiments for each cell line.

4.1. Cell Culture

Human OSCC cell line PCI-13 was obtained from the University of Pittsburgh Cancer Institute (UPCI, Pittsburgh, PA, USA) [27]. CD34+, c-kit+, and CD13+ human MC cell line LUVA was obtained from KERAFAST (Kerafast, Boston, MA, USA). PCI-13 cells were cultured in MEM with Earle's salts, 2.2 g/L NaHCO3, stable glutamine, and low endotoxin (Merck, Darmstadt, Germany), supplemented with 10% heat-inactivated fetal bovine serum (FBS) (Biochrom, Berlin, Germany), 1% nonessential amino acids (NEAA) (PAN Biotech, Aidenbach, Germany), 100 U/mL penicillin, and 100 µg/mL streptomycin (PAN Biotech), and incubated in a humidified chamber with 5% CO_2 at 37 °C. Human MC suspension cell line LUVA was cultivated in 20 mL of StemPro™-34 SFM medium (Thermo Fisher Scientific, Waltham, MA, USA) in upright T175 flasks and incubated in a humidified chamber with 5% CO_2 at 37 °C.

4.2. Preparation of Conditioned Cell Culture Media

An amount of 5×10^3 cells of the PCI-13 cell line was transferred to 10 mL StemPro™-34 SFM medium (Thermo Fisher Scientific, Waltham, MA, USA) and cultured in T175 flasks. After incubating for 48 h in a humidified chamber with 5% CO_2 at 37 °C, 20 mL of the stem cell medium per bottle were harvested and transferred to a Falcon tube. Cells remaining in the medium were removed by centrifugation at 1250 rpm at room temperature for 5 min. The medium was stored at −80 °C in 20 mL aliquots. An amount of 5×10^5 cells of the MC cell line LUVA was cultured in 20 mL of StemPro™-34 SFM medium (Thermo Fisher Scientific, Waltham, MA, USA). After 24 h, the medium was replaced with a fresh stem cell medium. Cells were cultivated in a humidified chamber with 5% CO_2 at 37 °C. Conditioned medium was harvested, transferred into a Falcon tube, and centrifuged for 5 min at 1000 rpm at room temperature. The supernatant was separated from the LUVA cell pellet and stored at −80 °C in 20 mL aliquots.

4.3. Mast Cell–Tumor Cell Co-Cultures

OSCC cell line PCI-13 was transferred into StemPro™-34 SFM medium (Thermo Fisher Scientific, Waltham, MA, USA) and cultured in T175 flasks to confluence (minimum 48 h incubation, Figure 2A). Twenty-four hours after attachment, the medium was replaced with 20 mL of StemPro™ medium, and 5×10^3 LUVA cells were added per flask. Medium and 5×10^3 cells were harvested and served as the control. The rest of the PCI-13 cells were divided (5×10^3 cells) into new T175 flasks. Cells were co-cultured, ranging from 48 to 72 h (Figure 2B). The medium was collected and centrifuged at $200\times g$ for 10 min at room temperature to collect LUVA cells grown in suspension. After collecting LUVA cells by separation from the medium, the PCI-13 cell line growing in monolayer was trypsinized and collected as cell pellets. Collected media (control and after co-culture) were centrifuged at $750\times g$ for 10 min, transferred into new falcon tubes, and again centrifuged at $1500\times g$ for 10 min. All media and cell pellets were stored at −80 °C in aliquots.

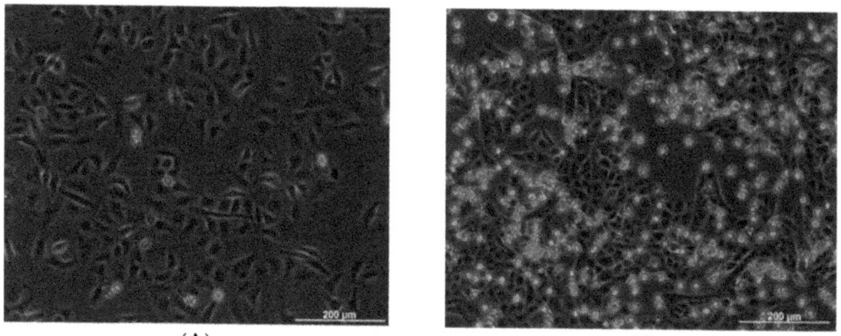

(A) **(B)**

Figure 2. Cell line cultivation: (**A**) PCI-13 monoculture and (**B**) LUVA/PCI-13 co-culture.

4.4. BrdU Cell Proliferation Assay

Amounts of 5×10^3 cells of the PCI-13 cell line and 1.5×10^4 cells of the LUVA cell line were seeded per well of a 96-well plate in 100 µL cell culture medium and incubated for 24 h. Cells were incubated for 4 h with bromodeoxyuridine (BrdU) at a final concentration of 10 µL. According to the manufacturer's instructions, proliferation analyses were performed using a BrdU-Cell Proliferation ELISA kit (Roche, Penzberg, Germany). The absorbance was measured using a microplate reader (BioRad, Feldkirchen, Germany) at 450 nm (control wavelength 655 nm).

4.5. Tumor Cell Invasion Assays

Corning®® BioCoat™ growth factor reduced matrigel invasion chamber with an 8.0 μm PET membrane and Corning®® BioCoat™ control inserts with an 8.0 μm PET membrane were used (Corning, Corning, NY, USA). Before the experiment, 500 μL of warm (37 °C) serum-free culture medium was added to the interior lumen of the inserts and incubated for 2 h at 37 °C for rehydration. The medium was carefully removed from the inserts, and 7×10^4 cells in a culture medium containing 0.1% BSA were added per insert. After 10 min incubation at 37 °C, 600 μL of chemoattractant (20% FBS in culture medium) was added to each well. Then, cells were incubated for 24 h at 37 °C in a humidified chamber with 5% CO_2. After 24 h, the medium and the remaining cells that had not migrated through the membrane pores were removed using cotton tip swabs. Inserts were incubated with 70% ethanol for 10 min to allow for cell fixation. Ethanol was removed, and the membrane was dried at room temperature for 15 min. Inserts were incubated with DAPI in 0.1% Triton X-100/PBS for 10 min at room temperature to visualize cells that had migrated through the membrane. Inserts were dipped twice in PBS and left in fresh PBS in wells, and three pictures of different areas of the membrane in each insert were taken using a fluorescence microscope (Zeiss, Oberkochen, Germany). Based on pictures of stained nuclei, the number of migrated cells was semi-automatically counted using the FIJI software [28] (Figure 3).

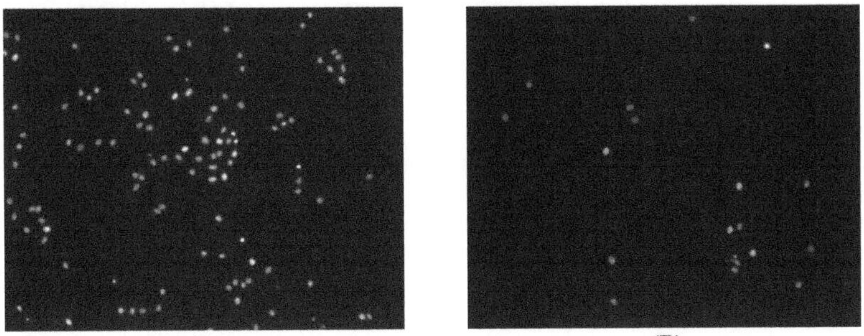

(A) (B)

Figure 3. Tumor cell invasion: (**A**) Invasive PCI-13 cells without indirect MC stimulation and (**B**) Invasive PCI-13 cells after indirect MC stimulation (MCM).

4.6. Multiplex ELISA Array

An individual multiplex ELISA assay (Quantibody; RayBiotech Inc., Peachtree Corners, GA, USA) was designed with MC/tumor cell interaction partners already known from the literature [19]: CXCL1, IL-6, IL-8, IL-10, CCL3, MMP-2, MMP-9, OX40L, CCL5, stem cell factor (SCF), TGF-β1, TNF-α, VEGF, and CCL2.

The conditioned media of the PCI-13 and mast cell lines (LUVA) and LUVA/PCI-13 co-cultures were compared accordingly. The concentration of each soluble factor was determined by RayBiotech Inc. using their Quantibody service. An unconditioned cell culture medium served as the control.

4.7. Statistical Analysis

Statistical analysis of all in vitro experiments was performed using independent Student's t-tests and one-way ANOVA. All tests were performed at a significance level of $\alpha = 5\%$ using the Prism 9 statistical software (GraphPad, La Jolla, CA, USA).

5. Conclusions

MC/OSCC interactions affect tumor cell characteristics, and thus, tumor progression, making them interesting candidates for targeted tumor therapy. In this study, we identified CCL2 for the first time in OSCC as a potential mediator of this interaction. Data suggest that CCL2 may promote tumor cell proliferation. Further studies should characterize the functional relationships.

Author Contributions: Conceptualization, B.H. and P.B.; methodology, L.R., T.K. and P.B.; software, P.B. and B.W.; validation, B.H., H.S. and P.B.; formal analysis, L.R.; investigation, B.H. and P.B.; resources, P.B.; data curation, L.R.; writing—original draft preparation, B.H. and P.B.; writing—review and editing, T.K. and H.S.; visualization, T.K. and P.B.; supervision, P.B.; project administration, P.B.; funding acquisition, B.H. and H.S. All authors have read and agreed to the published version of the manuscript.

Funding: We acknowledge support by the Open Access Publication Funds of the Goettingen University.

Institutional Review Board Statement: Not applicable.

Informed Consent Statement: Not applicable.

Data Availability Statement: All data are available through the corresponding author.

Conflicts of Interest: The authors declare no conflict of interest.

References

1. Gilfillan, A.M.; Beaven, M.A. Regulation of mast cell responses in health and disease. *Crit. Rev. Immunol.* **2011**, *31*, 475–529. [CrossRef] [PubMed]
2. Paolino, G.; Corsetti, P.; Moliterni, E.; Corsetti, S.; Didona, D.; Albanesi, M.; Mattozzi, C.; Lido, P.; Calvieri, S. Mast cells and cancer. *Ital. J. Dermatol. Venereol.* **2019**, *154*, 650–668. [CrossRef]
3. Johansson, A.; Rudolfsson, S.; Hammarsten, P.; Halin, S.; Pietras, K.; Jones, J.; Stattin, P.; Egevad, L.; Granfors, T.; Wikstrom, P.; et al. Mast cells are novel independent prognostic markers in prostate cancer and represent a target for therapy. *Am. J. Pathol.* **2010**, *177*, 1031–1041. [CrossRef] [PubMed]
4. de Souza Junior, D.A.; Santana, A.C.; da Silva, E.Z.; Oliver, C.; Jamur, M.C. The Role of Mast Cell Specific Chymases and Tryptases in Tumor Angiogenesis. *Biomed. Res. Int.* **2015**, *2015*, 142359. [CrossRef] [PubMed]
5. Roberts, R.; Govender, D. Gene of the month: KIT. *J. Clin. Pathol.* **2015**, *68*, 671–674. [CrossRef]
6. Ammendola, M.; Sacco, R.; Donato, G.; Zuccala, V.; Russo, E.; Luposella, M.; Vescio, G.; Rizzuto, A.; Patruno, R.; De Sarro, G.; et al. Mast cell positivity to tryptase correlates with metastatic lymph nodes in gastrointestinal cancer patients treated surgically. *Oncology* **2013**, *85*, 111–116. [CrossRef]
7. Somasundaram, R.; Connelly, T.; Choi, R.; Choi, H.; Samarkina, A.; Li, L.; Gregorio, E.; Chen, Y.; Thakur, R.; Abdel-Mohsen, M.; et al. Tumor-infiltrating mast cells are associated with resistance to anti-PD-1 therapy. *Nat. Commun.* **2021**, *12*, 346. [CrossRef]
8. Reddy, S.M.; Reuben, A.; Barua, S.; Jiang, H.; Zhang, S.; Wang, L.; Gopalakrishnan, V.; Hudgens, C.W.; Tetzlaff, M.T.; Reuben, J.M.; et al. Poor Response to Neoadjuvant Chemotherapy Correlates with Mast Cell Infiltration in Inflammatory Breast Cancer. *Cancer Immunol. Res.* **2019**, *7*, 1025–1035. [CrossRef]
9. Gaje, P.N.; Amalia Ceausu, R.; Jitariu, A.; Stratul, S.I.; Rusu, L.C.; Popovici, R.A.; Raica, M. Mast Cells: Key Players in the Shadow in Oral Inflammation and in Squamous Cell Carcinoma of the Oral Cavity. *Biomed. Res. Int.* **2016**, *2016*, 9235080. [CrossRef]
10. Mohtasham, N.; Babakoohi, S.; Salehinejad, J.; Montaser-Kouhsari, L.; Shakeri, M.T.; Shojaee, S.; Sistani, N.S.; Firooz, A. Mast cell density and angiogenesis in oral dysplastic epithelium and low- and high-grade oral squamous cell carcinoma. *Acta Odontol. Scand* **2010**, *68*, 300–304. [CrossRef]
11. Shrestha, A.; Keshwar, S.; Raut, T. Evaluation of Mast Cells in Oral Potentially Malignant Disorders and Oral Squamous Cell Carcinoma. *Int. J. Dent.* **2021**, *2021*, 5609563. [CrossRef] [PubMed]
12. Ansari, F.; Asif, M.; Kiani, M.N.; Zareef, A.; Rashid, F.; ud Din, H.; Ansar, F. Relationship between Mast Cell Density and Microvessel Density in Oral Squamous Cell Carcinoma and Normal Oral Mucosa: Immunohistochemical Analysis using CD117 and CD34 Antibodies. *Int. J. Pathol.* **2022**, 114–120.
13. Teofilo, C.R.; Ferreira Junior, A.E.C.; Batista, A.C.; Fechini Jamacaru, F.V.; Sousa, F.B.; Lima Mota, M.R.; Silva, M.F.E.; Barros Silva, P.G.; Alves, A. Mast Cells and Blood Vessels Profile in Oral Carcinogenesis: An Immunohistochemistry Study. *Asian Pac. J. Cancer Prev.* **2020**, *21*, 1097–1102. [CrossRef] [PubMed]
14. Michailidou, E.Z.; Markopoulos, A.K.; Antoniades, D.Z. Mast cells and angiogenesis in oral malignant and premalignant lesions. *Open Dent. J.* **2008**, *2*, 126–132. [CrossRef] [PubMed]
15. Rojas, I.G.; Spencer, M.L.; Martinez, A.; Maurelia, M.A.; Rudolph, M.I. Characterization of mast cell subpopulations in lip cancer. *J. Oral. Pathol. Med.* **2005**, *34*, 268–273. [CrossRef] [PubMed]
16. Ishikawa, K.; Yagi-Nakanishi, S.; Nakanishi, Y.; Kondo, S.; Tsuji, A.; Endo, K.; Wakisaka, N.; Murono, S.; Yoshizaki, T. Expression of interleukin-33 is correlated with poor prognosis of patients with squamous cell carcinoma of the tongue. *Auris Nasus Larynx* **2014**, *41*, 552–557. [CrossRef]

17. Attramadal, C.G.; Kumar, S.; Gao, J.; Boysen, M.E.; Halstensen, T.S.; Bryne, M. Low Mast Cell Density Predicts Poor Prognosis in Oral Squamous Cell Carcinoma and Reduces Survival in Head and Neck Squamous Cell Carcinoma. *Anticancer Res.* **2016**, *36*, 5499–5506. [CrossRef] [PubMed]
18. Brockmeyer, P.; Kling, A.; Schulz, X.; Perske, C.; Schliephake, H.; Hemmerlein, B. High mast cell density indicates a longer overall survival in oral squamous cell carcinoma. *Sci. Rep.* **2017**, *7*, 14677. [CrossRef]
19. Lichterman, J.N.; Reddy, S.M. Mast Cells: A New Frontier for Cancer Immunotherapy. *Cells* **2021**, *10*, 1270. [CrossRef] [PubMed]
20. Vossen, D.M.; Verhagen, C.V.M.; Verheij, M.; Wessels, L.F.A.; Vens, C.; van den Brekel, M.W.M. Comparative genomic analysis of oral versus laryngeal and pharyngeal cancer. *Oral Oncol.* **2018**, *81*, 35–44. [CrossRef]
21. Jin, J.; Lin, J.; Xu, A.; Lou, J.; Qian, C.; Li, X.; Wang, Y.; Yu, W.; Tao, H. CCL2: An Important Mediator Between Tumor Cells and Host Cells in Tumor Microenvironment. *Front. Oncol.* **2021**, *11*, 722916. [CrossRef] [PubMed]
22. Gorzalczany, Y.; Merimsky, O.; Sagi-Eisenberg, R. Mast Cells Are Directly Activated by Cancer Cell-Derived Extracellular Vesicles by a CD73- and Adenosine-Dependent Mechanism. *Transl. Oncol.* **2019**, *12*, 1549–1556. [CrossRef] [PubMed]
23. Iamaroon, A.; Pongsiriwet, S.; Jittidecharaks, S.; Pattanaporn, K.; Prapayasatok, S.; Wanachantararak, S. Increase of mast cells and tumor angiogenesis in oral squamous cell carcinoma. *J. Oral. Pathol. Med.* **2003**, *32*, 195–199. [CrossRef]
24. Khazaie, K.; Blatner, N.R.; Khan, M.W.; Gounari, F.; Gounaris, E.; Dennis, K.; Bonertz, A.; Tsai, F.-N.; Strouch, M.J.; Cheon, E. The significant role of mast cells in cancer. *Cancer Metastasis Rev.* **2011**, *30*, 45–60. [CrossRef] [PubMed]
25. Cai, H.; Li, J.; Zhang, Y.; Liao, Y.; Zhu, Y.; Wang, C.; Hou, J. LDHA Promotes Oral Squamous Cell Carcinoma Progression Through Facilitating Glycolysis and Epithelial-Mesenchymal Transition. *Front. Oncol.* **2019**, *9*, 1446. [CrossRef]
26. Theoharides, T.C. Mast cells and pancreatic cancer. *N. Engl. J. Med.* **2008**, *358*, 1860. [CrossRef]
27. Heo, D.S.; Snyderman, C.; Gollin, S.M.; Pan, S.; Walker, E.; Deka, R.; Barnes, E.L.; Johnson, J.T.; Herberman, R.B.; Whiteside, T.L. Biology, cytogenetics, and sensitivity to immunological effector cells of new head and neck squamous cell carcinoma lines. *Cancer Res.* **1989**, *49*, 5167–5175.
28. Schindelin, J.; Arganda-Carreras, I.; Frise, E.; Kaynig, V.; Longair, M.; Pietzsch, T.; Preibisch, S.; Rueden, C.; Saalfeld, S.; Schmid, B.; et al. Fiji: An open-source platform for biological-image analysis. *Nat. Methods* **2012**, *9*, 676–682. [CrossRef]

International Journal of
Molecular Sciences

MDPI

Article

miR-125b-5p, miR-155-3p, and miR-214-5p and Target *E2F2* Gene in Oral Squamous Cell Carcinoma

Karolina Gołąbek [1,*], Dorota Hudy [1], Agata Świętek [1,2], Jadwiga Gaździcka [1], Natalia Dąbrowska [3], Katarzyna Miśkiewicz-Orczyk [4], Natalia Zięba [4], Maciej Misiołek [4] and Joanna Katarzyna Strzelczyk [1]

1 Department of Medical and Molecular Biology, Faculty of Medical Sciences in Zabrze, Medical University of Silesia in Katowice, 19 Jordana St., 41-808 Zabrze, Poland
2 Silesia LabMed Research and Implementation Center, Medical University of Silesia in Katowice, 19 Jordana St., 41-808 Zabrze, Poland
3 Strathclyde Institute of Pharmacy and Biomedical Sciences, University of Strathclyde, 161 Cathedral Street, Glasgow G4 0RE, UK
4 Department of Otorhinolaryngology and Oncological Laryngology, Faculty of Medical Sciences in Zabrze, Medical University of Silesia in Katowice, 10 C Skłodowska St., 41-800 Zabrze, Poland
* Correspondence: kgolabek@sum.edu.pl

Abstract: It is known that E2F2 (E2F transcription factor 2) plays an important role as controller in the cell cycle. This study aimed to analyse the expression of the *E2F2* gene and E2F2 protein and demonstrate *E2F2* target microRNAs (miRNAs) candidates (miR-125b-5p, miR-155-3p, and miR-214-5p) in oral squamous cell carcinoma tumour and margin samples. The study group consisted 50 patients. The *E2F2* gene and miRNAs expression levels were assessed by qPCR, while the E2F2 protein was assessed by ELISA. When analysing the effect of miRNAs expression on *E2F2* gene expression and E2F2 protein level, we observed no statistically significant correlations. miR-125b-5p was downregulated, while miR-155-3p, and miR-214-5p were upregulated in tumour samples compared to margin. We observed a difference between the miR-125b-5p expression level in smokers and non-smokers in margin samples. Furthermore, HPV-positive individuals had a significantly higher miR-125b-5p and miR-214-5p expression level compared to HPV-negative patients in tumour samples. The study result showed that the *E2F2* gene is not the target for analysed miRNAs in OSCC. Moreover, miR-155-3p and miR-125b-5p could play roles in the pathogenesis of OSCC. A differential expression of the analysed miRNAs was observed in response to tobacco smoke and HPV status.

Keywords: oral squamous cell carcinoma; OSCC; E2F2; miR-125b-5p; miR-155-3p; miR-214-5p; tumour; margin

Citation: Gołąbek, K.; Hudy, D.; Świętek, A.; Gaździcka, J.; Dąbrowska, N.; Miśkiewicz-Orczyk, K.; Zięba, N.; Misiołek, M.; Strzelczyk, J.K. miR-125b-5p, miR-155-3p, and miR-214-5p and Target *E2F2* Gene in Oral Squamous Cell Carcinoma. *Int. J. Mol. Sci.* **2023**, *24*, 6320. https://doi.org/10.3390/ijms24076320

Academic Editors: Marko Tarle and Ivica Lukšić

Received: 13 March 2023
Revised: 26 March 2023
Accepted: 27 March 2023
Published: 28 March 2023

1. Introduction

Oral squamous cell carcinoma (OSCC) is considered one of the most common cancers in the head and neck squamous cell carcinoma (HNSCC) region. More than 300,000 new cases were reported worldwide in 2020 according to GLOBOCAN 2020 analysis [1]. It is also worth adding that this type of cancer is characterized by a 5 year survival rate ranging only from 45 to 50% [2,3]. It is believed that 80% of squamous cell carcinoma cases are due to alcohol consumption and smoking as risk factors [4,5]. However, the genetic background of this cancer type seems still insufficiently understood. Therefore, it seems reasonable to search for new biomarkers for an improved diagnosis and prognosis of the disease.

The E2F family of transcription factors includes eight proteins (E2F1–E2F8). These factors play an important role in cell proliferation and cell-cycle progression, regulate autophagy, mitochondrial functions, and the DNA damage response [6,7]. Pocket proteins, such as hypophosphorylated retinoblastoma protein Rb, and related proteins p107 and p130 can critically control E2F activity [6]. Changes in the *E2F* gene expression were analysed in several types of cancer—breast cancer, gastric cancer, liver cancer, and non-small-cell lung cancer [6,8–11]. The higher *E2F2* expression levels were significantly associated with poor prognosis in patients with non-small-cell lung cancer [6,8].

MicroRNAs (miRNAs) are a class of small, non-coding RNAs with about 18–22 nucleotides. The action mechanism of miRNA is based on binding to the 3′-UTR of mRNAs and silencing them [12,13]. These types of RNA are involved in the post-transcriptional regulation of approximately 60% of human genes [14]. miRNAs play an important role in modulating processes such as embryogenesis, cellular development, cell proliferation, cell metabolism, and homeostasis [13]. The importance of miRNAs in cancer biology was first demonstrated by Calin et al. [15] in a study to determine frequent deletions and downregulation of miR15 and miR16 in chronic lymphocytic leukaemia [15]. Currently, many studies on miRNAs focus on how these molecules affect gene expression in carcinogenesis. miRNAs are tissue-specific and may be seen as oncogenic (OncomiRs) when involved in the repression of tumour suppressor gene expression. In addition, miRNAs as tumour suppressors (oncosuppressor miRs) can also participate in the downregulation of oncogenes [16,17]. Some studies examine the role of miRNA in various cancers, such as pancreatic [18], colon [19], prostate [20,21], renal [22], bladder [23], breast [24], cervical [25], ovarian [26], lung [27], and HNSCC [28]. To date, analyses of the role of miRNAs in HNSCC pathogenesis are focused generally on studies of miRNAs, such as miR-375, miR-1234, miR-103, miR-638, miR-200b-3p, miR-191-5p, miR-24-3p, miR-572, miR-483-5p, miR-20a, miR-22, miR-29a, miR-29b, mir-let-7c, miR-17, miR-374b-5p, miR-425-5p, miR-122, miR-134, miR-184, miR 191, miR-412, miR-512, miR-8392, miR-21, miR-31, miR-155, miR-196a, miR-196b, miR-9, miR-29c, miR-223, miR-187, Let-7a, miR- 27, miR-34, miR-92, miR-124, miR-125a, miR-136, miR-139, miR-145, miR-146a, miR-200, miR-195, and miR-205 [29–33].

This study aimed to analyse the expression of the *E2F2* gene and E2F2 protein and demonstrate *E2F2* target miRNA candidates (miR-125b-5p, miR-155-3p, and miR-214-5p) in oral squamous cell carcinoma tumour and margin samples.

2. Results

2.1. Patient Sociodemographic and Clinical Characteristics

In the patient cohort group, the median age was 62.5 years (range: 27–87 years). There were 38 (76%) men and 12 (24%) women; 27 (54%) reported alcohol consumption; 28 (56%) patients who were smokers; and 17 (34%) who were both smokers and alcohol users. HPV 16 DNA was found in 13 of 50 samples (26%). The 3 year survival rate for all patients was approximately 24%. Clinical parameters of the OSCC group are shown in Table 1.

Table 1. Clinical parameters of the OSCC group.

Clinical Parameters	Patients, *n* (%)
Histological grading	
G1 (Well differentiated)	9 (18)
G2 (Moderately differentiated)	23 (46)
G3 (Poorly differentiated)	18 (36)
T classification	
T1	10 (20)
T2	23 (46)
T3	16 (32)
T4	1 (2)
Nodal status	
N0	24 (48)
N1	2 (4)
N2	20 (40)
N3	4 (8)
Patient status at 3 years	
Alive	12 (24)
Dead	38 (76)

2.2. E2F2 Gene Expression and E2F2 Protein Expression in Tumour Samples Compared to Margin Samples

We found no statistically significant differences in the *E2F2* expression gene level and E2F2 protein level in tumour samples compared to margin samples. The median *E2F2* relative gene expression in the tumour was 0.263 (0.145–0.578) and 0.47 (0.051–0.784) in the margin. While the median E2F2 protein level in the tumour was 0.129 ng/µg (0.051–0.238) and 0.082 ng/µg (0.047–0.282) in the margin (Figure 1). We also showed no effect of gene expression on protein expression in the examined tissues.

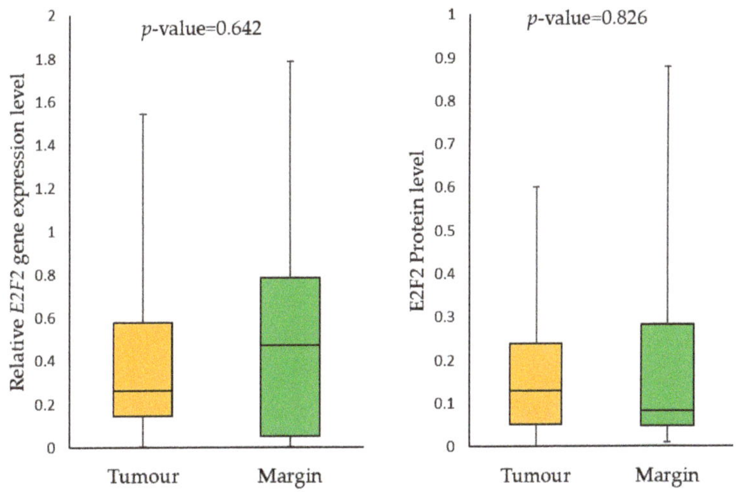

Figure 1. The *E2F2* mRNA expression and E2F2 protein level in tumour and margin samples.

2.3. miR-125b-5p, miR-155-3p, and miR-214-5p Expression in Tumour Samples Compared to Margin Samples

Analysis of the relative expression levels of the tested miRNAs demonstrated statistically significant levels for only one (miR-155-3p) of the tested miRNAs when comparing tumour versus margin samples. The tests showed that miR-125b-5p (*p*-value = 0.235) was downregulated, while miR-155-3p (*p*-value = 0.013), and miR-214-5p (*p*-value = 0.368) were upregulated in tumour samples compared to the margin samples (Figure 2).

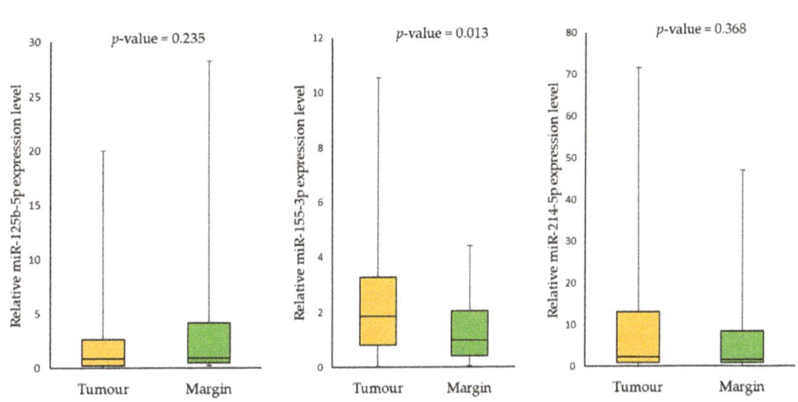

Figure 2. The relative expression levels of tested miRNAs in tumour samples compared to margin samples.

2.4. Correlation of E2F2 Gene Expression and E2F2 Protein Concentration with miRNAs Expression

When analysing the effect of miRNAs expression on *E2F2* gene expression and E2PF2 protein level, we observed no statistically significant difference in the tumour samples. We showed a similar observation in margin samples. Figure 3 presents the correlation between the expressions of *E2F2* gene, E2F2 protein, and the tested miRNAs in tumour and margin samples.

Tumour			
Spearman's rank correlation coefficient	125b-5p	155-3p	214-5p
E2F2 gene	−0.02	0.07	−0.13
E2F2 protein	0.07	0.25	−0.06
Margin			
Spearman's rank correlation coefficient	125b-5p	155-3p	214-5p
E2F2 gene	−0.04	−0.28	−0.07
E2F2 protein	0.10	0.21	0.04

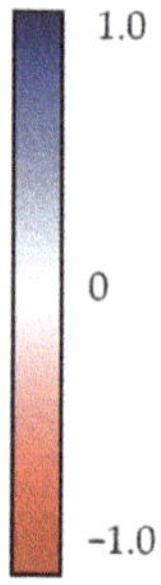

Tumour			
p-value	125b-5p	155-3p	214-5p
E2F2 gene	0.91	0.68	0.47
E2F2 protein	0.70	0.17	0.77
Margin			
p-value	125b-5p	155-3p	214-5p
E2F2 gene	0.81	0.08	0.69
E2F2 protein	0.64	0.31	0.85

Figure 3. Correlation between the expressions of *E2F2* gene, E2F2 protein, and the tested miRNAs in tumour and margin samples.

2.5. Correlations between E2F2 Gene Expression and Sociodemographic and Clinicopathological Features

No association was found between the *E2F2* gene expression levels, age, gender, smoking, alcohol consumption, HPV status and clinical parameters (N and G) in tumour and margin samples, except T parameter. The patients with T1 had a significantly higher gene expression level of *E2F2* than patients with T2 (0.581 vs. 0.237; *p*-value = 0.019) and T3 (0.581 vs. 0.145; *p*-value = 0.004) in tumour samples. Furthermore, we noticed that high *E2F2* gene expression levels in the margin could contribute to a lower 3 year survival rate (*p*-value = 0.026).

2.6. Correlations between E2F2 Protein Expression and Sociodemographic and Clinicopathological Features

No association was found between the E2F2 protein expression levels, age, gender, smoking, alcohol consumption, and clinical parameters (T and G) in tumour and margin samples, except N parameter. The patients with N0 had a significantly lower protein level of E2F2 than patients with N3 (0.125 vs. 0.581; *p*-value = 0.022) in tumour samples. At the same time, protein expression was lower in HPV-positive individuals compared to HPV-negative patients (0.035 vs. 0.164; *p*-value = 0.002) in tumour samples (Figure 4).

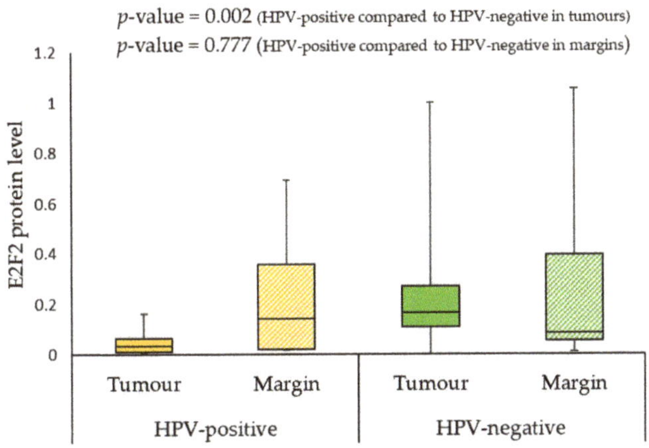

Figure 4. E2F2 protein level in HPV-positive compared to HPV-negative patients.

2.7. *Correlation of miRNAs Expression Level with Sociodemographic and Clinicopathological Variables*

We also assessed the correlation of the expression levels of selected miRNAs with demographics and clinical characteristics of the patients. When analysing the effect of smoking on miRNAs expression, we observed a statistically significant difference between the miR-125b-5p expression level in smokers and non-smokers (0.568 vs. 2.194; *p*-value = 0.009) in margin samples. In addition, the patients with G2 had a significantly lower miR-125b-5p expression level than patients with G3 (0.507 vs. 0.992, *p*-value = 0.008) in tumour samples. Furthermore, HPV-positive individuals had significantly higher miR-125b-5p and miR-214-5p expression levels in tumour samples compared to HPV-negative patients (2.629 vs. 0.627; *p*-value = 0.035 and 7.942 vs 1.684; *p*-value = 0.039, respectively). Figures 5–7 present the expressions of the tested miRNAs in HPV-positive compared to HPV-negative patients.

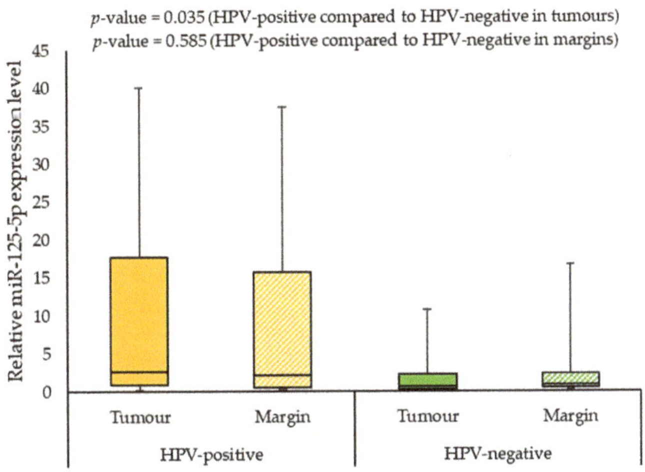

Figure 5. The relative expression level of miR-125b-5p in HPV-positive compared to HPV-negative patients.

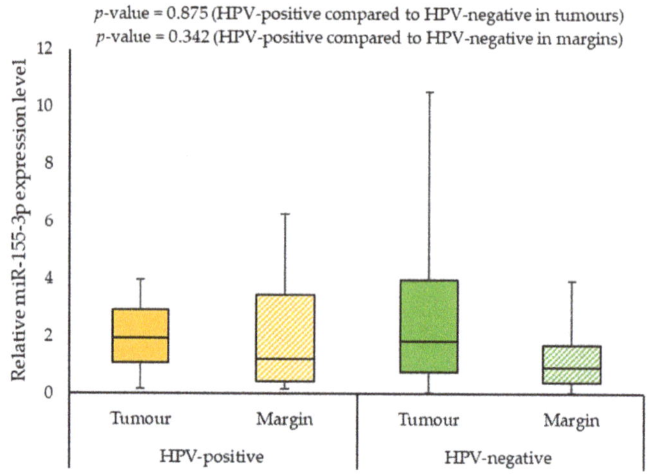

Figure 6. The relative expression level of miR-155-3p in HPV-positive compared to HPV-negative patients.

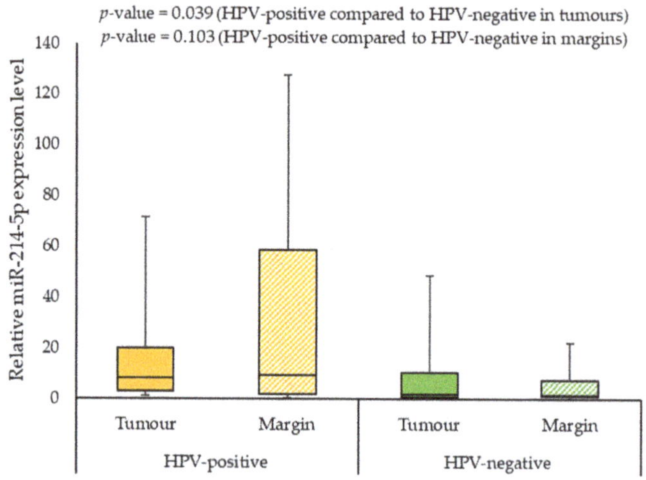

Figure 7. The relative expression level of miR-214-5p in HPV-positive compared to HPV-negative patients.

3. Discussion

It is known that E2F2 plays an important role as a controller in the cell cycle [6]. Our study demonstrated no statistically significant differences in the *E2F2* expression gene level and the E2F2 protein level in tumour samples compared to margin samples. Still, we found a higher expression of *E2F2* gene in the margin samples, while E2F2 protein level was higher in the tumour specimens. Furthermore, we noticed that the tumour progression could be associated with a decrease in gene expression. High *E2F2* gene expression levels in the margin could contribute to a lower 3 year survival rate. Moreover, the patients with N0 had a significantly lower protein expression level of E2F2 than patients with N3 in tumour samples. At the same time, protein concentration was lower in HPV-positive individuals compared to HPV-negative patients in tumour samples. Perhaps these results are related to the ambiguous role of E2F2 as a transcription factor in cell cycle regulation. This protein can act as both a promoter of cell division and a suppressor. Furthermore, changes in gene expression profile in normal samples could be explained by Slaughter's model of "field cancerization". According to this idea, in the samples of the margin without a trace of the tumour, cells genetically altered by the action of carcinogens could be present [34,35]. It is also noteworthy that E7 is a well-known HPV oncogene that plays a critical role in cellular growth control pathways. E7 targets the retinoblastoma protein Rb of tumour suppressor for proteasome-mediated degradation, and this protein can critically control the E2F family of transcription factors activity [6,36].

For many years, there has been interest in research with regard to the use of miRNAs as potential diagnostic and prognostic biomarkers in many types of cancers. Based on several studies, it can be assumed that miRNAs (for example microRNA-let-7a, miR-125b, miR-146b-3p, miR-638, miR-31, miR-218, miR-454-3p and miRNA-936) could play an important role in targeting *E2F2* expression. The analyses concerned with types of cancer, such as breast cancer, ovarian cancer, colon cancer, gastric cancer, prostate cancer, hepatocellular carcinoma, non-small cell lung cancer cell, glioma, and laryngeal cancer, suggested that miRNAs, by targeting *E2F2*, could be involved in cancer progression, overall survival of patients, and response to radiochemotherapy [37–46]. Moreover, circ_RPPH1/miR-146b-3p/*E2F2* axis could promote the progression of breast cancer and circCUL2/miR-214-5p/*E2F2* axis-suppressed retinoblastoma cells [46,47]. When analysing the effect of miRNAs expression on *E2F2* gene expression and E2F2 protein concentration, we observed no statistically significant differences in the OSCC tumour samples. However, we showed a similar observation in margin samples.

The miR-125 family is highly conserved and composed of a few homologs (e.g., miR-125a-3p, miR-125a-5p, miR-125b-1 and miR-125b-2) [48]. Some studies showed miR-125b could be downregulated in many types of tumours. Decreased miRNA expression was found in carcinomas of bladder [49], breast [50,51], liver [52,53], ovary [54,55], as well as Ewing's sarcoma [56]. Upregulation of miR-125b is also known to reverse the effects of drug resistance in ovarian cancer cells and nasopharyngeal carcinoma cells [57,58]. In this work, we demonstrated that miR-125b-5p was downregulated in tumour samples but not at statistically significant levels. However, it is noteworthy that the patients with G2 had a significantly lower miR-125b-5p expression level than patients with G3 in tumour samples. This result confirms previous analyses. The study by Shiiba [59] and others has shown a downregulated expression of miR-125b in OSCC-derived cell lines and OSCC samples. Furthermore, forced expression of miR-125b has been observed to enhance radiosensitivity in OSCC cells. Moreover, miR-125b expression is correlated with OSCC tumour staging and survival [59]. Our tests showed a statistically significant difference between the miR-125b-5p expression level in smokers and non-smokers in margin samples. The Doukas et al. [60] analysis demonstrated that tobacco could play a role in miRNA expression modification in HNSCC. The tobacco-specific nitrosamine—NNK (4-(methylnitrosamino)-1-(3-pyridyl)-1-butanone) has been identified as an important inducing factor in the upregulation of miR-21 and miR-155 and in the downregulation of miR-422 [60]. Perhaps miR-125b-5p expression is also regulated by NNK. Furthermore, HPV-positive individuals had a significantly higher miR-125b-5p expression level in tumour samples compared to HPV-negative patients. Our observation thus confirms the result of another study. The analysis of miRNA expression in cells transfected with HPV 11, 16, and 45 showed that this virus could be a modifier of miRNAs expression. It is noteworthy that the most upregulated miRNA is miR-125a-5p in cancers such as head and neck and gastric cancer [61].

The miR-155 host gene (MIR155HG) produces two different miRNA strands: miR155-5p and miR-155-3p [62]. In our study, we showed a statistically significant increased expression of miR-155-3p in tumour samples compared to margin samples. Several studies reported higher miR-155-5p expression in OSCC tumour samples [63–65]. Furthermore, miR-155-5p overexpression was associated with ESCC (oesophageal squamous cell carcinoma) tumour aggressiveness [66] and lymph node metastases and relapse OSCC [64,65]. It is worth adding that a meta-analysis based on eight studies including 709 HNSCC patients (279 presenting OSCC) showed that the OSSC subgroup had a worsening survival for patients with a high expression of miR-155-5p in tumour samples [33].

In our study, the last of the miRNAs analysed was miR-214-5p. miR-214-5p is known as a tumour-suppressive miRNA that plays a role in the pathogenesis of cancers such as osteosarcoma [67], hepatocellular carcinoma [68], and pancreatic cancer [69]. It is also noteworthy that miR-214-5p was upregulated in the tongue squamous cell carcinoma cisplatin-resistant subline [70]. Yao and others [71] demonstrated that miR-214-5p expression had a negative correlation with *E2F2* expression in pancreatic cancer tissue samples [71]. Our study showed no association between miR-214-5p level and *E2F2* expression, but HPV-positive individuals had a significantly higher miR-214-5p expression compared to HPV-negative patients in tumour samples. However, the role of miR-214-5p in HPV replication has not been reported. Interestingly, Patil et al.'s [72] study indicated that miR-214-5p regulates viral replications of hepatitis E virus [72].

In summary, one of the main limitations of this study is the small sample size. In addition, our results should be confirmed in studies using OSCC cell lines.

4. Materials and Methods

4.1. Patient and Samples

In total, 50 paired tumour and matching margin specimens were collected from patients with OSCC. The tissues were obtained following surgical resection at the Department of Otorhinolaryngology and Oncological Laryngology, Faculty of Medical Sciences in Zabrze, Medical University of Silesia in Katowice. Tumour staging was based on the American Joint Committee on Cancer (AJCC, version 2007) [73,74] and the WHO Classification of Head and Neck Tumours [75]. The normal tissues (margins) were checked and classified as cancer-free by pathologists. The main inclusion criteria were: written informed consent to participate in the study, age over 18 years, no metabolic diseases (e.g., diabetes, hypertension) or no chronic inflammatory diseases, a diagnosis of primary tumours, and no history of preoperative radio- or chemotherapy. All laboratory analyses were performed at the Department of Medical and Molecular Biology, Faculty of Medical Sciences in Zabrze, Medical University of Silesia in Katowice. The samples were transported to the Department on ice. The study was approved by the Bioethics Committee of the Medical University of Silesia (approval no. KNW/022/KB1/49/16 and no. KNW/002/KB1/49/II/16/17).

4.2. RNA and miRNAs Extraction and Quantification

The methodology for the extraction was presented in a previous study [76]. All tissue samples were homogenized with FastPrep®-24 homogenizer (MP Biomedicals, Solon, CA, USA) with ceramic beads Lysing Matrix D (MP Biomedicals, Solon, CA, USA). The RNA and miRNAs were extracted using the RNA isolation kit (catalog number RIK 001, BioVendor, Brno, Czech Republic) to the standard instruction. The concentration and purity of the isolated RNA was determined using spectrophotometry in NanoPhotometer Pearl UV/Vis Spectrophotometer (Implen, Munich, Germany) [76].

4.3. Selection of Candidate MicroRNAs to E2F2 Target

The target miRNAs of the *E2F2* gene were predicted by miRCode (version 11) [77], miRDB (version 6.0) [78], and TargetScan (version 7.2) [79] online databases.

4.4. Complementary DNA (cDNA) Synthesis

The methodology for the cDNA synthesis was presented in a previous study [76]. Total RNA (5 ng) was reverse-transcribed into cDNA using a high capacity cDNA reverse transcription kit with RNase inhibitor (Applied Biosystems, Foster City, CA, USA) according to manufacturer's protocol. The compound mix was prepared in a 20 μL volume containing: 2 μL of 10× Buffer RT; 0.8 μL of 25× dNTP mix (100 mM); 2 μL of 10× RT random primers; 1 μL of MultiScribe® reverse transcriptase; 1 μL of RNase inhibitor; 3.2 μL of nuclease-free H_2O; and 10 μL of previously isolated RNA. The reaction was processed in Mastercycler personal (Eppendorf, Hamburg, Germany) with the following thermal profile: 25 °C for 10 min, 37 °C for 120 min, 85 °C for 5 min, and 4 °C–∞ [76].

Furthermore, the obtained RNA (5 ng) was reverse-transcribed using TaqMan® Advanced miRNA cDNA synthesis kit (Applied Biosystems, Foster City, CA, USA) according to manufacturers' protocol. The whole procedure consisted four reactions with different profiles, which are presented in Table 2. The reactions were prepared in Mastercycler personal (Eppendorf, Hamburg, Germany).

Table 2. cDNA synthesis procedure using TaqMan® Advanced miRNA cDNA synthesis kit (Applied Biosystems, Foster City, CA, USA) according to manufacturer's protocol.

	Reaction Composition			
	Component	**Volume**		
Perform the poly(A) tailing reaction	10× Poly(A) Buffer	0.5 µL		
	ATP	0.5 µL		
	Poly(A) enzyme	0.3 µL		
	RNA sample	2 µL		
	RNase-free water	1.7 µL		
	Thermal Profile			
	Step	**Temperature**	**Time**	
	Polyadenylation	37 °C	45 min	
	Stop reaction	65 °C	10 min	
	Hold	4 °C	Hold	
	Reaction Composition			
	Component	**Volume**		
Perform the adaptor ligation reaction	5× DNA Ligase Buffer	3 µL		
	50% PEG 8000	4.5 µL		
	25× Ligation Adaptor	0.6 µL		
	RNA Ligase	1.5 µL		
	Poly(A) tailing reaction product	5 µL		
	RNase-free water	0.4 µL		
	Thermal Profile			
	Step	**Temperature**	**Time**	
	Ligation	16 °C	60 min	
	Hold	4 °C	Hold	
	Reaction Composition			
	Component	**Volume**		
Perform the reverse transcription (RT) reaction	5× RT Buffer	6 µL		
	dNTP Mix (25 mM each)	1.2 µL		
	20× Universal RT primer	1.5 µL		
	10× RT enzyme mix	3 µL		
	Adaptorligation reaction product	15 µL		
	RNase-free water	3.3 µL		
	Thermal Profile			
	Step	**Temperature**	**Time**	
	Reverse transcription	42 °C	15 min	
	Stop reaction	85 °C	5 min	
	Hold	4 °C	Hold	
	Reaction Composition			
	Component	**Volume**		
Perform the miR-Amp reaction	2× miR-Amp master mix	25 µL		
	20× miR-Amp primer mix	2.5 µL		
	RT reaction product	5 µL		
	RNase-free water	17.5 µL		
	Thermal Profile			
	Step	**Temperature**	**Time**	**Cycles**
	Enzyme activation	95 °C	5 min	1
	Denature	95 °C	3 s	14
	Anneal/extend	60 °C	30 s	
	Stop reaction	99 °C	10 min	1
	Hold	4 °C	Hold	1

4.5. E2F2 Gene and miRNAs Expression Analysis

The methodology for the *E2F2* gene expression analysis was presented in a previous study [35]. The relative gene expression (RQ) analysis was performed by Real-Time PCR (qPCR) using TaqMan® gene expression assays, QuantStudio 5 Real-Time PCR System, and Analysis Software v1.5.1 (Applied Biosystems, Foster City, CA, USA). The kit was supplied with primers and fluorescently marked molecular probes. The glyceraldehyde-3-phosphate dehydrogenase gene (*GAPDH*) was used as an endogenous control. Five surgical margin samples were used as a calibrator. The comparative threshold cycle (Ct) method $2^{-\Delta\Delta Ct}$ was used to determine the RQ. The qPCR was performed in a volume of 20 μL using 1 μL of cDNA, 10 μL of TaqMan® fast advanced master mix (Applied Biosystems, Foster City, CA, USA), 1 μL of TaqMan® gene expression assays (Assay ID: Hs00914334_m1 for *E2F2*, and Assay ID: Hs03929097_g1 for *GAPDH*), and 8 μL of nuclease-free H_2O (EURx, Gdańsk, Poland). Thermal cycle for all analysed genes was: 95 °C for 20 s, followed by 40 cycles of 95 °C for 1 s, and 60 °C for 20 s [76].

The relative expression (RQ) of miR-125b-5p, miR-155-3p, and miR-214-5p were assessed based on the guidelines by the TaqMan® advanced miRNA assays (Applied Biosystems, Foster City, CA, USA). The kit was supplied with primers and fluorescently marked molecular probes. All reactions were performed in QuantStudio 5 Real-Time PCR System and Analysis Software v1.5.1 (Applied Biosystems, Foster City, CA, USA). The housekeeping miR-361-5p was used for normalizing the expression. Five surgical margin samples were used as a calibrator. RQ was calculated using $2^{-\Delta\Delta Ct}$ after normalization with the reference miRNA. The qPCR was performed in a volume of 20 μL using 5 μL of cDNA (1:10 dilution), 10 μL of TaqMan® fast advanced master mix (Applied Biosystems, Foster City, CA, USA) and 1 μL of TaqMan® advanced miRNA assay (assay ID: 477885_mir for miR-125b-5p, assay ID: 477926_mir for miR-155-3p, assay ID: 478768_mir for miR-214-5p, and assay ID: 478056_mir for miR-361-5p). Thermal cycle for all analysed miRNAs was: 95 °C for 20 s, followed by 40 cycles of 95 °C for 1 s, and 60 °C for 20 s. Table 3 presents the sequence of the tested miRNAs.

Table 3. Sequences of analysed miRNAs.

miRNA	Mature miRNA Sequence
miR-125b-5p	UCCCUGAGACCCUAACUUGUGA
miR-155-3p	CUCCUACAUAUUAGCAUUAACA
miR-214-5p	UGCCUGUCUACACUUGCUGUGC
miR-361-5p (Housekeeping control)	UUAUCAGAAUCUCCAGGGGUAC

4.6. E2F2 and Total Protein Concentration Determinations

The tumour and margin tissue samples were homogenized with a homogenizer Bio-Gen PRO200 (PRO Scientific Inc., Oxford, CT, USA) at a speed 10,000 RPM (5 times 1 min at 2 min intervals) in nine volumes of cold PBS (EURx, Gdańsk, Poland). Then, the suspensions were sonicated with the ultrasonic processor UP100H (Hilscher, Teltow, Germany).

Enzyme-linked immunosorbent assay (ELISA) technique was used to evaluate E2F2 protein concentrations in tissue homogenates. Enzyme-linked immunosorbent assay kit (Assay ID: SEJ182Hu, Cloud-Clone Corp., Houston, TX, USA) was used for the tests according to the manufacturer's instructions. Absorbance was recorded at 450 nm wavelength and calibrated according to the standard curve in Synergy H1 microplate reader (BioTek, Winooski, VT, USA) and results were calculated with Gen5 2.06 software (BioTek, Winooski, VT, USA). The sensitivity of this assay was 0.059 ng/mL. Precision-measured as the coefficient of variation was <10% (intra-assay) and <12% (inter-assay).

The quantified total protein was performed using AccuOrange™ protein quantitation kit (Biotium, Fremont, CA, USA) according to the standard instructions. The samples were assayed in a 100-fold dilution. The detection range of the assay was 0.1–15 μg/mL protein. The fluorescence was measured with excitation/emission at 480/598 nm (SYNERGY H1 microplate reader; BIOTEK, Winooski, VT, USA). The E2F2 protein concentrations for each sample were normalized to the total amount of protein in the tissue lysates. Values were expressed in ng/μg protein.

4.7. HPV 16 Detection

DNA was extracted from tissue samples using a gene matrix tissue DNA purification kit (EURx, Gdansk, Poland) according to the manufacturer's instructions. The concentration and purity of the isolated DNA was prepared using spectrophotometry in NanoPhotometer Pearl UV/Vis Spectrophotometer (Implen, Munich, Germany). HPV was detected using AmpliSens® HPV 16/18-FRT PCR kit (InterLabService, Moscow, Russia) according to manufacturers' protocol. The PCR was performed in a volume of 25 μL using 7 μL of PCR-mix-1-FEP/FRT HPV; 8 μL mixture of PCR-buffer-FRT, TaqF polymerase, and 10 μL of DNA. The amplification program was as follows: 95 °C for 20 s, followed by 45 cycles of 95 °C for 20 s, and 60 °C for 1 min. All PCR reactions were performed using in QuantStudio 5 Real-Time PCR System (Applied Biosystems, Foster City, CA, USA).

4.8. Statistical Analyses

The Shapiro–Wilk test evaluated the distribution of variables. The median with interquartile range (25–75%) was used to describe miRNAs expression, *E2F2* gene expression, and E2F2 protein concentration. The Mann–Whitney U test was used to compare the sociodemographic and clinical characteristics, miRNAs, *E2F2* gene, and E2F2 protein level. Correlations between miRNAs, *E2F2* gene, and E2F2 protein concentration were calculated using Spearman's rank correlation analysis. The level of statistical significance was set at 0.05. The statistical software STATISTICA version 13 (TIBCO Software Inc., Palo Alto, CA, USA) was used to perform all the analyses.

5. Conclusions

The study result showed that the *E2F2* gene is not the target for analysing miRNAs in OSCC. Moreover, miR-155-3p and miR-125b-5p could play roles in the pathogenesis of OSCC. A differential expression of the analysed miRNAs in response to tobacco smoke and HPV status was observed.

Author Contributions: Conceptualization, K.G.; methodology, K.G.; collection of samples, K.M.-O. and N.Z.; RNA extraction, cDNA synthesis, gene and miRNAs expression analyses, K.G.; protein level analyses and HPV detection, A.Ś., K.G. and J.G.; data analysis and interpretation, K.G., D.H. and N.D.; writing—original draft preparation, K.G.; supervision, M.M. and J.K.S. All authors have read and agreed to the published version of the manuscript.

Funding: This research was funded from the grant by the Medical University of Silesia (PCN-1-025/N/1/O).

Institutional Review Board Statement: The study was conducted in accordance with the Declaration of Helsinki and approved by the Bioethics Committee of the Medical University of Silesia (approval no. KNW/022/KB1/49/16 and no. KNW/002/KB1/49/II/16/17).

Informed Consent Statement: Informed consent was obtained from all subjects involved in the study.

Data Availability Statement: The data used to support the findings of this study are available from the corresponding author upon request.

Acknowledgments: We would like to thank Krzysztof Biernacki, for help with HPV detection.

Conflicts of Interest: The authors declare no conflict of interest. The funders had no role in the design of the study, in the collection, analyses, or interpretation of data, in the writing of the manuscript, or in the decision to publish the results.

References

1. Sung, H.; Ferlay, J.; Siegel, R.L.; Laversanne, M.; Soerjomataram, I.; Jemal, A.; Bray, F. Global Cancer Statistics 2020: GLOBOCAN Estimates of Incidence and Mortality Worldwide for 36 Cancers in 185 Countries. *CA Cancer J. Clin.* **2021**, *71*, 209–249. [CrossRef]
2. Golusinski, P.; Di Maio, P.; Pehlivan, B.; Colley, S.; Nankivell, P.; Kong, A.; Hartley, A.; Mehanna, H. Evidence for the approach to the diagnostic evaluation of squamous cell carcinoma occult primary tumors of the head and neck. *Oral Oncol.* **2019**, *88*, 145–152. [CrossRef]
3. Aghiorghiesei, O.; Zanoaga, O.; Raduly, L.; Aghiorghiesei, A.I.; Chiroi, P.; Trif, A.; Buiga, R.; Budisan, L.; Lucaciu, O.; Pop, L.A.; et al. Dysregulation of miR-21-5p, miR-93-5p, miR-200c-3p and miR-205-5p in Oral Squamous Cell Carcinoma: A Potential Biomarkers Panel? *Curr. Issues Mol. Biol.* **2022**, *44*, 1754–1767. [CrossRef]
4. Siegel, R.L.; Miller, K.D.; Jemal, A. Cancer statistics, 2016. *CA Cancer J. Clin.* **2016**, *66*, 7–30. [CrossRef]
5. Dioguardi, M.; Caloro, G.A.; Laino, L.; Alovisi, M.; Sovereto, D.; Crincoli, V.; Aiuto, R.; Coccia, E.; Troiano, G.; Lo Muzio, L. Circulating miR-21 as a Potential Biomarker for the Diagnosis of Oral Cancer: A Systematic Review with Meta-Analysis. *Cancers* **2020**, *12*, 936. [CrossRef]
6. Emmrich, S.; Pützer, B.M. Checks and balances: E2F-microRNA crosstalk in cancer control. *Cell Cycle* **2010**, *9*, 2555–2567. [CrossRef]
7. Wang, H.; Wang, X.; Xu, L.; Zhang, J.; Cao, H. Integrated analysis of the E2F transcription factors across cancer types. *Oncol. Rep.* **2020**, *43*, 1133–1146. [CrossRef]
8. Gao, Z.; Shi, R.; Yuan, K.; Wang, Y. Expression and prognostic value of E2F activators in NSCLC and subtypes: A research based on bioinformatics analysis. *Tumour Biol.* **2016**, *37*, 14979–14987. [CrossRef]
9. Li, Y.; Huang, J.; Yang, D.; Xiang, S.; Sun, J.; Li, H.; Ren, G. Expression patterns of E2F transcription factors and their potential prognostic roles in breast cancer. *Oncol. Lett.* **2018**, *15*, 9216–9230. [CrossRef]
10. Manicum, T.; Ni, F.; Ye, Y.; Fan, X.; Chen, B.C. Prognostic values of E2F mRNA expression in human gastric cancer. *Biosci. Rep.* **2018**, *38*, BSR20181264. [CrossRef]
11. Huang, Y.L.; Ning, G.; Chen, L.B.; Lian, Y.F.; Gu, Y.R.; Wang, J.L.; Chen, D.M.; Wei, H.; Huang, Y.H. Promising diagnostic and prognostic value of E2Fs in human hepatocellular carcinoma. *Cancer Manag. Res.* **2019**, *11*, 1725–1740. [CrossRef]
12. Kabzinski, J.; Maczynska, M.; Majsterek, I. MicroRNA as a Novel Biomarker in the Diagnosis of Head and Neck Cancer. *Biomolecules* **2021**, *11*, 844. [CrossRef]
13. Thomaidou, A.C.; Batsaki, P.; Adamaki, M.; Goulielmaki, M.; Baxevanis, C.N.; Zoumpourlis, V.; Fortis, S.P. Promising Biomarkers in Head and Neck Cancer: The Most Clinically Important miRNAs. *Int. J. Mol. Sci.* **2022**, *23*, 8257. [CrossRef] [PubMed]
14. Avram, E.G.; Moatar, I.A.; Miok, V.; Baderca, F.; Samoila, C.; Alexa, A.; Andreescu, I.N.; Podariu, A.; Marian, C.; Sirbu, I.O. Gene network analysis of the transcriptome impact of methylated microRNAs on oral squamous cell carcinoma. *Adv. Clin. Exp. Med.* **2022**, *31*, 1231–1242. [PubMed]
15. Calin, G.A.; Dumitru, C.D.; Shimizu, M.; Bichi, R.; Zupo, S.; Noch, E.; Aldler, H.; Rattan, S.; Keating, M.; Rai, K.; et al. Frequent deletions and down-regulation of micro-RNA genes miR15 and miR16 at 13q14 in chronic lymphocytic leukemia. *Proc. Natl. Acad. Sci. USA* **2002**, *99*, 15524–15529. [CrossRef]
16. Di Leva, G.; Garofalo, M.; Croce, C.M. MicroRNAs in cancer. *Annu. Rev. Pathol.* **2014**, *9*, 287–314. [CrossRef]
17. Ali Syeda, Z.; Langden, S.S.S.; Munkhzul, C.; Lee, M.; Song, S.J. Regulatory Mechanism of MicroRNA Expression in Cancer. *Int. J. Mol. Sci.* **2020**, *21*, 1723. [CrossRef]
18. Kent, O.A.; Fox-Talbot, K.; Halushka, M.K. RREB1 repressed miR-143/145 modulates KRAS signaling through downregulation of multiple targets. *Oncogene* **2013**, *32*, 2576–2585. [CrossRef]
19. Wang, C.; Shi, Z.; Hong, Z.; Pan, J.; Chen, Z.; Qiu, C.; Zhuang, H.; Zheng, X. MicroRNA-1276 Promotes Colon Cancer Cell Proliferation by Negatively Regulating LACTB. *Cancer Manag. Res.* **2020**, *12*, 12185–12195. [CrossRef]
20. Coarfa, C.; Fiskus, W.; Eedunuri, V.K.; Rajapakshe, K.; Foley, C.; Chew, S.A.; Shah, S.S.; Geng, C.; Shou, J.; Mohamed, J.S.; et al. Comprehensive proteomic profiling identifies the androgen receptor axis and other signaling pathways as targets of microRNAs suppressed in metastatic prostate cancer. *Oncogene* **2016**, *35*, 2345–2356. [CrossRef] [PubMed]
21. Takayama, K.I.; Misawa, A.; Inoue, S. Significance of microRNAs in Androgen Signaling and Prostate Cancer Progression. *Cancers* **2017**, *9*, 102. [CrossRef] [PubMed]
22. Wang, X.J.; Yan, Z.J.; Luo, G.C.; Chen, Y.Y.; Bai, P.M. miR-26 suppresses renal cell cancer via down-regulating coronin-3. *Mol. Cell. Biochem.* **2020**, *463*, 137–146. [CrossRef] [PubMed]
23. Li, X.; Chen, W.; Li, R.; Chen, X.; Huang, G.; Lu, C.; Wen, Z.; Peng, X.; Liu, K.; Zhang, C.; et al. Bladder cancer diagnosis with a four-miRNA panel in serum. *Future Oncol.* **2022**, *18*, 3311–3322. [CrossRef]
24. Gao, S.; Shi, P.; Tian, Z.; Yang, X.; Liu, N. Overexpression of miR-1225 promotes the progression of breast cancer, resulting in poor prognosis. *Clin. Exp. Med.* **2021**, *21*, 287–296. [CrossRef] [PubMed]
25. Gao, C.; Zhou, C.; Zhuang, J.; Liu, L.; Liu, C.; Li, H.; Liu, G.; Wei, J.; Sun, C. MicroRNA expression in cervical cancer: Novel diagnostic and prognostic biomarkers. *J. Cell. Biochem.* **2018**, *119*, 7080–7090. [CrossRef]
26. Wei, L.; He, Y.; Bi, S.; Li, X.; Zhang, J.; Zhang, S. miRNA-199b-3p suppresses growth and progression of ovarian cancer via the CHK1/E-cadherin/EMT signaling pathway by targeting ZEB1. *Oncol. Rep.* **2021**, *45*, 569–581. [CrossRef]

27. Liang, G.; Meng, W.; Huang, X.; Zhu, W.; Yin, C.; Wang, C.; Fassan, M.; Yu, Y.; Kudo, M.; Xiao, S.; et al. miR-196b-5p-mediated downregulation of TSPAN12 and GATA6 promotes tumor progression in non-small cell lung cancer. *Proc. Natl. Acad. Sci. USA* **2020**, *117*, 4347–4357. [CrossRef]
28. Wan, Y.; Hoyle, R.G.; Xie, N.; Wang, W.; Cai, H.; Zhang, M.; Ma, Z.; Xiong, G.; Xu, X.; Huang, Z.; et al. A Super-Enhancer Driven by FOSL1 Controls miR-21-5p Expression in Head and Neck Squamous Cell Carcinoma. *Front. Oncol.* **2021**, *11*, 656628. [CrossRef]
29. Patil, S.; Warnakulasuriya, S. Blood-based circulating microRNAs as potential biomarkers for predicting the prognosis of head and neck cancer-a systematic review. *Clin. Oral Investig.* **2020**, *24*, 3833–3841. [CrossRef]
30. Al Rawi, N.; Elmabrouk, N.; Abu Kou, R.; Mkadmi, S.; Rizvi, Z.; Hamdoon, Z. The role of differentially expressed salivary microRNA in oral squamous cell carcinoma. A systematic review. *Arch. Oral Biol.* **2021**, *125*, 105108. [CrossRef]
31. Dioguardi, M.; Cantore, S.; Sovereto, D.; La Femina, L.; Caloro, G.A.; Spirito, F.; Scacco, S.; Di Cosola, M.; Lo Muzio, L.; Troiano, G.; et al. Potential Role of miR-196a and miR-196b as Prognostic Biomarkers of Survival in Head and Neck Squamous Cell Carcinoma: A Systematic Review, Meta-Analysis and Trial Sequential Analysis. *Life* **2022**, *12*, 1269. [CrossRef]
32. Dioguardi, M.; Spirito, F.; Caloro, G.A.; Lo Muzio, L.; Cantore, S.; Ballini, A.; Scacco, S.; Malcangi, A.; Sembronio, S.; Cascardi, E.; et al. Is the Non-Coding RNA miR-195 a Biodynamic Marker in the Pathogenesis of Head and Neck Squamous Cell Carcinoma? A Prognostic Meta-Analysis. *J. Pers. Med.* **2023**, *13*, 275. [CrossRef] [PubMed]
33. Dioguardi, M.; Spirito, F.; Sovereto, D.; La Femina, L.; Campobasso, A.; Cazzolla, A.P.; Di Cosola, M.; Zhurakivska, K.; Cantore, S.; Ballini, A.; et al. Biological Prognostic Value of miR-155 for Survival Outcome in Head and Neck Squamous Cell Carcinomas: Systematic Review, Meta-Analysis and Trial Sequential Analysis. *Biology* **2022**, *11*, 651. [CrossRef]
34. Slaughter, D.P.; Southwick, H.W.; Smejkal, W. Field cancerization in oral stratified squamous epithelium; clinical implications of multicentric origin. *Cancer* **1953**, *6*, 963–968. [CrossRef] [PubMed]
35. Braakhuis, B.J.; Tabor, M.P.; Kummer, J.A.; Leemans, C.R.; Brakenhoff, R.H. A genetic explanation of Slaughter's concept of field cancerization: Evidence and clinical implications. *Cancer Res.* **2003**, *63*, 1727–1730. [PubMed]
36. Roman, A.; Munger, K. The papillomavirus E7 proteins. *Virology* **2013**, *445*, 138–168. [CrossRef] [PubMed]
37. Dong, Y.; Zou, J.; Su, S.; Huang, H.; Deng, Y.; Wang, B.; Li, W. MicroRNA-218 and microRNA-520a inhibit cell proliferation by downregulating E2F2 in hepatocellular carcinoma. *Mol. Med. Rep.* **2015**, *12*, 1016–1022. [CrossRef]
38. Li, T.; Luo, W.; Liu, K.; Lv, X.; Xi, T. miR-31 promotes proliferation of colon cancer cells by targeting E2F2. *Biotechnol. Lett.* **2015**, *37*, 523–532. [CrossRef]
39. Zhang, Y.; Han, D.; Wei, W.; Cao, W.; Zhang, R.; Dong, Q.; Zhang, J.; Wang, Y.; Liu, N. MiR-218 Inhibited Growth and Metabolism of Human Glioblastoma Cells by Directly Targeting E2F2. *Cell. Mol. Neurobiol.* **2015**, *35*, 1165–1173. [CrossRef]
40. Wang, H.; Zhang, X.; Liu, Y.; Ni, Z.; Lin, Y.; Duan, Z.; Shi, Y.; Wang, G.; Li, F. Downregulated miR-31 level associates with poor prognosis of gastric cancer and its restoration suppresses tumor cell malignant phenotypes by inhibiting E2F2. *Oncotarget* **2016**, *7*, 36577–36589. [CrossRef]
41. Fang, Z.Q.; Li, M.C.; Zhang, Y.Q.; Liu, X.G. MiR-490-5p inhibits the metastasis of hepatocellular carcinoma by down-regulating E2F2 and ECT2. *J. Cell. Biochem.* **2018**, *119*, 8317–8324. [CrossRef] [PubMed]
42. Zhou, X.; Tao, H. Overexpression of microRNA-936 suppresses non-small cell lung cancer cell proliferation and invasion via targeting E2F2. *Exp. Ther. Med.* **2018**, *16*, 2696–2702. [CrossRef] [PubMed]
43. Cui, X.; Xiao, D.; Cui, Y.; Wang, X. Exosomes-Derived Long Non-Coding RNA HOTAIR Reduces Laryngeal Cancer Radiosensitivity by Regulating microRNA-454-3p/E2F2 Axis. *OncoTargets Ther.* **2019**, *12*, 10827–10839. [CrossRef] [PubMed]
44. Lin, Q.Y.; Wang, J.Q.; Wu, L.L.; Zheng, W.E.; Chen, P.R. miR-638 represses the stem cell characteristics of breast cancer cells by targeting E2F2. *Breast Cancer* **2020**, *27*, 147–158. [CrossRef]
45. Miyamoto, M.; Sawada, K.; Nakamura, K.; Yoshimura, A.; Ishida, K.; Kobayashi, M.; Shimizu, A.; Yamamoto, M.; Kodama, M.; Hashimoto, K.; et al. Paclitaxel exposure downregulates miR-522 expression and its downregulation induces paclitaxel resistance in ovarian cancer cells. *Sci. Rep.* **2020**, *10*, 16755. [CrossRef]
46. Feng, H.; Sun, S.Z.; Cheng, F.; Zhang, N.Q. Mediation of circ_RPPH1 on miR-146b-3p/E2F2 pathway to hinder the growth and metastasis of breast carcinoma cells. *Aging* **2021**, *13*, 20552–20568. [CrossRef]
47. Zhang, H.; Qiu, X.; Song, Z.; Lan, L.; Ren, X.; Ye, B. CircCUL2 suppresses retinoblastoma cells by regulating miR-214-5p/E2F2 Axis. *Anticancer Drugs* **2022**, *33*, e218–e227. [CrossRef]
48. Yin, H.; Sun, Y.; Wang, X.; Park, J.; Zhang, Y.; Li, M.; Yin, J.; Liu, Q.; Wei, M. Progress on the relationship between miR-125 family and tumorigenesis. *Exp. Cell Res.* **2015**, *339*, 252–260. [CrossRef]
49. Huang, L.; Luo, J.; Cai, Q.; Pan, Q.; Zeng, H.; Guo, Z.; Dong, W.; Huang, J.; Lin, T. MicroRNA-125b suppresses the development of bladder cancer by targeting E2F3. *Int. J. Cancer* **2011**, *128*, 1758–1769. [CrossRef] [PubMed]
50. Feliciano, A.; Castellvi, J.; Artero-Castro, A.; Leal, J.A.; Romagosa, C.; Hernández-Losa, J.; Peg, V.; Fabra, A.; Vidal, F.; Kondoh, H.; et al. miR-125b acts as a tumor suppressor in breast tumorigenesis via its novel direct targets ENPEP, CK2-α, CCNJ, and MEGF9. *PLoS ONE* **2013**, *8*, e76247. [CrossRef]
51. Zhang, Y.; Yan, L.X.; Wu, Q.N.; Du, Z.M.; Chen, J.; Liao, D.Z.; Huang, M.Y.; Hou, J.H.; Wu, Q.L.; Zeng, M.S.; et al. miR-125b is methylated and functions as a tumor suppressor by regulating the ETS1 proto-oncogene in human invasive breast cancer. *Cancer Res.* **2011**, *71*, 3552–3562. [CrossRef] [PubMed]
52. Jia, H.Y.; Wang, Y.X.; Yan, W.T.; Li, H.Y.; Tian, Y.Z.; Wang, S.M.; Zhao, H.L. MicroRNA-125b functions as a tumor suppressor in hepatocellular carcinoma cells. *Int. J. Mol. Sci.* **2012**, *13*, 8762–8774. [CrossRef]

53. Gong, J.; Zhang, J.P.; Li, B.; Zeng, C.; You, K.; Chen, M.X.; Yuan, Y.; Zhuang, S.M. MicroRNA-125b promotes apoptosis by regulating the expression of Mcl-1, Bcl-w and IL-6R. *Oncogene* **2013**, *32*, 3071–3079. [CrossRef] [PubMed]
54. Guan, Y.; Yao, H.; Zheng, Z.; Qiu, G.; Sun, K. MiR-125b targets BCL3 and suppresses ovarian cancer proliferation. *Int. J. Cancer* **2011**, *128*, 2274–2283. [CrossRef] [PubMed]
55. He, J.; Xu, Q.; Jing, Y.; Agani, F.; Qian, X.; Carpenter, R.; Li, Q.; Wang, X.R.; Peiper, S.S.; Lu, Z.; et al. Reactive oxygen species regulate ERBB2 and ERBB3 expression via miR-199a/125b and DNA methylation. *EMBO Rep.* **2012**, *13*, 1116–1122. [CrossRef] [PubMed]
56. Li, J.; You, T.; Jing, J. MiR-125b inhibits cell biological progression of Ewing's sarcoma by suppressing the PI3K/Akt signalling pathway. *Cell Prolif.* **2014**, *47*, 152–160. [CrossRef]
57. Kong, F.; Sun, C.; Wang, Z.; Han, L.; Weng, D.; Lu, Y.; Chen, G. miR-125b confers resistance of ovarian cancer cells to cisplatin by targeting pro-apoptotic Bcl-2 antagonist killer 1. *J. Huazhong Univ. Sci. Technol. Med. Sci.* **2011**, *31*, 543. [CrossRef]
58. Yuan, T.Z.; Zhang, H.H.; Lin, X.L.; Yu, J.X.; Yang, Q.X.; Liang, Y.; Deng, J.; Huang, L.J.; Zhang, X.P. microRNA-125b reverses the multidrug resistance of nasopharyngeal carcinoma cells via targeting of Bcl-2. *Mol. Med. Rep.* **2017**, *15*, 2223–2228. [CrossRef]
59. Shiiba, M.; Shinozuka, K.; Saito, K.; Fushimi, K.; Kasamatsu, A.; Ogawara, K.; Uzawa, K.; Ito, H.; Takiguchi, Y.; Tanzawa, H. MicroRNA-125b regulates proliferation and radioresistance of oral squamous cell carcinoma. *Br. J. Cancer* **2013**, *108*, 181721. [CrossRef]
60. Doukas, S.G.; Vagelim, D.P.; Lazopoulos, G.; Spandidos, D.A.; Sasaki, C.T.; Tsatsakis, A. The Effect of NNK, A Tobacco Smoke Carcinogen, on the miRNA and Mismatch DNA Repair Expression Profiles in Lung and Head and Neck Squamous Cancer Cells. *Cells* **2020**, *9*, 1031. [CrossRef]
61. Chawla, J.P.; Iyer, N.; Soodan, K.S.; Sharma, A.; Khurana, S.K.; Priyadarshni, P. Role of miRNA in cancer diagnosis, prognosis, therapy and regulation of its expression by Epstein-Barr virus and human papillomaviruses: With special reference to oral cancer. *Oral Oncol.* **2015**, *51*, 731–737. [CrossRef]
62. Mycko, M.P.; Cichalewska, M.; Cwiklinska, H.; Selmaj, K.W. miR-155-3p Drives the Development of Autoimmune Demyelination by Regulation of Heat Shock Protein 40. *J. Neurosci.* **2015**, *35*, 16504–16515. [CrossRef]
63. Manikandan, M.; Deva Magendhra Rao, A.K.; Rajkumar, K.S.; Rajaraman, R.; Munirajan, A.K. Altered levels of miR-21, miR-125b-2*, miR-138, miR-155, miR-184, and miR-205 in oral squamous cell carcinoma and association with clinicopathological characteristics. *J. Oral Pathol. Med.* **2015**, *44*, 792–800. [CrossRef] [PubMed]
64. Baba, O.; Hasegawa, S.; Nagai, H.; Uchida, F.; Yamatoji, M.; Kanno, N.I.; Yamagata, K.; Sakai, S.; Yanagawa, T.; Bukawa, H. MicroRNA-155-5p is associated with oral squamous cell carcinoma metastasis and poor prognosis. *J. Oral Pathol. Med.* **2016**, *45*, 248–255. [CrossRef] [PubMed]
65. Wu, M.; Duan, Q.; Liu, X.; Zhang, P.; Fu, Y.; Zhang, Z.; Liu, L.; Cheng, J.; Jiang, H. MiR-155-5p promotes oral cancer progression by targeting chromatin remodeling gene ARID2. *Biomed. Pharm.* **2020**, *122*, 109696. [CrossRef] [PubMed]
66. Zheng, Y.J.; Liang, T.S.; Wang, J.; Zhao, J.Y.; Zhai, S.N.; Yang, D.K.; Wang, L.D. MicroRNA-155 acts as a diagnostic and prognostic biomarker for oesophageal squamous cell carcinoma. *Artif. Cells Nanomed. Biotechnol.* **2020**, *48*, 977–982. [CrossRef]
67. Zhang, M.; Wang, D.; Zhu, T.; Yin, R. miR-214-5p Targets ROCK1 and Suppresses Proliferation and Invasion of Human Osteosarcoma Cells. *Oncol. Res.* **2017**, *25*, 75–81. [CrossRef]
68. Li, H.; Wang, H.; Ren, Z. MicroRNA-214-5p Inhibits the Invasion and Migration of Hepatocellular Carcinoma Cells by Targeting Wiskott-Aldrich Syndrome Like. *Cell. Physiol. Biochem.* **2018**, *46*, 757–764. [CrossRef]
69. Cao, T.H.; Ling, X.; Chen, C.; Tang, W.; Hu, D.M.; Yin, G.J. Role of miR-214-5p in the migration and invasion of pancreatic cancer cells. *Eur. Rev. Med. Pharmacol. Sci.* **2018**, *22*, 7214–7221.
70. Yu, Z.W.; Zhong, L.P.; Ji, T.; Zhang, P.; Chen, W.T.; Zhang, C.P. MicroRNAs contribute to the chemoresistance of cisplatin in tongue squamous cell carcinoma lines. *Oral Oncol.* **2010**, *46*, 317–322. [CrossRef]
71. Yao, Z.; Chen, Q.; Ni, Z.; Zhou, L.; Wang, Y.; Yang, Y.; Huang, H. Long Non-Coding RNA Differentiation Antagonizing Nonprotein Coding RNA (DANCR) Promotes Proliferation and Invasion of Pancreatic Cancer by Sponging miR-214-5p to Regulate E2F2 Expression. *Med. Sci. Monit.* **2019**, *25*, 4544–4552. [CrossRef] [PubMed]
72. Patil, R.N.; Karpe, Y.A. Uncovering the Roles of miR-214 in Hepatitis E Virus Replication. *J. Mol. Biol.* **2020**, *432*, 5322–5342. [CrossRef] [PubMed]
73. Brunner, M.; Ng, B.C.; Veness, M.J.; Clark, J.R. Comparison of the AJCC N staging system in mucosal and cutaneous squamous head and neck cancer. *Laryngoscope* **2014**, *124*, 1598–1602. [CrossRef]
74. Rodrigues, P.C.; Miguel, M.C.; Bagordakis, E.; Fonseca, F.P.; de Aquino, S.N.; Santos-Silva, A.R.; Lopes, M.A.; Graner, E.; Salo, T.; Kowalski, L.P.; et al. Clinicopathological prognostic factors of oral tongue squamous cell carcinoma: A retrospective study of 202 cases. *Int. J. Oral Maxillofac. Surg.* **2014**, *43*, 795–801. [CrossRef] [PubMed]
75. El-Naggar, A.K.; Chan, J.K.C.; Grandis, J.R.; Takata, T.; Slootweg, P.J. *WHO Classification of Head and Neck Tumours International Agency for Research on Cancer (IARC)*, 4th ed.; IARC Publications: Lyon, France, 2017.
76. Gołąbek, K.; Rączka, G.; Gaździcka, J.; Miśkiewicz-Orczyk, K.; Zięba, N.; Krakowczyk, Ł.; Misiołek, M.; Strzelczyk, J.K. Expression Profiles of CDKN2A, MDM2, E2F2 and LTF Genes in Oral Squamous Cell Carcinoma. *Biomedicines* **2022**, *10*, 3011. [CrossRef]
77. miRCode. Available online: http://www.mircode.org (accessed on 14 September 2022).

78. miRDB. Available online: http://mirdb.org (accessed on 14 September 2022).
79. TargetScan. Available online: http://www.targetscan.org/vert_72 (accessed on 14 September 2022).

International Journal of *Molecular Sciences*

MDPI

Article

Combinations of PRI-724 Wnt/β-Catenin Pathway Inhibitor with Vismodegib, Erlotinib, or HS-173 Synergistically Inhibit Head and Neck Squamous Cancer Cells

Robert Kleszcz *, Mikołaj Frąckowiak, Dawid Dorna and Jarosław Paluszczak

Department of Pharmaceutical Biochemistry, Poznan University of Medical Sciences, 4, Święcickiego Str., 60-781 Poznań, Poland; mikfrackowiak97@gmail.com (M.F.); dawid.dorna97@gmail.com (D.D.); paluszcz@ump.edu.pl (J.P.)

* Correspondence: kleszcz@ump.edu.pl

Abstract: The Wnt/β-catenin, EGFR, and PI3K pathways frequently undergo upregulation in head and neck squamous carcinoma (HNSCC) cells. Moreover, the Wnt/β-catenin pathway together with Hedgehog (Hh) signaling regulate the activity of cancer stem cells (CSCs). The aim of this study was to investigate the effects of the combinatorial use of the Wnt/β-catenin and Hh pathway inhibitors on viability, cell cycle progression, apoptosis induction, cell migration, and expression of CSC markers in tongue (CAL 27) and hypopharynx (FaDu) cancer cells. Co-inhibition of Wnt signaling with EGFR or PI3K pathways was additionally tested. The cells were treated with selective inhibitors of signaling pathways: Wnt/β-catenin (PRI-724), Hh (vismodegib), EGFR (erlotinib), and PI3K (HS-173). Cell viability was evaluated by the resazurin assay. Cell cycle progression and apoptosis induction were tested by flow cytometric analysis after staining with propidium iodide and Annexin V, respectively. Cell migration was detected by the scratch assay and CSC marker expression by the R-T PCR method. Mixtures of PRI-724 and vismodegib affected cell cycle distribution, greatly reduced cell migration, and downregulated the transcript level of CSC markers, especially *POU5F1* encoding OCT4. Combinations of PRI-724 with erlotinib or HS-173 were more potent in inducing apoptosis.

Keywords: Wnt pathway; hedgehog pathway; β-catenin; PRI-724; vismodegib; erlotinib; HS-173; head and neck cancer; cancer stem cells; synergism

Citation: Kleszcz, R.; Frąckowiak, M.; Dorna, D.; Paluszczak, J. Combinations of PRI-724 Wnt/β-Catenin Pathway Inhibitor with Vismodegib, Erlotinib, or HS-173 Synergistically Inhibit Head and Neck Squamous Cancer Cells. *Int. J. Mol. Sci.* **2023**, *24*, 10448. https://doi.org/10.3390/ijms241310448

Academic Editors: Marko Tarle and Ivica Lukšić

Received: 23 May 2023
Revised: 19 June 2023
Accepted: 20 June 2023
Published: 21 June 2023

1. Introduction

Head and neck squamous cell carcinomas (HNSCCs) are a diverse group of tumors that share common clinical risk factors, including smoking tobacco, often with concomitant abuse of high-proof alcohol, or oncogenic virus infection (mainly the human papilloma virus, HPV, or the Epstein–Barr virus, EBV). On the other hand, HNSCCs are characterized by heterogeneous genetic and molecular abnormalities, including the most frequently occurring mutations of *TP53*, and mutations/alterations in other cell cycle regulators or epigenetic changes [1]. According to the Global Cancer Statistics 2020, new cases of lip and oral cavity cancers amounted to 2.0%, followed by other head and neck localizations: larynx (1.0%), nasopharynx (0.7%), oropharynx (0.5%), and hypopharynx (0.4%). Lip and oral cavity cancers had the highest incidence rate per 100,000 in the male population of Melanesia (22.2), South Central Asia (13.3), and Eastern Europe (9.2) [2].

The rapid development of pharmaceutical and medical sciences has resulted in translational 'bench to bedside' studies allowing for more robust treatment of oncological disorders. Since epidermal growth factor receptor (EGFR) is commonly overexpressed among HNSCC patients, EGF signaling was thought to be a good target for HNSCC treatment. Unfortunately, despite the dysregulation of EGFR expression reaching 90% of cases, only 10–30% of patients respond to monotherapy based on EGFR inhibitors like cetuximab, a chimeric mouse-human IgG1 antibody against the extracellular domain of EGFR [3]. It has been suggested that EGFR-directed therapies can be improved by the concurrent targeting of EGFR-related PI3K/Akt signaling and by searching for combination therapies with other molecular targets important for the growth of HNSCC [4,5]. In this regard, our earlier study showed that the effects of erlotinib, a small-molecule inhibitor of EGFR, can be augmented by the concurrent use of inhibitors of KDM4 or KDM6 histone lysine demethylases [6].

In previous years, an idea arose to pharmacologically target/inhibit the Wnt canonical (β-catenin-dependent) signaling pathway because its dysregulation, also based on epigenetic mechanisms, can be observed as early as at the pre-cancerous stage, like oral submucous fibrosis [7]. The dysregulation in Wnt/β-catenin signaling stimulates HNSCC cell proliferation, supports the avoidance of apoptosis, and improves cell migration [8,9]. Wnt canonical signaling can be inhibited at various levels of signal transduction, starting from the maturation of Wnt ligands, through pathway activation at the cell membrane, further secondary transduction of signals through the cytoplasm, and finally to the modulation of TCF/LEF transcription factor activity in the nucleus. In fact, both synthetic and natural compounds can affect particular targets [10–14]. Our previous research on six HNSCC cell lines allowed for the identification of two suitable protein targets: Porcupine, the *O*-acyltransferase required for the maturation of Wnt ligands, and the interaction of β-catenin with CBP, which is crucial for the activation of transcription of Wnt signaling target genes [15]. In the first case, the inhibition has an influence on both canonical and non-canonical Wnt signaling, but the second target selectively attenuates the Wnt/β-catenin pathway.

Stem cells (SCs) play an indispensable role in hierarchical development during embryogenesis and remain active in adult tissues to maintain their self-renewal ability. Moreover, it is now widely acknowledged that tumors contain a population of so-called cancer stem cells (CSCs), which can support phenotypically diverse tumor mass growth and create resistance to standard therapy [16]. The presence of CSCs was also detected in HNSCCs, and targeting this subpopulation of cells has become a potential new therapeutic strategy [9,10,14,17,18]. Importantly, Wnt/β-catenin pathway inhibition had anti-stemness potential in HNSCC cells [19]. Indeed, this pathway maintains the activity of both normal and cancer stem cells [10]. Hedgehog (Hh) is another pathway responsible for the viability and function of normal SCs and CSCs, and it is active in different types of head and neck cancers [20]. Thus, Wnt/β-catenin and Hh pathways can both be involved in the promotion of CSCs in HNSCC, which can potentiate the development of cancer. There is crosstalk between these pathways, and recently, the GSK-3β kinase activity state was shown to be important for both Wnt and Hh signaling control [21]. Moreover, EGFR and PI3K/Akt signaling are able to accelerate the tumorigenic potential of HNSCC cells and present crosstalk with Wnt and Hh pathways [22]. Currently, there are limited data about the potential usefulness and benefits of targeting the Hh pathway in HNSCC. Vismodegib (GDC-0449) is a small, orally administrable molecule that inhibits the Hh pathway and was approved by the U.S. Food and Drug Administration for the treatment of basal cell carcinoma (BCC) [23]. However, evidence regarding its biological activity in HNSCC is scarce.

Considering the above data and our previous research, we aimed to analyze the influence of Wnt/β-catenin pathway inhibition by PRI-724 and Hedgehog pathway inhibition by vismodegib, individually and in combinations, on the viability, cell cycle progression, apoptosis induction, and cell migration of squamous cell carcinoma of the tongue (CAL 27) and hypopharynx (FaDu) cancer cells. The results were compared to the effects of the co-inhibition of Wnt/β-catenin and better-known molecular targets in HNSCC, particularly the EGF receptor (targeted by erlotinib) and PI3 kinase (targeted by HS-173). Furthermore, we evaluated the influence of PRI-724 and vismodegib on the expression of selected genes related to CSC to preliminarily check the potential of Wnt and Hh pathway inhibition in modulating their levels in CAL 27 and FaDu cells. All combinations demonstrated beneficial effects in HNSCC cells, but the profile of biological activity differed. The mixtures of PRI-724 and vismodegib were especially interesting because of their ability to accumulate cells in the G1/G0 phase, greatly reduce cell migration, and downregulate the transcript level of genes expressed by cancer stem cells.

2. Results

2.1. Expression of the Components of the Wnt/β-Catenin Pathway Is Increased in Higher Grade HNSCC Tumors

We have previously tested the value of the inhibition of canonical Wnt signaling to treat HNSCC cells [15], and we hypothesized that the effects of Wnt pathway inhibition could be further augmented by co-treatment with chemicals targeting other key signaling pathways. Indeed, the analysis of TCGA data corroborated that the Wnt pathway is frequently dysregulated in HNSCC, and the changes increase with tumor grade (Figure 1). Figure 1A contains data on the expression of several genes related to the first step of Wnt/β-catenin signaling activation. These initial events are based on the attachment of the Wnt ligand to the Frizzled (FZD) receptor. Further, a co-receptor (LRP) and the cytoplasmic protein Dishevelled (DVL) bind together to form a Wnt-FZD-LRP-DVL complex, which leads to downstream effects.

Figure 1B presents data on the expression of the essential elements of the nuclear part of canonical Wnt signal transduction, especially β-catenin and CREB binding protein (CBP). PRI-724, the small-molecule inhibitor of the Wnt/β-catenin pathway used in this study, blocks the interaction between β-catenin and CBP, which is crucial for their transcriptional activity. A complex of β-catenin and CBP binds to and activates transcription factors (TCF1, TCF3, TCF4, LEF1) and promotes the expression of canonical Wnt signaling target genes, e.g., the anti-apoptotic survivin (*BIRC5*) and claudin 1 (*CLDN1*)—a component of tight junction complexes.

In general, the expression of Wnt/β-catenin pathway-related genes was higher in HNSCC samples than in normal epithelium samples and showed growth with the increase in tumor grade. This suggests that the progression of HNSCC relies on the elevated activity of Wnt/β-catenin signaling. Thus, in this study, the inhibition of the Wnt/β-catenin pathway was considered the central and starting point of co-treatment strategies of HNSCC cells with combinations of PRI-724 and inhibitors targeting other molecular pathways.

2.2. Vismodegib and PRI-724 Reduce the Viability of CAL 27 and FaDu Cells

We performed the resazurin assay to establish the influence of vismodegib, an inhibitor of the Hedgehog pathway, on the viability of CAL 27 cells (tongue cancer) and FaDu cells (hypopharyngeal cancer). The sub-toxic effect (IC25) was reached for both CAL 27 and FaDu cells at a similar level. However, at concentrations above 20 µM CAL 27 cells were more sensitive to vismodegib in comparison to FaDu cells (Figure 2A).

In the same assay, PRI-724 showed similar effects on both tongue and hypopharynx cancer cells. However, around the IC50 value, once again, CAL 27 cells were more affected than FaDu cells (Figure 2B).

Table 1 shows the concentrations of vismodegib and PRI-724, which reduced cell viability by 25% (IC25) or by 50% (IC50) in CAL 27 and FaDu cells. The IC25 and IC50 values for erlotinib and HS-173 were established in our previous research [6] and are also shown in Table 1 with an asterisk.

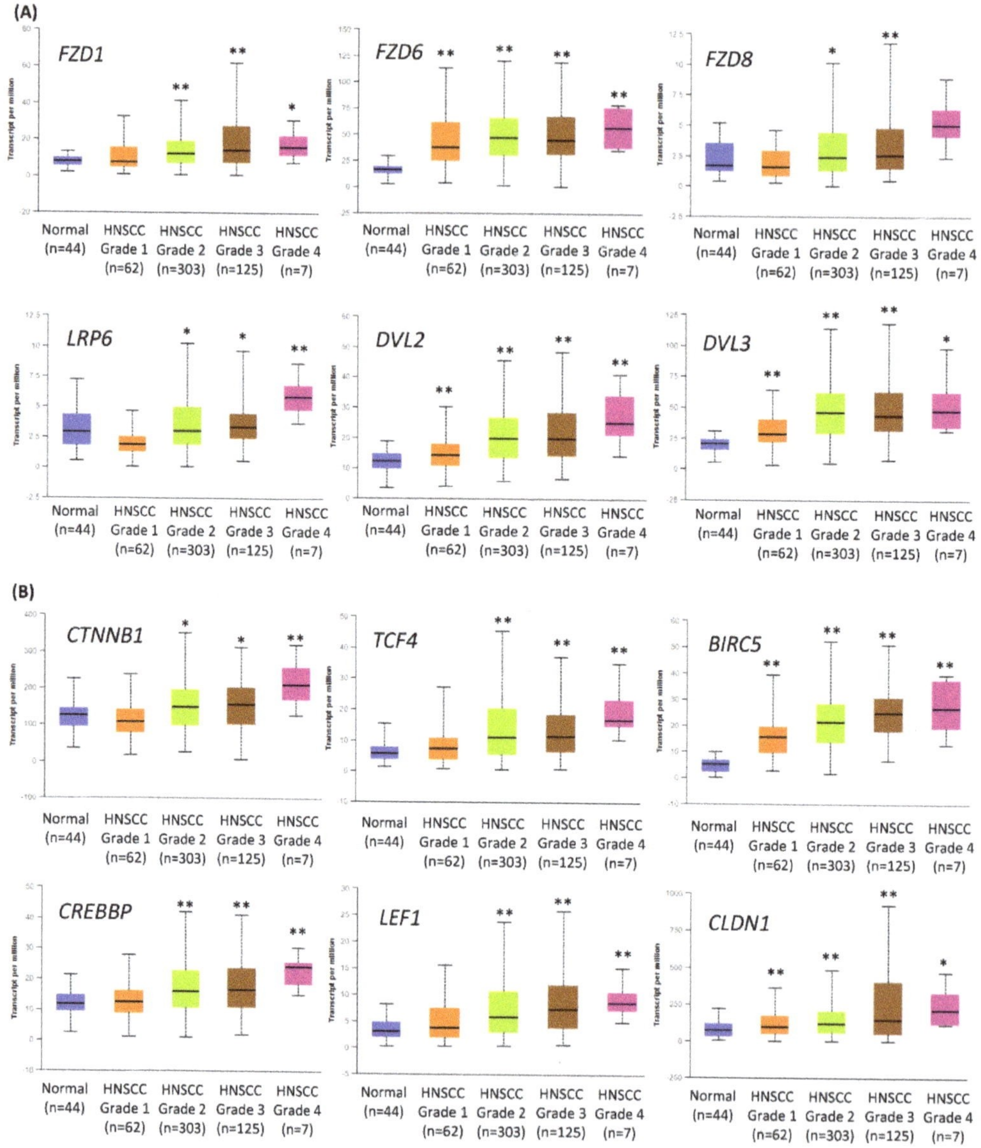

Figure 1. The results of the analysis of Wnt/β-catenin pathway-related gene expression data available from The Cancer Genome Atlas using the UALCAN tool. The differences in the level of gene expression depending on tumor grade (grade 1—well-differentiated, grade 4—undifferentiated), compared with normal epithelium, are shown. The asterisk (*) above the bar denotes statistically significant changes in comparison to normal control samples, * $p < 0.05$, ** $p < 0.01$. (**A**) Exemplary genes related to the transduction of the signal from Wnt ligand to cytoplasm: Frizzled receptors (*FZD1*, *FZD6*, *FZD8*), *LRP6* co-receptor, and cytoplasmic protein Dishevelled (*DVL2*, *DVL3*) that relays Wnt signals from receptors to downstream effectors. (**B**) Genes related to the nucleic part of Wnt signal transduction: β-catenin (*CTNNB1*) creating complexes with CREB binding protein (*CREBBP*), exemplary transcription factors (transcription factor 4—*TCF4*, lymphoid enhancer binding factor 1—*LEF1*), and target genes of Wnt/β-catenin pathway (survivin—*BIRC5*, claudin 1—*CLDN1*).

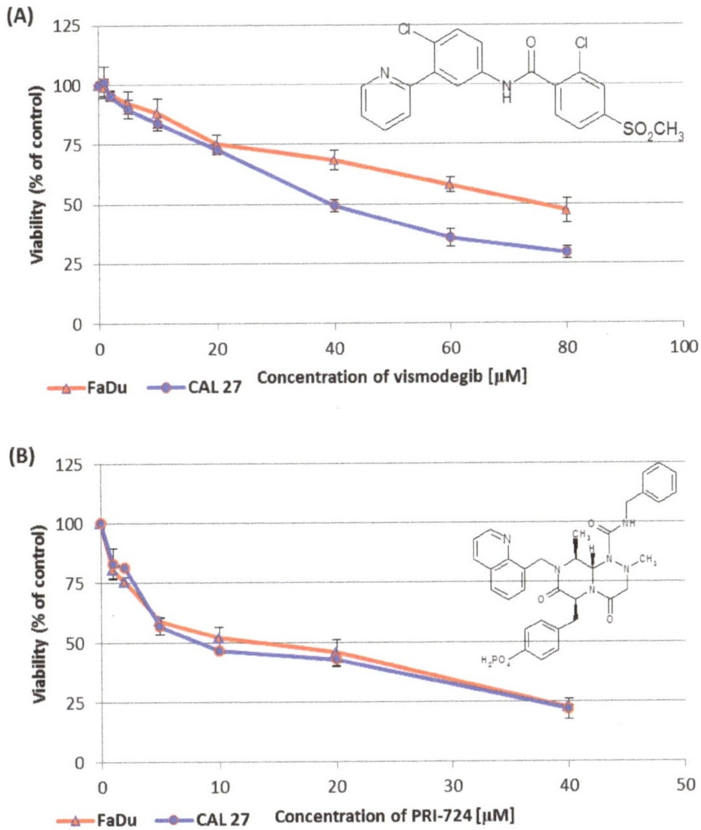

Figure 2. The effect of vismodegib (**A**) and PRI-724 (**B**) on the viability of CAL 27 and FaDu cells after 48 h of incubation, as determined by the resazurin assay. The chemical structure of the compounds is also presented. The results are the mean values from three independent experiments with four technical repeats ± SD.

Table 1. The IC25 and IC50 values for CAL 27 and FaDu cells based on the resazurin assay.

Compound	CAL 27		FaDu	
	IC25 [μM]	IC50 [μM]	IC25 [μM]	IC50 [μM]
PRI-724	2.6	8.3	2.1	14.6
vismodegib	18.0	39.4	21.0	74.8
erlotinib	0.3 *	2.9 *	0.6 *	7.0 *
HS-173	0.09 *	0.2 *	0.125 *	0.8 *

* IC25 and IC50 values determined by the resazurin assay and previously reported [6].

2.3. *Combinations of PRI-724 with Other Inhibitors Present Better Synergistic Effects in FaDu Cells*

In this research, we wanted to compare the effects of the inhibition of Wnt canonical signaling by PRI-724 with the inhibitors of three other important pathways—Hedgehog, EGFR, and PI3K. Firstly, we evaluated the effects of the combinations of inhibitors on the viability of CAL 27 and FaDu cells. Detailed information about the concentrations and proportions of chemicals as well as the effects on viability reduction can be found in Supplementary Table S1.

The collected data were analyzed using the CompuSyn software, version 1.0 (downloaded from the website www.combosyn.com on 31 May 2021). This software can be used to calculate single-drug and drug-combined pharmacodynamics. The unique mathematical system analysis for dose-effect dynamics led to the discovery of the median-effect equation (MEE), the unified biodynamics, pharmacodynamics, and bioinformatics general principle. This unified dynamics algorithm allows using a few dose data points to create an automated quantitative simulation, unlike the traditional, expensive experimental approach that uses many dose data points to fit an empirical curve.

The results of analyses refer to the 'Combination Index' (CI). There are three general conclusions concerning the CI value. CI = 1 denotes that the experimental result of the drug combination compared to the effects of individually used compounds is additional (additive effect). A CI value below 1 reflects better experimental effects than just the mathematically calculated addition of single compound activity and is called synergism. Conversely, a CI above 1 suggests the loss of some of the effects associated with the action of individual compounds (antagonism).

When the proportions between concentrations of mixed compounds are changeable, only the CI for a particular mixture can be calculated. However, when this proportion is stable, e.g., 1:1, CompuSyn software creates plots showing CI (the character of interaction) in a broad concentration range, extrapolating experimental data. On the 0X axis, the parameter 'fraction affected' (Fa) is used. Fa means the intensity of the effect, in this case, the reduction of cell viability. Fa = 0 denotes a lack of viability reduction, and Fa = 1 is a synonym for total cell death.

We showed dose–effect curves for individual PRI-724 and vismodegib, which were evaluated by the CompuSyn software for the first time (Figure 3A). Figure 3B presents dose-effect curves for PRI-724 combined with either vismodegib, erlotinib, or HS-173. The Combination Index calculated for each mixture in the form of plots showing the character of interaction between two inhibitors in the function of Fa is shown in Figure 3C.

Based on the analysis of the interaction between the compounds, it can be stated that the combination of PRI-724 and HS-173 synergistically reduced the viability of FaDu cells (Figure 3C). In other cases, synergism was detected for a part of the effect range. Two mixtures in FaDu cells needed higher concentrations of compounds to reach synergistic effects, namely, Fa > 0.45 for the combination with vismodegib and Fa > 0.50 for the combination with erlotinib. In CAL 27 cells, the best results were observed for the mixture of PRI-724 and erlotinib, where synergism appeared for Fa > 0.30. In turn, data for the combinations of PRI-724 with vismodegib (Fa < 0.80) and HS-173 (Fa < 0.70) suggest weak synergism below the indicated Fa.

In all further experiments, we used the concentrations of compounds presented in Table 1.

2.4. *Signaling Inhibitors Affect Proliferation Mostly by Cell Cycle Arrest in the G1/G0 Phase*

We performed an analysis of the cell cycle distribution of CAL 27 and FaDu cells to establish the possible influence of mixtures of chemicals on the induction of cell cycle arrest (Figure 4). In CAL 27 cells (Figure 4A), PRI-724 at IC25 and both concentrations of vismodegib induced the accumulation of cells in the G1/G0 phase. The same effect was observed previously for erlotinib [6]. Interestingly, the treatment of cells with PRI-724 at IC50 caused the opposite effect, i.e., the reduction of the G1/G0 population of CAL 27 cells. Such a result was also present in PRI-724 at IC50 combined with vismodegib at IC25, suggesting that the activity of Wnt/β-catenin inhibitor was dominant. However, both mixtures of erlotinib and PRI-724 were able to arrest cells in G1/G0 phases.

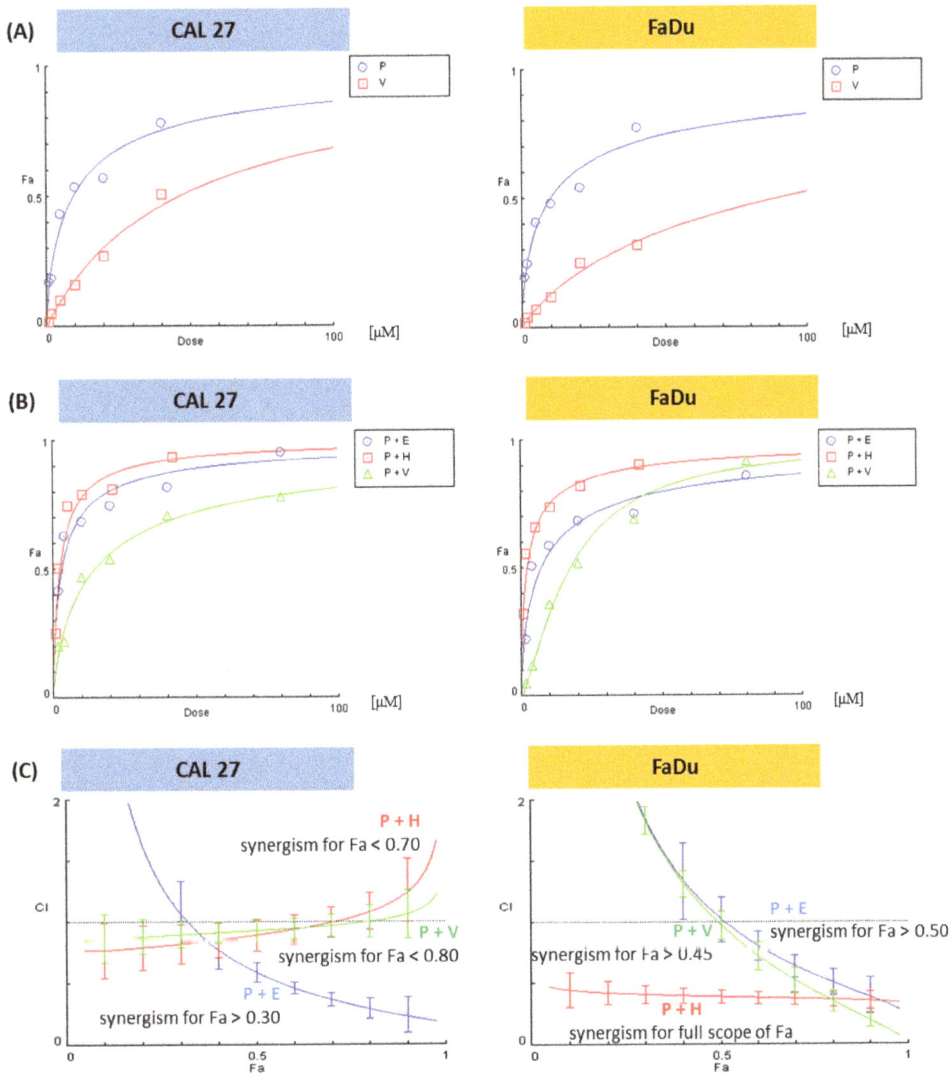

Figure 3. The results of the analysis of the combinatorial effects between PRI-724 and vismodegib, erlotinib, or HS-173 on cell viability by the resazurin assay. CAL 27 and FaDu cells were treated with increasing concentrations (Supplementary Table S1) of the individual compounds and their combinations for 48 h. Control cells were treated with vehicle (DMSO). Mean values from three independent experiments were used in calculations using the CompuSyn software (version 1.0). Dose-effect curves for individual compounds (**A**) or their combinations (**B**) were generated. Plots (**C**) represent the evaluation of the Combination Index (CI), where CI < 1 (the area below the dotted line in plots) denotes a synergistic effect between compounds. Fa—Fraction affected: viability reduction from lack of effect (0) to maximal effect (1; viability = 0%), E—erlotinib, H—HS-173, P—PRI-724, V—vismodegib.

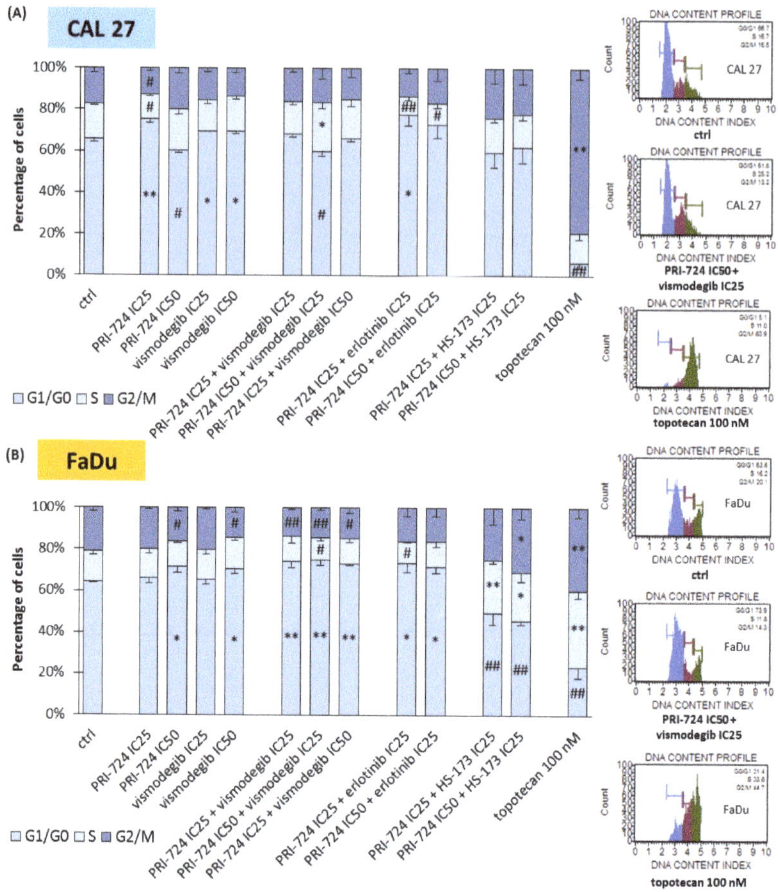

Figure 4. The effect of PRI-724, vismodegib, erlotinib, HS-173, and their combinations on the cell cycle distribution in CAL 27 (**A**) and FaDu (**B**) cells after 48 h of incubation. The cell cycle distribution (G1/G0, S, and G2/M phases) was measured by flow cytometric analysis of cells after propidium iodide staining. DMSO-vehicle-treated cells were used as a negative control, while topotecan (100 nM) was used as a positive control for cell cycle arrest. Exemplary flow cytometry plots are shown on the right side. Mean values ± SD from three independent experiments are shown. The asterisk (*) inside the bars denotes a statistically significant increase in cell population between the analyzed compound used alone or in combination, and the control (ctrl), * $p < 0.05$, ** $p < 0.01$; (#) inside the bars denotes a statistically significant decrease in cell population between the analyzed compound used alone or in combination, and the control (ctrl), # $p < 0.05$, ## $p < 0.01$.

The accumulation of FaDu cells in G1/G0 phases was the main effect for all the combinations of PRI-724 with vismodegib and erlotinib (Figure 4B). A significant change for individually used PRI-724 or vismodegib was found only at IC50 concentrations. Surprisingly, mixtures of PRI-724 with HS-173 significantly reduced the G1/G0 population of cells with the concomitant accumulation of cells in S and/or G2/M phases, although HS-173 at IC25 [6] and PRI-724 at IC25 individually had no effect or even showed the opposite effect, like in the case of PRI-724 at IC50.

2.5. Combinations of PRI-724 with Erlotinib or HS-173 Exert Better Pro-Apoptotic Effects

In the next step, we evaluated whether the changes in cell cycle distribution were also followed by the induction of apoptosis (Figure 5). Both CAL 27 and FaDu cells were susceptible to a slight induction of apoptosis after individual exposure to PRI-724 and vismodegib, except PRI-724 at IC25 in CAL 27 cells. The same scale of action was previously observed for erlotinib and HS-173 [6]. The combination of PRI-724 with vismodegib failed to improve the effects. In turn, combinations of PRI-724 with erlotinib and HS-173 enriched the population of apoptotic cells. Discrimination between early and late phases of apoptosis points to the appearance of the early stages of apoptosis after 48 h of incubation with the evaluated compounds, including a 100 nM concentration of topotecan—the positive control for apoptosis.

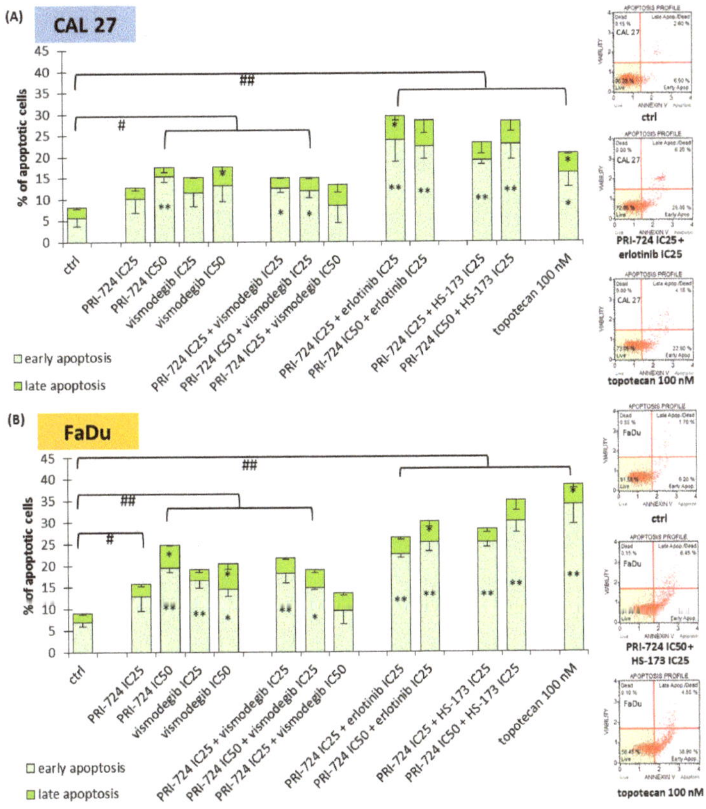

Figure 5. The effect of PRI-724, vismodegib, erlotinib, HS-173, and their combinations on the induction of apoptosis in CAL 27 (**A**) and FaDu (**B**) cells after 48 h of incubation. The apoptotic cells were detected by flow cytometric analysis after Annexin V and 7-Aminoactinomycin D staining. DMSO-vehicle-treated cells were used as a negative control, while topotecan (100 nM) was used as a positive control for apoptosis induction. Exemplary flow cytometry plots are shown on the right side. Mean values ± SD from three independent experiments are shown. The asterisk (*) inside the bars denotes a statistically significant increase in cell population between the analyzed compound used alone or in combination, and the control (ctrl) for early or late apoptotic cells, * $p < 0.05$, ** $p < 0.01$; (#) above the bars denotes a statistically significant increase in total apoptotic cells between the analyzed compound used alone or in combination, and the control (ctrl), # $p < 0.05$, ## $p < 0.01$.

2.6. PRI-724 Combined with Vismodegib or Erlotinib Synergistically Reduced Cell Migration

Besides cell cycle arrest and the induction of apoptosis, the inhibition of signaling pathways can reduce the migration rate of cancer cells. We introduced the scratch assay to check the potential benefits of combining PRI-724 with other inhibitors (Figure 6).

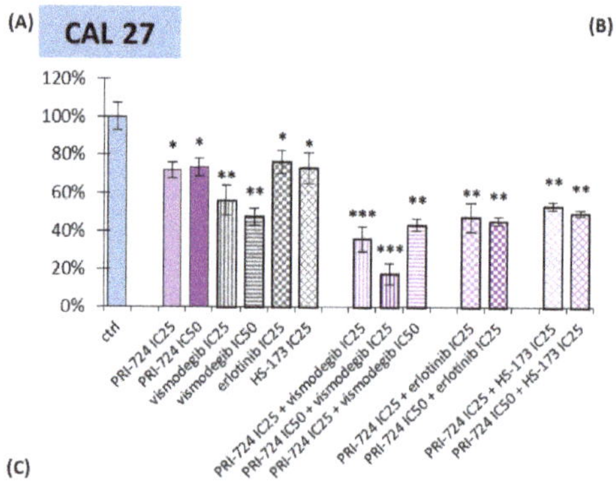

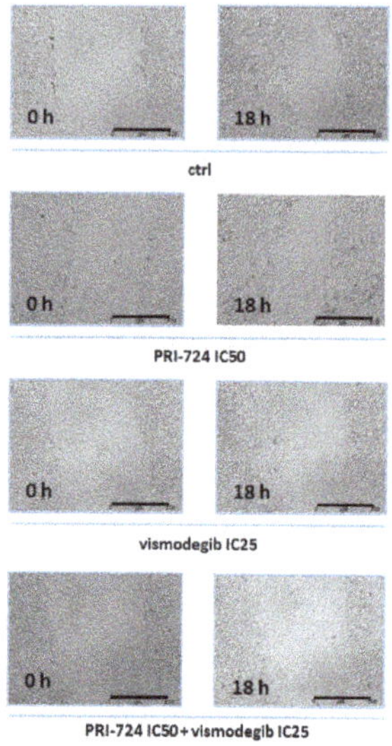

(C)

Interaction (CAL 27 cells)	vismodegib IC25	vismodegib IC50	erlotinib IC25	HS-173 IC25
PRI-724 IC25	1.07 (addition)	0.86 (addition)	1.17 (synergism)	1.15 (addition)
PRI-724 IC50	1.40 (synergism)	X	1.25 (synergism)	1.09 (addition)

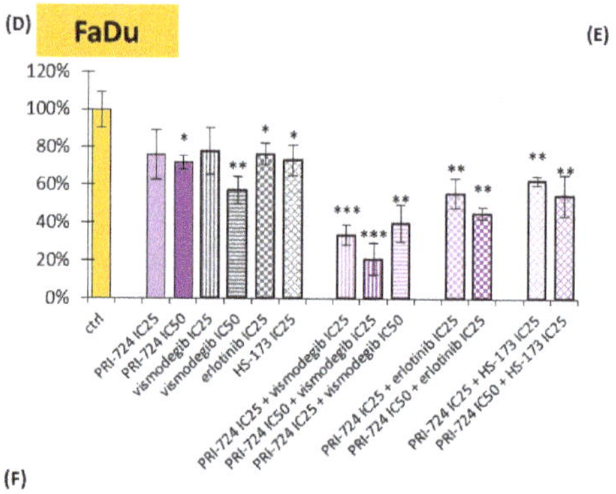

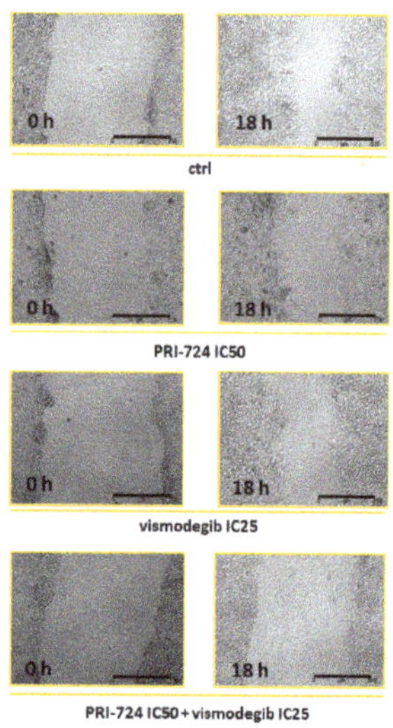

(F)

Interaction (FaDu cells)	vismodegib IC25	vismodegib IC50	erlotinib IC25	HS-173 IC25
PRI-724 IC25	1.62 (synergism)	1.07 (addition)	1.05 (addition)	0.85 (addition)
PRI-724 IC50	1.78 (synergism)	X	1.21 (synergism)	0.95 (addition)

Figure 6. The scratch assay (cell migration) was performed for PRI-724, vismodegib, erlotinib, HS-173, and their combinations in CAL 27 (**A–C**) and FaDu (**D–F**) cells. Results (mean values ± SD) were calculated from four experiments (**A**,**D**). The asterisk (*) above the bars denotes a statistically significant decrease in migration rate between the analyzed compound used alone or in combination, and the control (ctrl), * $p < 0.05$, ** $p < 0.01$, *** $p < 0.001$. Exemplary microscopic images of the scratch, which were taken at the beginning and after 18 h of incubation with the compounds, are shown (**B**,**E**). The scale bar represents 500 µm. The assessment of the type of interaction between compounds using the modified Bürgi formula is shown (**C**,**F**). The addition of effects ($0.85 \leq q \leq 1.15$) is highlighted in yellow, while synergistic effects ($q > 1.15$) are highlighted in green.

All individually used compounds decreased cell migration in both CAL 27 and FaDu cells, except PRI-724 and vismodegib at IC25 concentrations in FaDu cells (Figure 6D). Notably, strong effects, with a >40% reduction in migration rate, were detected for vismodegib. Mixtures of chemicals significantly decreased the migration of CAL 27 and FaDu cells. Excellent results, with a reduction of approximately 80%, were obtained for the combination of PRI-724 at IC50 with vismodegib at IC25.

Next, we performed an analysis of the type of interaction between chemicals with regard to their effect on cell migration (Figure 6C,F). PRI-724 mixed with vismodegib or erlotinib had a synergistic effect on cell migration, most prominently in the case of the mixture with vismodegib at IC25 in FaDu cells (Figure 6F). The single use of vismodegib IC50 presented a beneficial effect, and its combination with PRI-724 IC25 led to only additive inhibition of migration. Similarly, the mixture of PRI-724 and HS-173 showed additive effects.

2.7. *ALDH1A1, SOX2, and POU5F1 Genes Were Differentially Expressed among HNSCC Patients*

Cancer stem cells (CSCs) play an important role in tumor development, survival, recurrence, and metastasis. Thus, we retrieved data from The Cancer Genome Atlas (TCGA) and analyzed the expression profile of ALDH1 (*ALDH1A1*), SOX2 (*SOX2*), and OCT4 (*POU5F1*) genes related to CSC in HNSCC, using the UALCAN tool [24,25]. Transcript levels were compared between HNSCC cases (n = 520) and normal epithelium samples (n = 44). The expression of *ALDH1A1* and *SOX2* was significantly lower in the population of HNSCC patients, but *POU5F1* showed upregulation (Figure 7A).

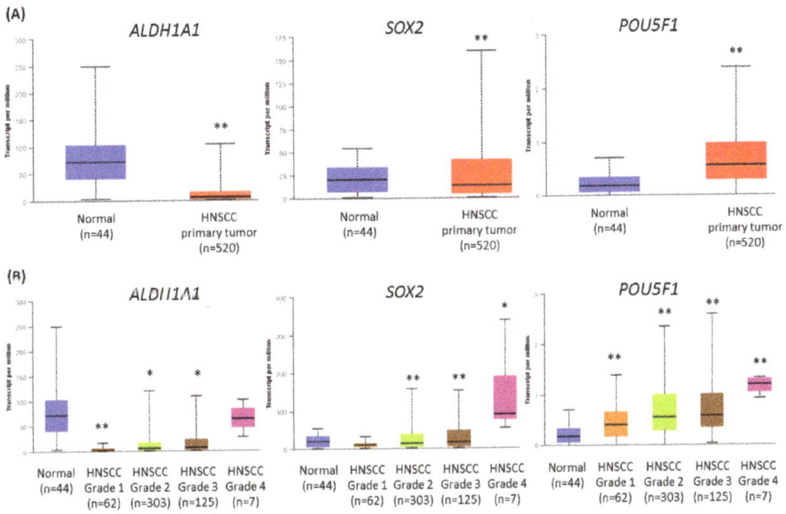

Figure 7. The results of the analysis of *ALDH1A1*, *SOX2*, and *POU5F1* gene expression data available from The Cancer Genome Atlas using the UALCAN tool. (**A**) The comparison of the level of expression between normal epithelium and HNSCC tumor samples. (**B**) The differences in the level of gene expression in relation to tumor grade (grade 1—well-differentiated, grade 4—undifferentiated), compared with normal epithelium. The asterisk (*) above the bar denotes statistically significant changes in comparison to normal control samples, * $p < 0.05$, ** $p < 0.01$.

Next, we analyzed the differences in gene expression levels depending on tumor grade (Figure 7B). The transcript level of *ALDH1* was strongly reduced in grade 1 tumors, and in grade 4, the level was similar to normal tissue. The expression of *SOX2* was significantly lower in grades 2 and 3, and upregulated in grade 4. Finally, the transcript level of *OCT4* gradually increased from grade 1 to grade 4 tumors. In general, the expression of CSC-related genes was higher in histologically more advanced HNSCC cases, where the role of CSC is probably increasing.

2.8. Vismodegib Effectively Reduced the Expression of Cancer Stem Cells-Related Genes in CAL27 and FaDu Cells

Wnt and Hedgehog signaling pathways have an influence on the CSC population and can control each other's activities. Thus, we decided to compare the activity of Wnt and Hedgehog pathway inhibitors against the *ALDH1A1*, *SOX2*, and *POU5F1* genes.

On the one side, PRI-724 upregulated the expression of *ALDH1A1* and *SOX2* in CAL 27 cells (Figure 8A) and *SOX2* in FaDu cells (Figure 8B). In other cases, there was no significant change. On the other side, vismodegib in one or both concentrations was able to decrease the expression of the evaluated genes, with the exception of *ALDH1A1* in FaDu cells.

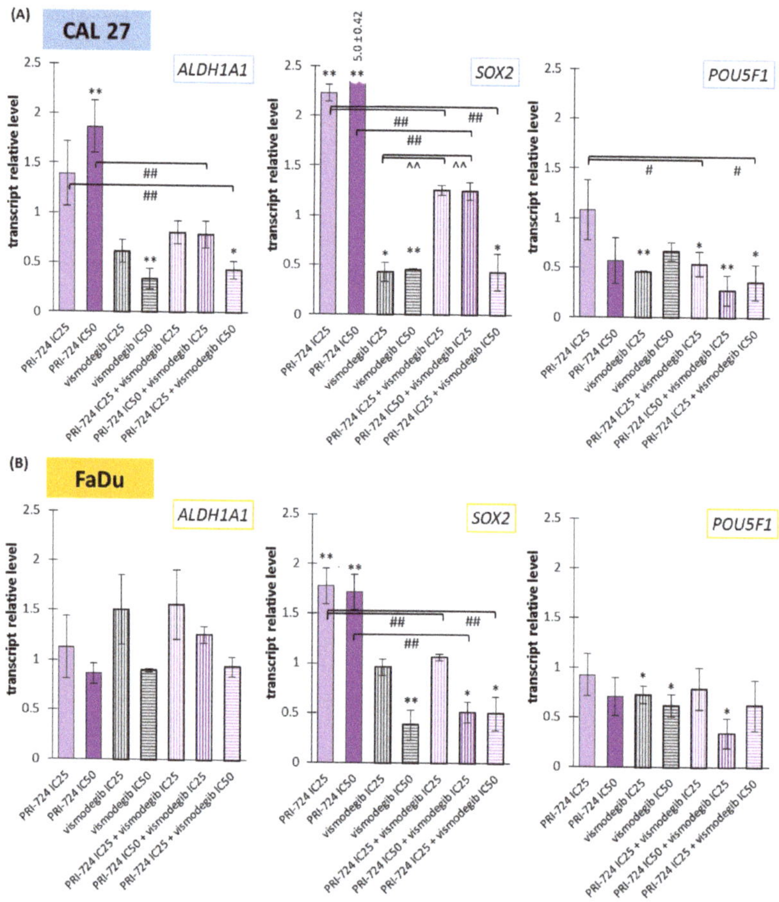

Figure 8. The effect of PRI-724 and vismodegib on the relative transcript levels of *ALDH1A1*, *SOX2*, and *POU5F1* genes in CAL 27 (**A**) and FaDu (**B**) cells. Mean values ± SD from three independent experiments with three replicates per R-T PCR reaction are shown. The level of DMSO-treated cells was considered to be 1. The asterisk (*) above the bar denotes statistically significant changes in comparison to control (* $p < 0.05$, ** $p < 0.01$), (#) denotes statistically significant changes in comparison to PRI-724 (# $p < 0.05$, ## $p < 0.01$), and (^) denotes statistically significant changes in comparison to vismodegib (^^ $p < 0.01$).

The expression of *ALDH1A1* was unchanged in FaDu cells, but in CAL27 cells, a reduction was present for the mixture of PRI-724 IC25 and vismodegib IC50. Two other combinations represented balanced effects on gene expression, i.e., between an induced level for PRI-724 and a decreased level for vismodegib. The co-treatment of CAL27 cells with PRI-724 IC25 and vismodegib IC50 decreased the expression of *SOX2* compared to the control. Due to intensively upregulated expression of *SOX2* under the influence of PRI-724 and significantly downregulated expression after vismodegib treatment, mixtures of PRI-724 in both concentrations with vismodegib IC25 resulted in an intermediate level of expression. However, the effect of vismodegib IC50 was dominant in mixtures. For FaDu cells, the effects of combinations were similar to those seen for vismodegib alone, but the mixture of PRI-724 IC50 with vismodegib IC25 presented the opposite action compared to PRI-724 used individually.

Finally, *POU5F1* expression was downregulated by approximately 70% after exposure of CAL 27 and FaDu cells to PRI-724 IC50 and vismodegib IC25.

3. Discussion

Molecularly targeted therapy based on the inhibition of EGFR signaling did not meet expectations for the improvement of the clinical fate of patients with HNSCC [26]. Thus, new potential targets have been intensively searched for. Wnt canonical signaling is considered a potential target, due to various genetic and epigenetic dysregulations affecting its activity, which are found in HNSCC cells, also at pre-clinical stages [8,10,27]. The inhibition of the nuclear interaction between CBP acetyltransferase and β-catenin translocated from the cytoplasm to the nucleus was described in our previous research as the best way to target this pathway [15]. Particularly, a small-molecule PRI-724 inhibitor was tested. Others have also reported the beneficial effects of this chemical. PRI-724 showed positive results in early-stage clinical trials with advanced ovarian cancer or pancreatic adenocarcinoma patients. Moreover, it showed therapeutic potential in soft tissue sarcomas, leading to a reduction in cancer cell viability, disruption of cell cycle progression, and promotion of apoptosis in pre-clinical tests [28]. Results from the same study also pointed to the synergistic activity of the combination of PRI-724 with standard chemotherapeutics such as doxorubicin or trabectedin. In other research, PRI-724 blocked the proliferation and formation of fibrolamellar hepatocellular carcinoma organoids [29]. In addition, the antitumor properties of PRI-724 were found in the cisplatin-resistant human embryonal carcinoma NTERA-2 cells [30] or in the human neuroendocrine tumor BON1, QCP-1, and NCI-H727 cells [31]. In acute myeloid leukemia, the *FLT3* gene (which encodes a class III receptor tyrosine kinase that regulates hematopoiesis) is frequently mutated, and *FLT3*-mutant cells are able to promote the Wnt/β-catenin pathway by activating Integrin αvβ3/PI3K/Akt/GSK-3β signaling [32]. The inhibition of FLT3 signaling by sorafenib or quizartinib with the concomitant use of PRI-724 to block the transcriptional activity of β-catenin improved the effects against acute myeloid leukemia stem cells [33]. Indeed, monotherapy based on PRI-724 and other Wnt pathway inhibitors is insufficient in molecularly diverse tumor cells, and thus PRI-724 should rather be combined with chemicals affecting other molecular targets.

Targeting the Wnt/β-catenin pathway exerted better effects in HPV-positive than in HPV-negative HNSCC tumors, in which a combinatorial treatment could have more prominent effects [34]. Interestingly, stronger anti-neoplastic and radiosensitizing effects of β-catenin inhibition were shown in HPV-negative cells, but greater anti-migratory potential was detected in HPV-positive HNSCC cells [35]. The different profiles of action against HPV-positive and HPV-negative cancer cells might be related to the diverse molecular features of these etiologically distinct groups of tumors [36]. Moreover, we also detected therapeutic crosstalk between PI3K/Akt/GSK-3β signaling and the Wnt pathway in HNSCC. In this regard, the mixture of an Akt kinase inhibitor together with either a Porcupine inhibitor (IWP-O1) or an inhibitor of CBP/β-catenin interaction (PRI-724) potentiated cell viability reduction in tongue SCC cells growing in 3D-culture as spheroids [37].

Wnt signaling is one of the master regulators of stem cells during embryogenesis and in selected adult tissues, but also during carcinogenesis [38]. Indeed, targeting cancer stem cells by inhibiting the Wnt canonical pathway is one of the possibilities to cure colorectal cancer [39], but obviously it should also be tested in all Wnt signaling-dependent tumors. Hedgehog (Hh) signaling is another pathway controlling SC and CSC [38,39]. Since 2012, vismodegib, an inhibitor of the Hh pathway, has been registered for the treatment of basal cell carcinoma (BCC) [23]. Although BCC and HNSCC are different types of tumors, some molecular similarities can be observed. In a case of sporadic BCC in an 80-year-old man, both Wnt and Hh signaling pathways were overexpressed [40]. In addition, the insulin-like growth factor 2 mRNA-binding protein 1 (IGF2BP1), a target gene of Wnt signaling, was overexpressed and further promoted the transcription level of Gli1, a transcription factor in the Hh pathway. More than twenty years ago, Mullor et al. (2001) described the ability of Gli1 to activate the expression of several Wnt ligands in early frog embryos [41]. Moreover, in RTOG10 cells, Gli1 induced the transformation of epithelial cells via the induction of Snail, a repressor of E-cadherin, which released β-catenin from the cell membrane compartment and induced its translocation to the cell nucleus [42].

Interactions between Wnt and Hh pathways and their special role in cancer stem cells were the basis of the idea to evaluate the effects of the simultaneous treatment of HNSCC cells by PRI-724 and vismodegib. Targeting EGFR and related signaling pathways led to limited effects against HNSCC [3]. For this reason, we previously performed experiments on CAL 27 and FaDu cells to test the effects of erlotinib (an EGFR inhibitor) and HS-173 (a PI3K kinase inhibitor) separately and in combination with inhibitors of KDM4 and KDM6 histone demethylases [6]. Individual compounds had limited influence, e.g., on the induction of apoptosis. However, cell death was synergistically potentiated after the addition of KDM inhibitors. In the current study, we used erlotinib and HS-173 in mixtures with PRI-724 to compare their effects with the anti-neoplastic influence of the combined use of PRI-724 and vismodegib. Importantly, recent studies have shown that PRI-724, vismodegib, and erlotinib were less active in non-cancerous HaCaT keratinocytes, suggesting some selectivity of these chemicals towards cancer cells [43–45].

The sensitivity of tongue cancer-derived CAL 27 cells and hypopharyngeal cancer-derived FaDu cells to Wnt and Hh pathway inhibitors was similar at sub-toxic concentrations (IC25). In turn, lower concentrations of both chemicals were needed to reach a 50% reduction in viability in CAL 27 cells compared to FaDu cells. Interestingly, the combination of PRI-724 and vismodegib had a rather weak synergistic effect on CAL 27 cells viability, while this combination of compounds at higher concentrations showed synergism in FaDu cells. Thus, hypopharyngeal tumor cells were more susceptible to the dual inhibition of Wnt and Hh signaling. A similar correlation was seen for the mixture of PRI-724 and erlotinib, whereas PRI-724 and the PI3K kinase inhibitor HS-173 acted highly synergistically in the full range of concentrations.

The incubation of CAL 27 and FaDu cells with vismodegib for 48 h resulted in the enrichment of the G1/G0 population of cells with a concomitant slight induction of the percentage of apoptotic cells. These results are generally consistent with the data generated by Freitas et al. (2020). They compared the effects of Hh pathway inhibitors vismodegib and itraconazole and conventional chemotherapeutics doxorubicin (DOX) and 5-fluorouracil (5-FU) used individually. Uncombined vismodegib clearly reduced the viability of CAL 27 cells after 48 h of incubation, but pro-apoptotic and anti-proliferative effects were much weaker than in the case of DOX and 5-FU [46].

The effectiveness of vismodegib was previously assessed in the basal cell carcinoma line BCC-1 and in the tongue cancer line SCC-25 in combination with irradiation. In both cellular models, the treatment resulted in reduced cell proliferation and radiosensitization [47]. In another study, vismodegib mixed with docetaxel, cisplatin, or cetuximab additively enhanced the anti-neoplastic effects in HNSCC samples derived ex vivo [48]. In our study, mixtures of the Wnt/β-catenin pathway inhibitor with vismodegib caused the accumulation of hypopharyngeal cancer cells in G1/G0 phases. In CAL 27 cells, the combination of PRI-724 IC50 and vismodegib IC25 enriched rather S phase cells, similarly to the sole use of PRI-724 IC50. A more significant induction of apoptosis appeared upon individual exposure of cells to PRI-724 and vismodegib, and this effect was lost in the mixture with vismodegib at higher concentrations. We can assume that the combination of Wnt and Hh signaling inhibition has better anti-proliferative than pro-apoptotic effects. A higher induction of apoptosis was detected in the other tested groups. PRI-724 combined with erlotinib or HS-173 presented a significant increase in apoptotic cell populations, although its individual use had rather low efficacy [6]. In cell cycle analysis, erlotinib had a dominant influence in combination with PRI-724. However, despite no effect of individually applied HS-173, its combination with PRI-724 was able to block cell cycle in S and G2/M phases in FaDu cells. Because of the synergistic effect on the reduction of viability and the highest induction of apoptotic death of HNSCC cells (among the evaluated combinations), the simultaneous disruption of Wnt and PI3K pathways seems to be an interesting option for further research in the field of pharyngeal SCC tumors.

The inhibition of signaling pathways may also have an influence on cell migration. Thus, we performed the scratch assay for all the tested inhibitors used individually and in combinations. CAL 27 and FaDu cells were susceptible to the reduction of migration rate, and vismodegib demonstrated better activity than the other chemicals. In contrast, the inhibition was not so significant in lung SCC H1703 and H12170 cells [49]. Furthermore, co-treatment of HNSCC cells with Wnt and Hh, EGFR, or PI3K inhibitors significantly reduced their migration. PRI-724 with vismodegib at a lower concentration (IC25) exerted a highly synergistic reduction of migration rate, especially in FaDu cells. Therefore, although the joint inhibition of Wnt/β-catenin and Hh signaling is unable to strongly induce cell death, it can intensively affect HNSCC proliferation and migration. In addition, PRI-724 with erlotinib also acted in a synergistic way. Thus, the potential of EGFR inhibitors in HNSCC tumors can still be improved.

In HNSCC tumors, cancer stem cells are present and can be detected by increased expression of, e.g., ALDH1 (*ALDH1A1* gene), SOX2 (*SOX2* gene), and OCT4 (*POU5F1* gene) [50–52]. We checked the expression levels of these genes among HNSCC patients based on data available from The Cancer Genome Atlas. We observed a decreased mRNA level for ALDH1 and SOX2, but an increased transcript level for OCT4. Moreover, advanced grade 4 tumors (potentially richer in the CSC population) showed the highest expression of those genes. SOX2 and OCT4 mRNA expression was increased compared to normal tissue. We assumed that in cancer cells, which contain a sub-population of CSC, the downregulation of CSC markers should be more visible in the case of over-expressed transcripts, like OCT4 mRNA. We wanted to preliminary check if Wnt/β-catenin and/or Hedgehog signaling inhibitors are able to modulate the transcript level of those CSC-related genes in CAL 27 and FaDu cells. Indeed, in FaDu cells, *ALDH1A1* lacked any significant changes. Surprisingly, incubation with the Wnt signaling inhibitor induced the expression of those CSC markers, but in contrast, the inhibition of Hh decreased their transcript level. The opposite effect for PRI-724 probably results from differences in time to evoke and sustain molecular changes after Wnt or Hh pathway inhibition. Hypothetically, gene expression upregulation after exposure to PRI-724 might be a secondary effect after the initial decrease in expression because, in other research, CBP/β-catenin targeting had inhibitory effects in lung cancer stem cells [53]. However, the gene encoding the OCT4 protein, which was overexpressed in patient-derived samples, was importantly downregulated in response to single and combined inhibitors. The expression of OCT4 is directly regulated by β-catenin in HNSCC stem-like cells, and higher levels of both OCT4 and β-catenin correlate with the worst prognosis for patients [54], so our results from CAL 27 and FaDu cells point to beneficial effects of the applied combination of inhibitors. Vismodegib was shown to reduce OCT4 (*POU5F1*) expression in biliary tract cancer Mz-ChA-1 and Sk-ChA-1 cells [55]. What is noteworthy is that in our study, vismodegib potently counteracted the inducing effect of PRI-724 in relation to *ALDH1A1* and *SOX2* expression, and the combinations showed more beneficial effects. These results are in line with the synergistic effects of Wnt and Hh pathway co-inhibition with respect to cell migration, cell cycle disruption, and viability. However, in future studies, the direct impact of PRI-724 and vismodegib on the CSC subpopulation must be evaluated.

The balancing of the exerted effects and the potentialization of activity speak in favor of using the combinations of PRI-724 with not only vismodegib but also with erlotinib and HS-173, and they invite more detailed subsequent studies. It should also be remembered that the molecular landscape of cancer cells differs between patients and is dynamic. In the future, by working with, e.g., ex vivo cultured cancer cells derived from HNSCC patients, the different profiles/endotypes of tumors might be identified. Artificial neural network analysis [56] based on new data can help establish the association between tumor profiles and benefit from the combinations proposed in this article.

4. Materials and Methods

4.1. Cells and Culture Conditions

Commercially available HNSCC cells were used in the experiments: CAL 27 cells derived from tongue cancer and FaDu cells derived from hypopharyngeal cancer were both purchased from the American Type Culture Collection (ATCC).

The cells were grown in high-glucose DMEM medium (Biowest, Nuaillé, France), supplemented with 10% FBS (EURx, Gdańsk, Poland) and 1% antibiotic solution (penicillin and streptomycin; Biowest, Nuaillé, France), and were cultured under standard conditions (37 °C, 5% CO_2, 95% humidity) in an incubator (Memmert, Schwabach, Germany).

4.2. Chemicals and Cell Viability Assay

Four small-molecule inhibitors of signaling pathways were used in the research. The Wnt canonical signaling inhibitor PRI-724, the Hedgehog signaling inhibitor vismodegib, and the EGF receptor intracellular domain inhibitor erlotinib were ordered from Selleck Chemicals (Pittsburgh, PA, USA), while the inhibitor of the p110α domain of PI3K was purchased from Sigma-Aldrich (St. Louis, MO, USA). Stock solutions of the compounds were prepared in DMSO and stored in aliquots at −20 °C.

Cells (10^4/well) were seeded into black 96-well plates. After 24 h of pre-incubation, a fresh medium containing different concentrations of the compounds (single or in combination) was added. Control cells were treated with vehicle (DMSO < 0.2%). After 48 h, cells were washed with PBS buffer, and fresh medium containing 1 µg/mL resazurin (Sigma-Aldrich, St. Louis, MI, USA) was added. After 2 h of additional incubation, the fluorescence was measured (ex—530 nm, em—590 nm) using an Infinite M200 multiplate reader (Tecan, Grödig, Austria). Three independent experiments were performed, with four separate replicates per experiment.

The influence of the combination of PRI-724 inhibitor with other compounds in relation to cell viability was determined by the evaluation of the Combination Index (CI) using the CompuSyn software (downloaded from the website www.combosyn.com on 31 May 2021) [57]. The synergistic action of the chemicals in combinations was identified when CI < 1.

4.3. Analysis of the Cell Cycle Distribution

The effect of single compounds and combinations of PRI-724 with other inhibitors on cell cycle distribution was analyzed using the Muse® Cell Cycle Kit (Merck, Darmstadt, Germany) according to the manufacturer's protocol. Briefly, 2×10^5 cells per well were seeded in 6-well plates. After 24 h of pre-incubation, the growth medium was replaced with fresh medium (2 mL per well) containing IC25 and/or IC50 concentrations of the compounds, and the cells were incubated for an additional 48 h. The cells incubated with DMSO served as a negative control, while cells incubated with 100 nM topotecan (Sigma-Aldrich, St. Louis, MI, USA) served as a positive control for cell cycle arrest. After incubation, cells were collected by trypsinization, washed with PBS buffer, fixed in ice-cold 70% ethanol, and stored overnight at −20 °C. The next day, fixed cells were collected by centrifugation and washed with PBS buffer. The distribution of cells depending on cell cycle phase (G1/G0, S, G2/M) was analyzed with the Muse® Cell Analyzer (Merck, Darmstadt, Germany) after staining with propidium iodide solution in the presence of RNase A for 30 min. The data were analyzed using Muse® 1.5 Analysis software (Merck, Darmstadt, Germany). All the experiments were done in triplicate.

4.4. Analysis of Apoptosis

The externalization of phosphatidylserine was applied as a marker of apoptotic cells and analyzed using the Muse® Annexin V and Dead Cell Kit (Merck, Darmstadt, Germany) according to the manufacturer's protocol. The 7-aminoactinomycin D (7-AAD) stain was applied as a counterstain to Annexin V to discriminate between early and late apoptotic cells. Briefly, 2×10^5 cells per well were seeded in 6-well plates. After 24 h of pre-incubation, the growth medium was replaced with fresh medium (2 mL per well) containing IC25 and/or IC50 concentrations of the compounds, and the cells were incubated for an additional 48 h. The cells incubated with DMSO served as a negative control, while cells incubated with 100 nM topotecan (Sigma-Aldrich, St. Louis, MI, USA) served as a positive control for active apoptosis. Subsequently, the cells were collected and stained with Annexin V and 7-AAD in a culture medium solution. After 20 min of incubation, the cells were analyzed by flow cytometry on the Muse® Cell Analyzer (Merck, Darmstadt, Germany), and the data were further evaluated using Muse® 1.5 Analysis software (Merck, Darmstadt, Germany).

4.5. Analysis of Cell Migration Using the Scratch Wound Assay

Cell migration was assessed by the scratch assay. Cells (5×10^5) were seeded into 24-well plates and grown overnight to reach confluency. A scratch was performed using a 10 µL tip. Wells were rinsed twice with PBS buffer to remove detached cells, and fresh medium with a reduced FBS concentration (0.5%) containing IC25 and/or IC50 concentrations of the compounds was added. Subsequently, representative microscopic photographs of scratch areas were taken by a JuLI FL microscope (NanoEntek, Seoul, Republic of Korea) directly after the addition of compounds (0 h) and after 18 h. Area covered by cells (%) was assessed using JuLI FL software, and the difference in the coverage of the growth area by cells between 18 h and 0 h time points was calculated for each well. The experiment was repeated four times. The relative effect of the tested compounds on cell migration (*RM*) was calculated using the following formula:

$$RM = \frac{tested\ compound\ area\ after\ 18\ h - tested\ compound\ area\ after\ 0\ h}{negative\ control\ area\ after\ 18\ h - negative\ control\ area\ after\ 0\ h} \times 100\% \quad (1)$$

The combinatorial effects of the compounds on cell migration were evaluated using the modified Bürgi formula [58,59] in order to assess the type of interaction between chemicals used in IC25 and/or IC50 concentrations. The q factor was calculated using the equation:

$$q = \frac{P_{mix}}{(P_1 + P_2) - (P_1 \times P_2)} \quad (2)$$

where P_1 denotes the effect of PRI-724 treatment, P_2 denotes the effect of a second compound (vismodegib, erlotinib, or HS-173) treatment, and P_{mix} denotes the effect of a combination of chemicals. Antagonistic effects were detected when $q < 0.85$, while synergistic effects (potentiation of action) were detected when $q > 1.15$. The compounds were considered to act independently of each other (additive effects) if q was in the range 0.85–1.15.

4.6. Expression Analysis Based on TCGA

In Figures 1 and 7, we present the analysis of gene expression data available from The Cancer Genome Atlas (TCGA). We used the UALCAN tool (https://ualcan.path.uab.edu, accessed on 11 April 2023 and 7 June 2023) [24,25] to show differences in the expression of genes related to the Wnt signaling pathway between healthy controls and HNSCC patients depending on the histological cancer grade (Figure 1) or genes related to cancer stem cells (Figure 7) between healthy controls and HNSCC patients and among HNSCC patients depending on the histological cancer grade (1–4).

4.7. Isolation of RNA, Reverse Transcription, and Quantitative Real-Time PCR

Total RNA was isolated from cells treated with the compounds for 48 h using the Universal RNA Purification Kit (EURx, Gdańsk, Poland), and samples were subjected to reverse transcription by the NG dART RT Kit (EURx, Gdańsk, Poland), according to the manufacturer's instructions.

For the quantitative R-T PCR analyses, the SG qPCR Master Mix (EURx, Gdańsk, Poland) and LightCycler 96 (Roche, Basel, Switzerland) were used. The initial enzyme activation at 95 °C lasted 10 min and was followed by 40 three-step cycles consisting of denaturation at 95 °C for 15 s, primer annealing at 56 °C for 30 s, elongation at 72 °C for 30 s with fluorescence measurement, and subsequently followed by melting curve analysis. The relative mRNA expression of Aldehyde dehydrogenase 1—ALDH1 (*ALDH1A1* gene), SRY (sex determining region Y)-box 2—SOX2 (*SOX2* gene), and Octamer-binding transcription factor 4—OCT4 (*POU5F1* gene) was determined. The expression of the TATA-box-binding protein (*TBP* gene) was used to normalize the data. The ΔΔCt method was used for fold-change quantification. Three independent experiments were performed with three technical repeats for each sample during R-T PCR. The sequences of primers used in the research are listed in Table 2.

Table 2. Primers used in the R-T PCR.

Gene	Forward Primer	Reverse Primer
ALDH1A1	5′CTGTCCTACTCACCGATT	5′CCTCCTTATCTCCTTCTTCTA
POU5F1	5′GGTTCTATTTGGGAAGGTAT	5′CATGTTCTTGAAGCTAAGC
SOX2	5′ATGGTTGTCTATTAACTTGT	5′TCTCTCCTCTTCTTTCTC
TBP	5′GGCACCACTCCACTGTATC	5′GGGATTATATTCGGCGTTTCG

4.8. Statistical Analysis

To analyze the significance of differences between controls and signaling pathway inhibitors: PRI-724, vismodegib, erlotinib, and HS-173, a one-way ANOVA test with the Tukey post hoc test was performed, with $p < 0.05$ considered significant. The analyses were performed using STATISTICA software (version 11.0).

5. Conclusions

This in vitro study implicated new directions in the development of molecularly targeted treatment of head and neck squamous carcinoma. The active status of the Wnt/β-catenin pathway stimulates the progression of HNSCC cells, but as previously reported, anti-cancer effects should be improved by co-targeting other signaling pathways important for HNSCC carcinogenesis. According to our results, Wnt/β-catenin and Hh signaling can interact with each other, so their concomitant inhibition presented in this research might be a good strategy to attenuate the growth of HNSCC tumors. Simultaneous inhibition of the Wnt and Hh pathways caused pronounced effects concerning decreased proliferation and migration. CAL 27 and FaDu cells, although coming from different locations of HNSCC, were in general both sensitive to the combinatorial inhibition of Wnt/β-catenin and Hh pathways. Notably, the simultaneous blockade of the EGFR-related pathways and Wnt/β-catenin pathway also presented promising results. The migration of HNSCC cells was diminished by mixtures of PRI-724 and erlotinib, or HS-173, to a lesser extent. However, the anti-proliferative activity and more robust induction of apoptosis can be the basis for the improvement of the anti-neoplastic effects of EGFR and PI3K inhibitors.

The main concepts of signaling pathway co-inhibition and the findings of this research are summarized in Figure 9.

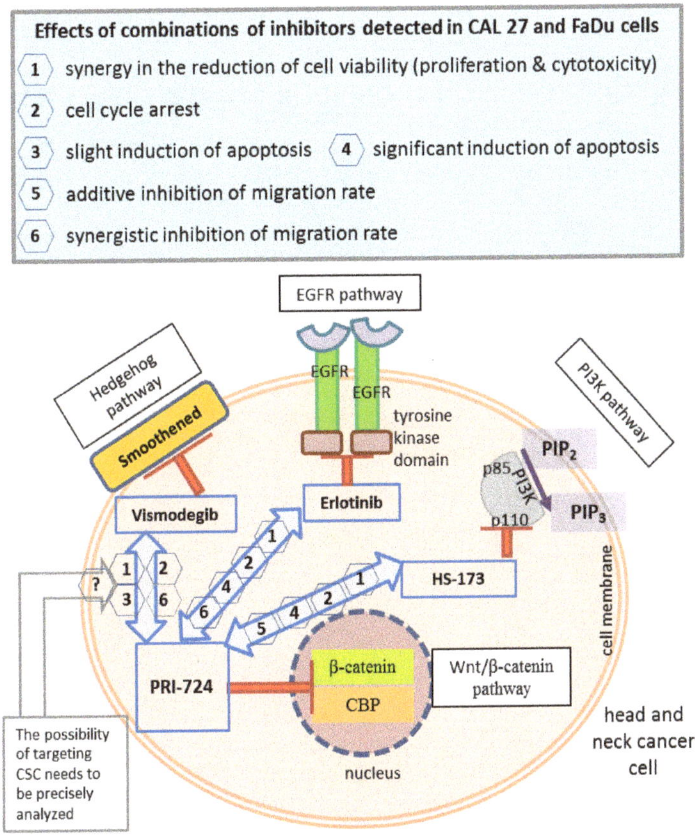

Figure 9. A summary of the main concepts and results of the study. Wnt/β-catenin signaling was inhibited by the PRI-724 small molecule, which targets the interaction between nuclear β-catenin and the CREB binding protein (CBP). PRI-724 was combined with the Hedgehog pathway inhibitor vismodegib, which blocks the Smoothened protein; the epidermal growth factor receptor (EGFR) pathway inhibitor erlotinib, which interacts with the cytoplasmic tyrosine kinase domains of EGFR; and the phosphoinositide 3-kinase (PI3K) inhibitor HS-173, which targets the p110α domain of PI3K. The effects detected in CAL 27 and FaDu cells after treatment with each combination of inhibitors used in this research are listed in the frame (upper panel), and appropriate numbers appear next to arrows denoting compound mixes in the head and neck cancer cell schematic representation. CSC, cancer stem cells; PIP2, phosphatidylinositol 4,5-bisphosphate; PIP3, phosphatidylinositol 3,4,5-trisphosphate.

The results are preliminary, and thus the full potential of the combinations of the studied chemicals should be further evaluated. The prospective research will cover testing the discussed molecularly targeted drug combinations in other cell lines to evaluate the generalizability of current results and the mechanism of action. More advanced in vitro models will be introduced, including three-dimensional cultures of cancer cells (spheroids, organoids) and co-cultures with fibroblasts to observe micro-environmental interactions between signaling pathways. Ex vivo culture of patient-derived cancer cells might be the final model for evaluating this treatment concept before in vivo experiments.

Wnt/β-catenin and Hh pathways are both related to the control of CSCs. The expression of exemplary CSC-related genes among HNSCC patients increases in parallel with tumor stage. Concomitant inhibition of Wnt/β-catenin and Hh pathways was able to partly reduce their transcript levels in CAL 27 and FaDu cells. Therefore, further experiments should also verify the usefulness of co-targeting those two signaling pathways for affecting CSCs in HNSCCs. Such an effect can be crucial for preventing cancer recurrence, which is thought to be tightly connected with the subpopulation of cancer stem cells resistant to current therapy.

Supplementary Materials: The following supporting information can be downloaded at: https://www.mdpi.com/article/10.3390/ijms241310448/s1.

Author Contributions: Conceptualization, R.K. and J.P.; methodology, R.K. and J.P.; software, R.K.; validation, R.K. and D.D.; formal analysis, R.K.; investigation, R.K., M.F., D.D., and J.P.; resources, R.K.; data curation, R.K.; writing—original draft preparation, R.K.; writing—review and editing, J.P.; visualization, R.K.; supervision, J.P.; project administration, R.K.; funding acquisition, R.K. and J.P. All authors have read and agreed to the published version of the manuscript.

Funding: This research was funded by Poznan University of Medical Sciences.

Institutional Review Board Statement: Not applicable.

Informed Consent Statement: Not applicable.

Data Availability Statement: Data are contained within the article and Supplementary Materials.

Acknowledgments: We would like to thank Agata Nowak for the technical support while performing real-time polymerase chain reactions.

Conflicts of Interest: The authors declare no conflict of interest.

References

1. Kirtane, K.; St. John, M.; Fuentes-Bayne, H.; Patel, S.P.; Mardiros, A.; Xu, H.; Ng, E.W.; Go, W.Y.; Wong, D.J.; Sunwoo, J.B.; et al. Genomic Immune Evasion: Diagnostic and Therapeutic Opportunities in Head and Neck Squamous Cell Carcinomas. *J. Clin. Med.* **2022**, *11*, 7259. [CrossRef]
2. Sung, H.; Ferlay, J.; Siegel, R.L.; Laversanne, M.; Soerjomataram, I.; Jemal, A.; Bray, F. Global Cancer Statistics 2020: GLOBOCAN Estimates of Incidence and Mortality Worldwide for 36 Cancers in 185 Countries. *CA Cancer J. Clin.* **2021**, *71*, 209–249. [CrossRef] [PubMed]
3. Byeon, H.K.; Ku, M.; Yang, J. Beyond EGFR inhibition: Multilateral combat strategies to stop the progression of head and neck cancer. *Exp. Mol. Med.* **2019**, *51*, 1–14. [CrossRef] [PubMed]
4. Xie, G.; Shan, L.; Liu, Y.; Wu, T.-C.; Gu, X. Antitumor Efficacy of EGFR-Targeted Recombinant Immunotoxin in Human Head and Neck Squamous Cell Carcinoma. *Biology* **2022**, *11*, 486. [CrossRef] [PubMed]
5. Tathineni, P.; Joshi, N.; Jelinek, M.J. Current State and Future Directions of EGFR-Directed Therapy in Head and Neck Cancer. *Curr. Treat. Options Oncol.* **2023**, *24*, 680–692. [CrossRef]
6. Kleszcz, R.; Skalski, M.; Krajka-Kuźniak, V.; Paluszczak, J. The inhibitors of KDM4 and KDM6 histone lysine demethylases enhance the anti-growth effects of erlotinib and HS-173 in head and neck cancer cells. *Eur. J. Pharm. Sci.* **2021**, *166*, 105961. [CrossRef]
7. Zhou, S.; Chen, L.; Mashrah, M.; Zhu, Y.; He, Z.; Hu, Y.; Xiang, T.; Yao, Z.; Guo, F.; Zhang, C. Expression and promoter methylation of Wnt inhibitory factor-1 in the development of oral submucous fibrosis. *Oncol. Rep.* **2015**, *34*, 2636–2642. [CrossRef] [PubMed]
8. Paluszczak, J. The Significance of the Dysregulation of Canonical Wnt Signaling in Head and Neck Squamous Cell Carcinomas. *Cells* **2020**, *9*, 723. [CrossRef]
9. Xie, J.; Huang, L.; Lu, Y.G.; Zheng, D.L. Roles of the Wnt Signaling Pathway in Head and Neck Squamous Cell Carcinoma. *Front. Mol. Biosci.* **2021**, *7*, 590912. [CrossRef]
10. Javed, Z.; Muhammad Farooq, H.; Ullah, M.; Zaheer Iqbal, M.; Raza, Q.; Sadia, H.; Pezzani, R.; Salehi, B.; Sharifi-Rad, J.; Cho, W.C. Wnt Signaling: A Potential Therapeutic Target in Head and Neck Squamous Cell Carcinoma. *Asian Pac. J. Cancer Prev.* **2019**, *20*, 995–1003. [CrossRef]
11. Majchrzak-Celińska, A.; Kleszcz, R.; Stasiłowicz-Krzemień, A.; Cielecka-Piontek, J. Sodium Butyrate Enhances Curcuminoids Permeability through the Blood-Brain Barrier, Restores Wnt/β-Catenin Pathway Antagonists Gene Expression and Reduces the Viability of Glioblastoma Cells. *Int. J. Mol. Sci.* **2021**, *22*, 11285. [CrossRef] [PubMed]
12. Oliveira, L.F.S.; Predes, D.; Borges, H.L.; Abreu, J.G. Therapeutic Potential of Naturally Occurring Small Molecules to Target the Wnt/β-Catenin Signaling Pathway in Colorectal Cancer. *Cancers* **2022**, *14*, 403. [CrossRef] [PubMed]
13. Majchrzak-Celińska, A.; Kleszcz, R.; Studzińska-Sroka, E.; Łukaszyk, A.; Szoszkiewicz, A.; Stelcer, E.; Jopek, K.; Rucinski, M.; Cielecka-Piontek, J.; Krajka-Kuźniak, V. Lichen Secondary Metabolites Inhibit the Wnt/β-Catenin Pathway in Glioblastoma Cells and Improve the Anticancer Effects of Temozolomide. *Cells* **2022**, *11*, 1084. [CrossRef] [PubMed]

14. Pećina-Šlaus, N.; Aničić, S.; Bukovac, A.; Kafka, A. Wnt Signaling Inhibitors and Their Promising Role in Tumor Treatment. *Int. J. Mol. Sci.* **2023**, *24*, 6733. [CrossRef] [PubMed]
15. Kleszcz, R.; Szymańska, A.; Krajka-Kuźniak, V.; Baer-Dubowska, W.; Paluszczak, J. Inhibition of CBP/β-catenin and porcupine attenuates Wnt signaling and induces apoptosis in head and neck carcinoma cells. *Cell. Oncol.* **2019**, *42*, 505–520. [CrossRef]
16. Cirillo, N.; Wu, C.; Prime, S.S. Heterogeneity of Cancer Stem Cells in Tumorigenesis, Metastasis, and Resistance to Antineoplastic Treatment of Head and Neck Tumours. *Cells* **2021**, *10*, 3068. [CrossRef]
17. Krishnamurthy, S.; Nör, J.E. Head and neck cancer stem cells. *J. Dent. Res.* **2012**, *91*, 334–340. [CrossRef]
18. Aminuddin, A.; Ng, P.Y. Promising Druggable Target in Head and Neck Squamous Cell Carcinoma: Wnt Signaling. *Front. Pharmacol.* **2016**, *7*, 244. [CrossRef]
19. Li, L.J.; Li, C.H.; Chang, P.M.; Lai, T.C.; Yong, C.Y.; Feng, S.W.; Hsiao, M.; Chang, W.M.; Huang, C.F. Dehydroepiandrosterone (DHEA) Sensitizes Irinotecan to Suppress Head and Neck Cancer Stem-Like Cells by Downregulation of WNT Signaling. *Front. Oncol.* **2022**, *12*, 775541. [CrossRef]
20. Chai, J.Y.; Sugumar, V.; Alshanon, A.F.; Wong, W.F.; Fung, S.Y.; Looi, C.Y. Defining the Role of GLI/Hedgehog Signaling in Chemoresistance: Implications in Therapeutic Approaches. *Cancers* **2021**, *13*, 4746. [CrossRef]
21. Yang, P.; Li, C.; Zhou, Q.; Zhang, X.; Kou, Y.; Feng, Q.; Wang, H.; Su, R.; Hasegawa, T.; Liu, H.; et al. Notum leads to potential pro-survival of OSCC through crosstalk between Shh and Wnt/β-catenin signaling via p-GSK3β. *Int. J. Biochem. Cell Biol.* **2022**, *153*, 106316. [CrossRef]
22. Carballo, G.B.; Honorato, J.R.; de Lopes, G.P.F.; Spohr, T.C.L.S.E. A highlight on Sonic hedgehog pathway. *Cell Commun. Signal.* **2018**, *16*, 11. [CrossRef] [PubMed]
23. Rudin, C.M. Vismodegib. *Clin. Cancer Res.* **2012**, *18*, 3218–3222. [CrossRef] [PubMed]
24. Chandrashekar, D.S.; Bashel, B.; Balasubramanya, S.A.H.; Creighton, C.J.; Ponce-Rodriguez, I.; Chakravarthi, B.V.S.K.; Varambally, S. UALCAN: A Portal for Facilitating Tumor Subgroup Gene Expression and Survival Analyses. *Neoplasia* **2017**, *19*, 649–658. [CrossRef] [PubMed]
25. Chandrashekar, D.S.; Karthikeyan, S.K.; Korla, P.K.; Patel, H.; Shovon, A.R.; Athar, M.; Netto, G.J.; Qin, Z.S.; Kumar, S.; Manne, U.; et al. UALCAN: An update to the integrated cancer data analysis platform. *Neoplasia* **2022**, *25*, 18–27. [CrossRef]
26. Xu, M.J.; Johnson, D.E.; Grandis, J.R. EGFR-targeted therapies in the post-genomic era. *Cancer Metastasis Rev.* **2017**, *36*, 463–473. [CrossRef] [PubMed]
27. Alamoud, K.A.; Kukuruzinska, M.A. Emerging Insights into Wnt/β-catenin Signaling in Head and Neck Cancer. *J. Dent. Res.* **2018**, *97*, 665–673. [CrossRef]
28. Martinez-Font, E.; Pérez-Capó, M.; Ramos, R.; Felipe, I.; Garcías, C.; Luna, P.; Terrasa, J.; Martín-Broto, J.; Vögler, O.; Alemany, R.; et al. Impact of Wnt/β-Catenin Inhibition on Cell Proliferation through *CDC25A* Downregulation in Soft Tissue Sarcomas. *Cancers* **2020**, *12*, 2556. [CrossRef]
29. Gulati, R.; Johnston, M.; Rivas, M.; Cast, A.; Kumbaji, M.; Hanlon, M.A.; Lee, S.; Zhou, P.; Lake, C.; Schepers, E.; et al. β-catenin cancer-enhancing genomic regions axis is involved in the development of fibrolamellar hepatocellular carcinoma. *Hepatol. Commun.* **2022**, *6*, 2950–2963. [CrossRef]
30. Schmidtova, S.; Kalavska, K.; Liskova, V.; Plava, J.; Miklikova, S.; Kucerova, L.; Matuskova, M.; Rojikova, L.; Cierna, Z.; Rogozea, A.; et al. Targeting of Deregulated Wnt/β-Catenin Signaling by PRI-724 and LGK974 Inhibitors in Germ Cell Tumor Cell Lines. *Int. J. Mol. Sci.* **2021**, *22*, 4263. [CrossRef]
31. Jin, X.-F.; Spöttl, G.; Maurer, J.; Nölting, S.; Auernhammer, C.J. Inhibition of Wnt/β-Catenin Signaling in Neuroendocrine Tumors In Vitro: Antitumoral Effects. *Cancers* **2020**, *12*, 345. [CrossRef]
32. Yi, H.; Zeng, D.; Shen, Z.; Liao, J.; Wang, X.; Liu, Y.; Zhang, X.; Kong, P. Integrin alphavbeta3 enhances β-catenin signaling in acute myeloid leukemia harboring Fms-like tyrosine kinase-3 internal tandem duplication mutations: Implications for microenvironment influence on sorafenib sensitivity. *Oncotarget* **2016**, *7*, 40387–40397. [CrossRef] [PubMed]
33. Jiang, X.; Mak, P.Y.; Mu, H.; Tao, W.; Mak, D.H.; Kornblau, S.; Zhang, Q.; Ruvolo, P.; Burks, J.K.; Zhang, W.; et al. Disruption of Wnt/β-Catenin Exerts Antileukemia Activity and Synergizes with FLT3 Inhibition in *FLT3*-Mutant Acute Myeloid Leukemia. *Clin. Cancer Res.* **2018**, *24*, 2417–2429. [CrossRef] [PubMed]
34. Brkic, F.F.; Stoiber, S.; Maier, T.; Gurnhofer, E.; Kenner, L.; Heiduschka, G.; Kadletz-Wanke, L. Targeting Wnt/Beta-Catenin Signaling in HPV-Positive Head and Neck Squamous Cell Carcinoma. *Pharmaceuticals* **2022**, *15*, 378. [CrossRef] [PubMed]
35. Maier, T.; Stoiber, S.; Gurnhofer, E.; Haas, M.; Kenner, L.; Heiduschka, G.; Kadletz-Wanke, L.; Brkic, F.F. Inhibition of beta-catenin shows therapeutic potential in head and neck squamous cell carcinoma in vitro. *Eur. Arch. Otorhinolaryngol.* **2023**, *280*, 399–408. [CrossRef] [PubMed]
36. Szyfter, K.; Kiwerska, K.; Wierzbicka, M. HPV-related HNC—New challenge and hope for head and neck cancer subjects. *J. Med. Sci.* **2018**, *87*, 112–116. [CrossRef]
37. Kleszcz, R.; Paluszczak, J. The combinatorial inhibition of Wnt signaling and Akt kinase is beneficial for reducing the survival and glycolytic activity of tongue cancer cells. *J. Oral Pathol. Med.* **2022**, *51*, 231–239. [CrossRef]
38. Katoh, M. Canonical and non-canonical WNT signaling in cancer stem cells and their niches: Cellular heterogeneity, omics reprogramming, targeted therapy and tumor plasticity (Review). *Int. J. Oncol.* **2017**, *51*, 1357–1369. [CrossRef] [PubMed]
39. Szaryńska, M.; Olejniczak, A.; Kobiela, J.; Spychalski, P.; Kmieć, Z. Therapeutic strategies against cancer stem cells in human colorectal cancer. *Oncol. Lett.* **2017**, *14*, 7653–7668. [CrossRef]

40. Takada, T. Activation of the Hedgehog and Wnt/β-Catenin Signaling Pathways in Basal Cell Carcinoma. *Case Rep. Dermatol.* **2021**, *13*, 506–512. [CrossRef]
41. Mullor, J.L.; Dahmane, N.; Sun, T.; Ruiz i Altaba, A. Wnt signals are targets and mediators of Gli function. *Curr. Biol.* **2001**, *11*, 769–773. [CrossRef]
42. Li, X.; Deng, W.; Lobo-Ruppert, S.M.; Ruppert, J.M. Gli1 acts through Snail and E-cadherin to promote nuclear signaling by beta-catenin. *Oncogene* **2007**, *26*, 4489–4498. [CrossRef] [PubMed]
43. Kleszcz, R.; Krajka-Kuźniak, V.; Paluszczak, J. Porcupine and CBP/β-catenin are the most suitable targets for the inhibition of canonical Wnt signaling in colorectal carcinoma cell lines. *Postepy Hig. Med. Dosw.* **2020**, *74*, 224–235. [CrossRef]
44. Ikarashi, N.; Kaneko, M.; Watanabe, T.; Kon, R.; Yoshino, M.; Yokoyama, T.; Tanaka, R.; Takayama, N.; Sakai, H.; Kamei, J. Epidermal Growth Factor Receptor Tyrosine Kinase Inhibitor Erlotinib Induces Dry Skin via Decreased in Aquaporin-3 Expression. *Biomolecules* **2020**, *10*, 545. [CrossRef]
45. Olesen, U.H.; Bojesen, S.; Gehl, J.; Haedersdal, M. Anticancer drugs and the regulation of Hedgehog genes GLI1 and PTCH1, a comparative study in nonmelanoma skin cancer cell lines. *Anticancer Drugs* **2017**, *28*, 1106–1117. [CrossRef] [PubMed]
46. Freitas, R.D.; Dias, R.B.; Vidal, M.T.A.; Valverde, L.F.; Gomes Alves Costa, R.; Damasceno, A.K.A.; Sales, C.B.S.; Siquara da Rocha, L.O.; Dos Reis, M.G.; Soares, M.B.P.; et al. Inhibition of CAL27 Oral Squamous Carcinoma Cell by Targeting Hedgehog Pathway with Vismodegib or Itraconazole. *Front. Oncol.* **2020**, *10*, 563838. [CrossRef] [PubMed]
47. Hehlgans, S.; Booms, P.; Güllülü, Ö.; Sader, R.; Rödel, C.; Balermpas, P.; Rödel, F.; Ghanaati, S. Radiation Sensitization of Basal Cell and Head and Neck Squamous Cell Carcinoma by the Hedgehog Pathway Inhibitor Vismodegib. *Int. J. Mol. Sci.* **2018**, *19*, 2485. [CrossRef]
48. Liebig, H.; Günther, G.; Kolb, M.; Mozet, C.; Boehm, A.; Dietz, A.; Wichmann, G. Reduced proliferation and colony formation of head and neck squamous cell carcinoma (HNSCC) after dual targeting of EGFR and hedgehog pathways. *Cancer Chemother. Pharmacol.* **2017**, *79*, 411–420. [CrossRef]
49. Yue, D.; Li, H.; Che, J.; Zhang, Y.; Tseng, H.H.; Jin, J.Q.; Luh, T.M.; Giroux-Leprieur, E.; Mo, M.; Zheng, Q.; et al. Hedgehog/Gli promotes epithelial-mesenchymal transition in lung squamous cell carcinomas. *J. Exp. Clin. Cancer Res.* **2014**, *33*, 34. [CrossRef]
50. Baillie, R.; Tan, S.T.; Itinteang, T. Cancer Stem Cells in Oral Cavity Squamous Cell Carcinoma: A Review. *Front. Oncol.* **2017**, *7*, 112. [CrossRef]
51. Kulsum, S.; Sudheendra, H.V.; Pandian, R.; Ravindra, D.R.; Siddappa, G.; Chevour, P.; Ramachandran, B.; Sagar, M.; Jayaprakash, A.; Mehta, A.; et al. Cancer stem cell mediated acquired chemoresistance in head and neck cancer can be abrogated by aldehyde dehydrogenase 1 A1 inhibition. *Mol. Carcinog.* **2017**, *56*, 694–711. [CrossRef] [PubMed]
52. Schulz, D.; Wirth, M.; Piontek, G.; Buchberger, A.M.; Schlegel, J.; Reiter, R.; Multhoff, G.; Pickhard, A. HNSCC cells resistant to EGFR pathway inhibitors are hypermutated and sensitive to DNA damaging substances. *Am. J. Cancer Res.* **2016**, *6*, 1963–1975.
53. Zhang, X.; Zheng, X.; Lou, Y.; Wang, H.; Xu, J.; Zhang, Y.; Han, B. β-catenin inhibitors suppress cells proliferation and promote cells apoptosis in PC9 lung cancer stem cells. *Int. J. Clin. Exp. Pathol.* **2017**, *10*, 11968–11978. [PubMed]
54. Lee, S.H.; Koo, B.S.; Kim, J.M.; Huang, S.; Rho, Y.S.; Bae, W.J.; Kang, H.J.; Kim, Y.S.; Moon, J.H.; Lim, Y.C. Wnt/β-catenin signalling maintains self-renewal and tumourigenicity of head and neck squamous cell carcinoma stem-like cells by activating Oct4. *J. Pathol.* **2014**, *234*, 99–107. [CrossRef] [PubMed]
55. Zuo, M.; Rashid, A.; Churi, C.; Vauthey, J.N.; Chang, P.; Li, Y.; Hung, M.C.; Li, D.; Javle, M. Novel therapeutic strategy targeting the Hedgehog signalling and mTOR pathways in biliary tract cancer. *Br. J. Cancer* **2015**, *112*, 1042–1051. [CrossRef]
56. Damiani, G.; Grossi, E.; Berti, E.; Conic, R.R.Z.; Radhakrishna, U.; Pacifico, A.; Bragazzi, N.L.; Piccinno, R.; Linder, D. Artificial neural networks allow response prediction in squamous cell carcinoma of the scalp treated with radiotherapy. *J. Eur. Acad. Dermatol. Venereol.* **2020**, *34*, 1369–1373. [CrossRef]
57. Chou, T.C. Drug combination studies and their synergy quantification using the Chou-Talalay method. *Cancer Res.* **2010**, *70*, 440–446. [CrossRef] [PubMed]
58. Jin, Z.J. About the evaluation of drug combination. *Acta Pharmacol. Sin.* **2004**, *25*, 146–147.
59. Tan, L.; Jia, X.; Jiang, X.; Zhang, Y.; Tang, H.; Yao, S.; Xie, Q. In vitro study on the individual and synergistic cytotoxicity of adriamycin and selenium nanoparticles against Bel7402 cells with a quartz crystal microbalance. *Biosens. Bioelectron.* **2009**, *24*, 2268–2272. [CrossRef]

International Journal of *Molecular Sciences*

MDPI

Review

Impact of Circulating Cell-Free DNA (cfDNA) as a Biomarker of the Development and Evolution of Periodontitis

Gaia Viglianisi [1], Simona Santonocito [1], Alessandro Polizzi [1], Giuseppe Troiano [2,*], Mariacristina Amato [1], Khrystyna Zhurakivska [2], Paolo Pesce [3] and Gaetano Isola [1]

1 Department of General Surgery and Surgical-Medical Specialties, School of Dentistry, University of Catania, 95124 Catania, Italy; gaia.viglianisi@gmail.com (G.V.); simonasantonocito.93@gmail.com (S.S.); alexpoli345@gmail.com (A.P.); gaetano.isola@unict.it (G.I.)

2 Department of Clinical and Experimental Medicine, University of Foggia, 71122 Foggia, Italy; khrystyna.zhurakivska@unifg.it

3 Department of Surgical Sciences and Integrated Diagnostics (DISC), University of Genoa, Ospedale S. Martino, 16148 Genoa, Italy

* Correspondence: giuseppe.troiano@unifg.it; Tel.: +39-0881588082

Abstract: In the last few decades, circulating cell-free DNA (cfDNA) has been shown to have an important role in cell apoptosis or necrosis, including in the development and evolution of several tumors and inflammatory diseases in humans. In this regard, periodontitis, a chronic inflammatory disease that can induce the destruction of supporting components of the teeth, could represent a chronic inflammatory stimulus linked to a various range of systemic inflammatory diseases. Recently, a possible correlation between periodontal disease and cfDNA has been shown, representing new important diagnostic–therapeutic perspectives. During the development of periodontitis, cfDNA is released in biological fluids such as blood, saliva, urine and other body fluids and represents an important index of inflammation. Due to the possibility of withdrawing some of these liquids in a non-invasive way, cfDNA could be used as a possible biomarker for periodontal disease. In addition, discovering a proportional relationship between cfDNA levels and the severity of periodontitis, expressed through the disease extent, could open the prospect of using cfDNA as a possible therapeutic target. The aim of this article is to report what researchers have discovered in recent years about circulating cfDNA in the development, evolution and therapy of periodontitis. The analyzed literature review shows that cfDNA has considerable potential as a diagnostic, therapeutic biomarker and therapeutic target in periodontal disease; however, further studies are needed for cfDNA to be used in clinical practice.

Keywords: periodontitis; circulating cell-free DNA; oral disease; periodontics; tooth loss: oral cancer; trials

Citation: Viglianisi, G.; Santonocito, S.; Polizzi, A.; Troiano, G.; Amato, M.; Zhurakivska, K.; Pesce, P.; Isola, G. Impact of Circulating Cell-Free DNA (cfDNA) as a Biomarker of the Development and Evolution of Periodontitis. *Int. J. Mol. Sci.* **2023**, *24*, 9981. https://doi.org/10.3390/ijms24129981

Academic Editors: Marko Tarle and Ivica Lukšić

Received: 14 May 2023
Revised: 7 June 2023
Accepted: 8 June 2023
Published: 10 June 2023

1. Introduction

Periodontitis is a chronic disease that affects 10% of the world's population [1]. It is characterized by the interaction among bacterial, inflammation and genetic factors. Specific virulent oral microbials cause the host immune response in patients with a genetic predisposition. The inflammation of the periodontal tissues could result, if not properly treated, in clinical attachment loss (CAL), the formation of periodontal pockets and alveolar bone resorption, which could finally lead to tooth loss [2,3]. Recent studies showed that the immune system cells release cfDNA during periodontal inflammation to promote alveolar bone resorption [4,5]. For this reason, cfDNA has captured the attention of the periodontal area.

Today, cell-free DNA (cfDNA) is commonly used as a biomarker in prenatal analysis and in the oncology field. Over the last years, cfDNA has caught the interest of scientists in other medical fields; for instance, cardiovascular disease [6], autoimmune diseases [7], sepsis [8], trauma [9] and others.

The term "liquid biopsy" specifies several body fluids that can be collected, such as blood and saliva. When high levels of biomarkers are found in saliva, they can be related to head and neck pathologies. Cell-free DNA (cfDNA) and mitochondrial cell-free DNA (mtDNA) are two markers that can be found in the body fluid of patients affected by oral conditions [10,11].

Several studies have found a greater concentration of cfDNA and mtDNA in the body fluids of patients affected by different cancer types than in healthy ones. For this reason, clinics have started to investigate the presence of the same circumstances in oral conditions, such as oral squamous cancer. Desai proposed the use of total cfDNA level as a screening marker for the early detection of oral precancer lesions and cancer [12]. A study conducted by Lin et al. [13] examined the cfDNA level in patients affected by oral squamous cell carcinoma (OSCC) compared to healthy ones. Their results showed that the cfDNA level was higher in patients affected by OSSC compared to the control group. These outcomes were similar to the results obtained in other studies that evaluated the same markers for solid cancers [14,15]. In particular, Lin et al. [13] obtained these outcomes in patients with extensive tumors, cervical lymph node metastasis and TNM (Tumor–Node–Metastasis) staging. The authors concluded that cfDNA is an independent indicator of cervical lymph node metastasis. According to these results, other researchers have investigated the concentration of these markers in the blood of patients affected by head and neck squamous cell carcinoma. Mazurek et al. [16] observed an increase of cfDNA in patients with N2-N3 lymph node metastasis affected by head and neck squamous cell carcinoma. They did not observe an increase in cfDNA level in patients with N0-N1 lymph node metastasis.

Sayal et al. [17] evaluated the cfDNA and mtDNA levels in patients affected by head and neck squamous cell carcinomas (HNSCCs). They observed higher levels of cfDNA and mtDNA in patients affected by HNSCCs compared to healthy ones. Moreover, they evaluated how these two markers change their level in the case of oral leukoplakia (precancer oral lesion). From this evaluation, it also emerged that in precancerous oral lesions, the cfDNA and mtDNA level changed compared to the healthy patients. The authors claim that the variation in the concentration of these markers could be used to estimate the grade of epithelial dysplasia and for surveillance among patients [17]. A recent study conducted by Sayal et al. [18] shows that the level of mtDNA is correlated with survival in patients affected by HNSCC. The higher concentration of cfDNA and mtDNA in body fluid can also be associated with other conditions, including inflammation and infection [19]. Therefore, cfDNA and mtDNA concentrations can vary in periodontitis, considering it is an inflammatory disease.

CfDNA was proposed as a new biomarker to study the disease's evolution and progression in the periodontal field. A different concentration of cfDNA was seen among healthy patients, periodontally affected and gingivitis-affected patients [20]. Moreover, a recent study has shown therapeutic results in treating periodontitis in mice using nanoparticles that remove cfDNA [4]. The aim of this article is to report what was discovered about the relationship between cfDNA and periodontitis in the last few years. Additionally, it will underline the possible uses of cfDNA as a marker in periodontitis for diagnosis and therapy.

2. Cell-Free DNA

In 1948, Mandel and Metais were the first to discover and describe cfDNA in the human plasma [21], as fragments of nucleic acids present in many fluids of the human body. The release of cfDNA is influenced by different variables such as age, smoking, physical exercise, sex, diet, infection, oxidative stress and pregnancy [22–24]. It originates from three main mechanisms:

- Apoptosis, in which the cell DNA is processed by endonucleases with the production of short fragments of DNA [25]. CfDNA originates from apoptosis and is formed by double-stranded fragments of about 150–200 base pairs [26].
- Necrosis is a mechanism of death common in cases of trauma and sepsis due to chemical or physical stimuli [27–29]. This mechanism [30] is correlated among Kilobase pairs of cfDNA [25]. cfDNA originating from necrosis has a longer length due to the increased time required to eliminate the necrotic cells, while the clearance of apoptotic cells requires less time [31].
- NETosis is a process that induces the neutrophil's death after its contact with exogenous agents [25] and represents an active source of cfDNA. It is a particular process based on the release of traps (NETs, neutrophil extracellular traps) by neutrophils to contrast and kill microbes [32]. NETs are composed of histones and DNA. During the NET mechanisms, DNA is released in two forms: vital and suicidal NETosis. In their vital form, neutrophils release DNA and perform their phagocytic activity against pathogens [33,34], while in suicidal NETosis, the programmed death of neutrophils occurs after their contact with a pathogen [35,36].

CfDNA can be found in different forms; for instance, in free fragments, linked to proteins or packed in extracellular vesicles [37]. A cfDNA fragment is defined when there is DNA alone without other molecules [38].

It is possible to identify three types of cfDNA in the human fluid: endogenous nuclear DNA (or genomic DNA), mitochondrial DNA (mDNA) and bacteria (bDNA) or viral DNA [39,40]. Genomic DNA and mDNA can be transported by extracellular vesicles (EVs) [41]. Recently, EVs were discovered as another form of active cfDNA release [22]. These extracellular vesicles originated from the fusion of intraluminal microvesicles and can carry DNA both in their lumen and on their surfaces [42]. There are three main types of extracellular vesicles: exosomes, microvesicles and apoptotic bodies [43]. In EVs, it is possible to find genomic DNA, mitochondrial DNA, RNA, proteins and lipids [44]. Different studies showed that extracellular vesicles carrying DNA play different functions in cellular communication, immune system control, homeostasis and material transportation [45–47].

Normally, in a healthy patient, the concentration of cfDNA in the plasma is less than 10 ng for mL [48]. In cases of trauma, systemic disease, heart disease, cancer and inflammation, cfDNA concentration increases [49]. An endogenous source of cfDNA is the fetal cell-free DNA present in the blood of pregnant individuals. This type of cfDNA can be detected through a non-invasive procedure (non-invasive prenatal testing), and it can be used to identify a possible mutation in the fetus's DNA. For example, using this marker, it is possible to search for the presence of trisomies [50]. In oncology cfDNA a blood sample can be used to search for a specific DNA methylation related to a specific cancer. Additionally, the analysis of specific DNA methylation present in the cancer's cells shows the presence of recurrence after the conclusion of the treatment or which type of therapy is better [25,51].

To maintain homeostasis, the cfDNA produced is typically removed by the endonucleases, such as DNase I. Endonucleases are enzymes capable of deleting nucleic acids. A system is defined as healthy when a balance exists between the release of cfDNA and the removal of cfDNA. CfDNA is digested by DNases and removed from the bloodstream through the liver, kidneys and spleen. The correct and rapid removal of cfDNA avoids the occurrence of an inflammatory process [52]. DNases are present in blood and saliva [53,54]. When free DNA is linked with EVs or with other molecules, it is more resistant to the activity of DNases [38].

3. CfDNA and Periodontitis

The presence of hyperactive polymorph nucleate neutrophils (PNMs), which characterize periodontitis [55,56], induces the NETs system's overstimulation. The NETs system, in the gingival sulcus of a healthy patient, allows the removal of bacterial, pathogen-associated molecular patterns (PAMPs) and damage-associated molecular patterns (DAMPs), releasing cfDNA and peptides [57,58]. DAMPs consist of intracellular components, such as proteins and nucleic acids, which the cells release during their necrosis process [59]. In the case of periodontitis, the level of the NETs system increases, causing the alteration of homeostasis and chronic inflammation [57,58].

Normally, during a proinflammatory immune process, the Toll-like receptors (TRLs) interact with different substances and allow the beginning of inflammation. In many inflammatory diseases, this process is altered, and TRL9 is involved [60]. It was discovered that the abnormal functioning of TRL9 plays a role in the development and establishment of periodontitis. An in vivo study showed that animals without TRL9 were resistant to the development of periodontitis. The same results were obtained in an in vitro study conducted by Kim et al. [61] and Crump et al. [62]. Moreover, a strong relationship was observed between TRL9 and periodontopathic bacteria [63]. TRL9 is one of the main receptors of cfDNA, and its interaction causes the beginning of the inflammatory process in alveolar bone inflammation [4]. TRL9 is normally present in the basement and sub-basement cells of the oral and pocket epitheliums [64]. In the periodontal pocket of patients affected by periodontitis, the TRL9 level is higher than that of healthy patients [63]. This discovery could be related to the active role of cfDNA in the development and progression of periodontitis [65]. In fact, a study conducted by Huang et al. [4] showed the relationship between high levels of cfDNA and elevated alveolar bone destruction in patients affected by periodontitis. In another study conducted by Huang et al. [66], it was found that cfDNA actively participates in bone resorption. The authors evaluated this activity by measuring the cfDNA level in GCF of patients during the post-operative 24 h in the sites where bone grafting was inserted. From the results of this evaluation, it was observed that the bone loss obtained after the alveolar bone grafting may be related to increased cfDNA levels in GCF [66].

The cfDNA in the mouth derivates from bacterial DNA (bDNA) [67,68], epithelial death cells of the periodontal tissue [69] and neutrophil extracellular traps (NETs) [70] (Figure 1). NETosis, in the mouth, physiologically avoids bacteria colonization on the gingival cells [71]. Excessive production of NETs interrupt homeostasis, allowing harmful periodontal bacterial entrance [57,58].

One of the sources of endogenous cfDNA is mtDNA. Correct mitochondrial function is fundamental for maintaining health. In the case of periodontitis, the dysfunction of mitochondria participates in the pathogenesis of the disease [72]. The role of dysfunctional mitochondria in the pathogenesis of periodontitis is probably related as mtDNA has similarities with bacterial DNA [73]. This characteristic underlines how mtDNA presence in the extracellular environment stimulates inflammation in many inflammation-related diseases [74]. In periodontitis, the presence of mtDNA in the extracellular space is caused by periodontal pathogens that stimulate the NETs activity [75,76]. In a study conducted by Liu et al. [74], it was demonstrated, for the first time, that in a culture of gingival fibroblasts affected by periodontitis, the exposition of periodontal pathogens has caused the release of mtDNA. Moreover, they observed an increase in mtDNA in mice affected by periodontitis compared to the control group [74]. In agreement with this study, it was proved that mtDNA outside the cells leads to bone resorption [77]. Furthermore, another study discovered that bDNA increases the extracellular mtDNA release, resulting in TRL9 activation [78].

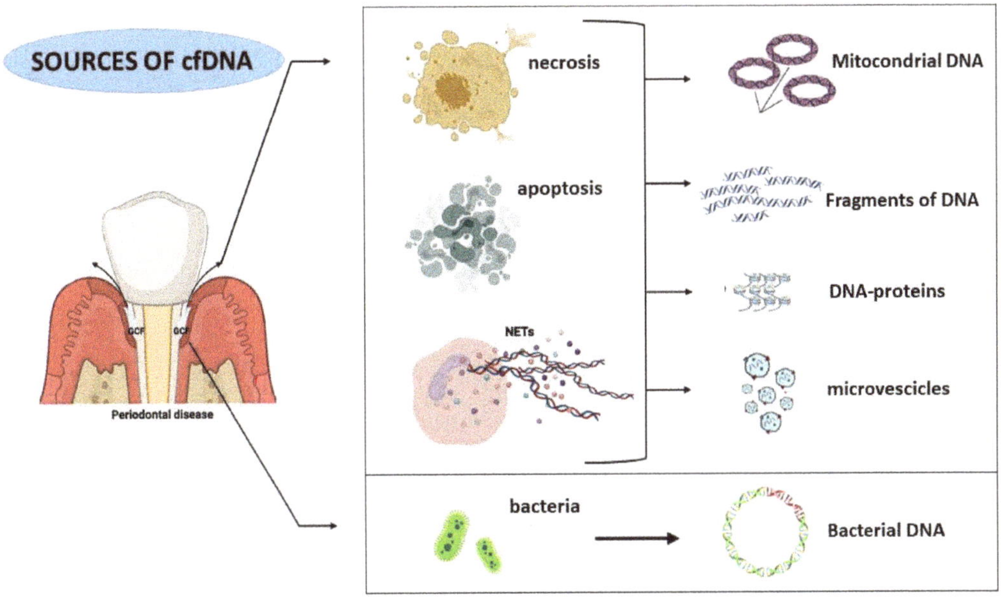

Figure 1. Description of the main mechanisms of origin of cfDNA in the organism and cfDNA's structural characteristics that each mechanism produces.

As mentioned before, cfDNA is normally removed from liquids due to the presence of DNases. DNases are a group of enzymes that hydrolyze cfDNA, allowing its removal from the body fluids. It could be possible that the incorrect functioning of the salivary DNases is another reason why the cfDNA level increases in periodontitis [79]. It was seen that periodontal bacteria could influence the activities of DNases [80]. Only one study has evaluated the activity of salivary DNases in periodontitis patients. This study did not show differences in the activity of DNases between patients affected by periodontitis and healthy patients. These results could be linked to the fact that the samplings were frozen and stored [79]. Therefore, it is not yet clear whether there is a correlation with cfDNA concentration. For these reasons, further studies are necessary for a better understanding. Additionally, further evaluation should analyze the DNases activity immediately after the levy.

CfDNA could be a new instrument to understand the status of periodontitis status. The short length of cfDNA can be a limit for its search, but due to different new technological methods, today, its detection is possible [25,81,82]. These methods are fluorescence [83], genomic sequencing [84] and polymerase chain reaction (PCR) [85]. In periodontology, cfDNA concentration was investigated in blood, saliva and gingival crevicular fluid (GCF) (Figure 2) [85]. Different studies have analyzed the level of cfDNA in periodontopathic patients and healthy patients in these different biofluids.

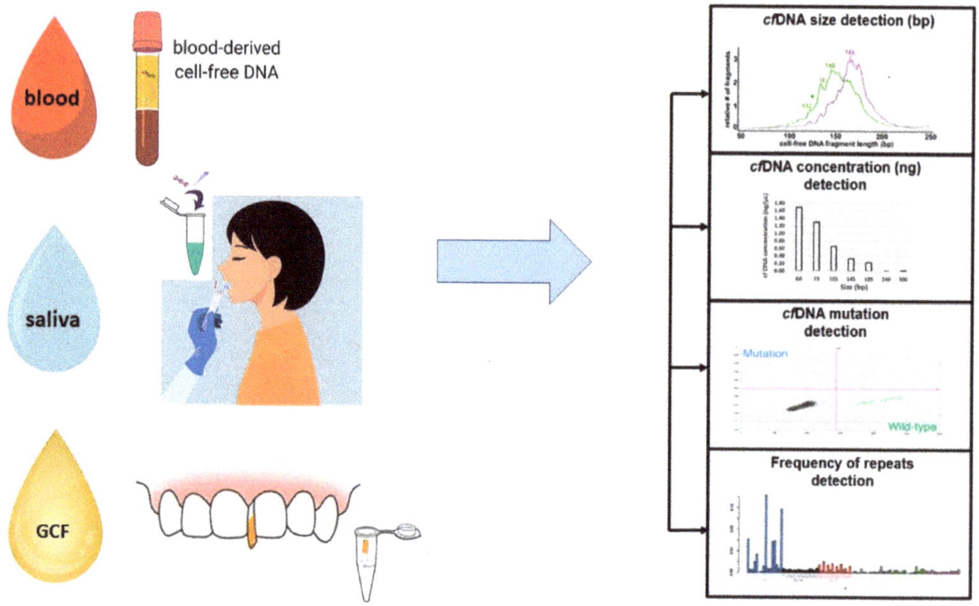

Figure 2. Description of the main methods of sampling biological fluids (blood, saliva and GCF) for research of the cfDNA level and of the analyses used for the study of cfDNA (cfDNA mutation, the variation of the cfDNA level and the size of the cfDNA). Partially modified and reproduced under permission of Creative Commons Licenses, from Hassan et al. [86].

3.1. Evaluation of the cfDNA Level in GCF

Two techniques can be used to collect gingival crevicular fluid (GCF): the washing technique [20,87] and the paper strips technique [88]. In the washing technique, the gingival pockets are washed with an isotonic solution, and the fluid that emerges from the pockets is aspirated. In the paper strips technique, three paper strips are used to collect the gingival crevicular fluid for 30 s each. Both techniques allow the collection of the GCF, but the paper strips technique is better because it does not require a long learning curve. In contrast, to collect GCF in the correct way with the washing technique, the operator needs to develop specific skills [89]. In a study conducted by Thaweboon et al. [89], GCF was collected for the evaluation of cfDNA in periodontopathic and healthy patients. It was seen that there was no statistical variation in the cfDNA concentration between the two techniques. Moreover, the authors observed little variation between these methods. The cfDNA level in patients affected by gingivitis was a little more concentrated using the paper strips than in the washing technique [89]. The same results were also obtained by Suwannagindra et al. [90]. Two studies evaluated the possible correlation between the cfDNA level in GCF and the periodontal clinical parameters (PD, BoP, PI plaque index). Suwannagindra et al. [90] collected the GCF in 20 patients affected by different degrees of periodontitis. After that, the concentration of cfDNA was evaluated, showing no correlation between the level of cfDNA and the periodontal parameters (PD, BoP and PI) [90]. In contrast, Zhu et al. [5] found a correlation between the level of cfDNA in GCF and periodontal parameters. The level of cfDNA increased based on the degree of the disease. In patients affected by gingivitis, the cfDNA levels were higher than in healthy patients, but in patients affected by periodontitis, the level of cfDNA was enhanced more than in patients affected by gingivitis. These results underline how the concentration of cfDNA in GCF is strongly correlated with the extent of the periodontal inflammation. Additionally, statistically predictive impacts of the cfDNA level in GCF and PD (pocket depth), BoP (bleeding on probing) and PI (plaque index) were shown [5]. The different results obtained from these two studies could be determined by the low number (only 20) of the patients evaluated in the study of Suwannagindra et al. [90] in contrast with the 114 patients in Zhu's study [5] (Table 1).

Table 1. The table above summarizes the results obtained in the clinical studies which have analyzed cfDNA in different biofluids.

Source	Type of Study	Results	Ref.
GCF	Evaluation on humans	The periodontopathic patients showed a higher level of cfDNA compared to the control group	[89]
	Evaluation on humans	A higher level of cfDNA was observed in periodontopathic patients	[90]
	Evaluation on humans	It was seen that the level of cfDNA was correlated with the degree of inflammation in patients with gingivitis, periodontitis, and healthy patients	[5]
Salivary	Evaluation on humans	It was observed that the level of cfDNA reflected the degree of the inflammation based on the presence of gingivitis, periodontitis, or oral health	[5]
	Evaluation on humans	From this study, the results showed the presence of high levels of cfDNA in patients affected with periodontitis compared to the healthy patients	[79]
Serum	Evaluation on humans	The results showed that the blood level of cfDNA was higher in patients with periodontitis, while healthy patients and patients affected with gingivitis did not have variations	[5]
	Evaluation on mice	Mice affected by periodontitis presented high blood levels of mtDNA compared to the healthy mice	[74]

3.2. Evaluation of the cfDNA Level in Saliva

In a sample of saliva, it is possible to detect a variety of biomarkers. Many factors, such as diet, disease and stress, can influence the elements of saliva [91]. In the periodontal field, using saliva allows us to evaluate the presence of cytokines, oxidative stress levels, antioxidants, periodontopathic bacteria and others [92–97]. The cfDNA in saliva comprises 70% of endogenous DNA and 30% of microbial DNA [98].

Zhun et al. [5] studied the cfDNA level variation in different biofluids, one of which was saliva. Their study showed that the cfDNA concentration was higher in patients affected by periodontitis and gingivitis compared to healthy patients. Moreover, they discovered a positive correlation between the cfDNA level and the clinical parameters; for instance, PD, BoP and PI [5]. Huang et al. [4] synthesized a type of nanoparticle to remove the cfDNA in the periodontal pockets to treat periodontitis in an animal model. To achieve their previous objective, they studied the mechanism between periodontitis and the increase of the cfDNA level in saliva and human blood. They observed that patients affected by periodontitis had a cfDNA concentration higher than patients affected by gingivitis or healthy ones.

Konečná et al. [79] studied the salivary cfDNA concentration in 25 periodontopathic and 29 healthy patients. The results of this study showed that the total salivary cfDNA level in patients with periodontitis was higher than in healthy patients. Despite these initial results, when the saliva was centrifugated to remove cells, the level of cfDNA in both groups did not differ. This study has demonstrated that the level of mtDNA in saliva was higher in patients affected by periodontitis than in the healthy group [79]. This result underlines mitochondria's important role in inflammation [99] (Table 1). Another study showed similar results in patients affected by periodontitis who had high cfDNA levels in saliva compared to the control group. Furthermore, in this study, the concentration of all the bacteria in saliva was not correlated with the salivary level of cfDNA in the periodontopathic patients [100].

It was recently discovered that methylation reaction products on the DNA chain can be detected in cfDNA. One of these methylation products is the global cytosine methylation (5 mC) found in breast, colorectal and prostate cancers and used as biomarkers [101]. Han et al. [102] researched the possible mutations of cfDNA that could be used in the periodontal field. They have researched the global epigenetic DNA present in the salivary small extracellular vesicle carrier DNA (sEVs) and in the genomic DNA (gDNA) among patients affected by gingivitis and periodontitis and healthy controls. The results showed that sEVs from the saliva of periodontopathic patients possess a significant increase of the 5 mC and m6dA (N6-methyl-2′-deoxyadenosine) methylation compared to the healthy group. The authors concluded that salivary sEV 5 mC methylation has a high sensitivity for discerning periodontitis patients from healthy ones [102]. However, further investigations are necessary on a huge cohort for a better understanding. The research of particular methylation in the cfDNA allowed us to understand from which tissue the cfDNA was released. Additionally, it was declared that the methylations present on the cfDNA are a valid method for cancer diagnosis [103,104].

3.3. Evaluation of cfDNA in Serum

As mentioned, it is possible to detect cfDNA in blood. In fact, two preclinical studies showed increased cfDNA levels in plasma after the injection of *Porphyromonas gingivalis* (*P. gingivalis*) in mice [105,106]. A study by Zhu et al. [5] evaluated the level of cfDNA in the serum of patients with periodontitis and gingivitis and healthy patients. This study showed that the cfDNA concentration was higher in the blood of the periodontopathic patients, while the cfDNA blood level was not different between the patients affected by gingivitis and the healthy patients. The authors concluded by saying that these results showed how the degree of inflammation in the periodontal tissue influenced the cfDNA blood concentration [5]. Furthermore, another study obtained similar results by investigating the cfDNA level in serum between patients affected by periodontitis and healthy patients. At the end of the study, the periodontopathic patients had a higher level of cfDNA in serum compared to the healthy patients. Additionally, they were the first to prove the strong correlation between the cfDNA level in serum and GCF and the progression of periodontitis [4]. In a study by Liu et al. [74], mice affected by periodontitis had an enhanced mtDNA level in serum compared to healthy mice. The same mechanism was replicated in human gingival fibroblastic culture cells affected by periodontitis in which the release of mtDNA was seen. Moreover, human gingival fibroblast culture cells without periodontitis started to release mtDNA when exposed to *P. gingivalis* [74]. These results evidenced how mtDNA actively contributes to the development of periodontitis (Table 1).

Most of the studies evaluated biomarkers in saliva, blood and GCF on freezing samples. For this reason, it is important to underline that plasma freezing causes free DNA liberation from exosomes [107]. This is an aspect that must also be considered in salivary sampling because freezing is part of the processes used in many studies.

3.4. Evaluation of cfDNA in Periodontitis and Oral Diseases

Many studies showed that cfDNA plays a central role in the development and progression of many diseases: for instance, rheumatoid arthritis, atherosclerosis and sepsis [65,108–110].

It can be seen that periodontal cfDNA is present in different biomaterials, such as serum [111], atherosclerotic plaque [112,113], synovial fluid [114] and intrauterine environment [115]. This underlines the possible relationship between periodontitis and systemic disease.

Over the years, different studies have evaluated the link between periodontitis and arthritis. Both pathologies share common inflammation mechanisms and lead to bone loss [116]. In a study conducted by Oliveira et al. [117], the cfDNA levels in serum and saliva were evaluated among different groups of patients: patients affected by initial arthritis with and without periodontitis, patients affected by prior arthritis with and without periodontitis and healthy patients. The results of this study showed that patients affected by initial and prior arthritis associated with periodontitis possessed high levels of cfDNA in saliva and serum compared to the patients without periodontitis and arthritis. Both pathologies are characterized by the increase of NET activity, which feeds the chronic inflammation. When both pathologies coexist in the same patient, the NETs level is overstimulated, and the cfDNA level in saliva and serum is very high [117].

In recent decades, numerous studies have focused on the possible correlation between periodontitis and cardiovascular disease. Periodontitis is one of the main risk factors for cardiovascular disease [118,119]. According to these studies, bDNA of periodontal pathogens has been seen in serum and cardiovascular tissue [120]. A study conducted by Wu et al. [121] evaluated the presence of *P. gingivalis* DNA in the cfDNA of saliva and serum between patients affected by acute myocardial infarction (AMI) and patients without coronary heart disease. The authors of this study support the idea that periodontitis pathogens actively participate in developing atherosclerosis [119]. This study showed that patients affected by AMI were positive for *P. gingivalis* DNA in the cfDNA of the serum withdrawal. Moreover, the positivity with Pg is associated with the severity of coronary inflammation. Furthermore, there was no statistically significant variation between the positivity of *P. gingivalis* in the saliva cfDNA between the group of patients without cardiovascular disease and those affected by IMA. The authors concluded that the invasion and establishment of periodontal pathogens in the endothelial tissues were one of the risk factors for acute myocardial infarction. Additionally, the presence of Pg in the cardiovascular tissue increases the host response [121].

In pregnant patients with a predisposition to periodontitis, adverse outcomes were seen during the pregnancy. This is related to the presence of periodontal pathogens and the increase of immune stimulus caused by their presence. Different studies have shown the presence of periodontal pathogens DNA in the plasma of pregnant patients affected by periodontitis [115].

Diabetes is another disease in which NETs play a crucial role. NETs has an important role in the physiopathology of diabetes and periodontitis. Hyperglycemia causes the activation of the NETs mechanism. In a study conducted by Carestia et al. [122], an increase in the NETosis level was observed in patients affected by diabetes compared to healthy patients. For this reason, it would be interesting to analyze the cfDNA level in both pathologies and see how their coexistence impacts the cfDNA level.

4. Strategy to Treat Periodontitis Removing the cfDNA

The discovery related to the presence of cfDNA in periodontitis has opened the possibility to a new therapy that uses cfDNA as a target, in particular for the treatment of bone loss [66] and inflammation in periodontitis. In a study conducted by Huang et al. [4], it was discovered that with the deletion of cfDNA in the periodontal pockets, the level of cfDNA in saliva and serum decreased. Furthermore, the intense relationship between the high level of cfDNA and elevated alveolar bone destruction was underlined. After this discovery, Huang et al. [4] formulated particular nanoparticles to remove cfDNA. These nanoparticles were firstly tested on cell cultures and subsequently on animals. The nanoparticles give better results when administered locally in the periodontal pockets instead of systemically. This study showed that the alveolar bone loss in the rats affected by periodontitis had a reduction. Further studies need to evaluate the efficacy and safety of these nanoparticles in humans. Despite the interesting results obtained, Huang's study was the first and only one that created and tested a new drug that used cfDNA as a target in periodontitis. The presence of high levels of cfDNA in other inflammatory diseases has stimulated researchers' interest in creating drugs against this target. Their results can lead to future studies about alternative treatments for periodontitis.

Many studies showed that different cation nanoparticles can scavenge cfDNA. Liu et al. [123] developed nanoparticles to scavenge the increase of cfDNA in sepsis. The cfDNA-scavenging nanoparticles [20] were composed of cationic polyethyleneimine (PEI), which was loaded with zeolitic imidazolate framework-8 (PEI-g-ZIF). This nanosystem was tested in an in vitro model. The results of this study showed a decrease in the cfDNA, confirming the ability of these nanoparticles to bind and remove cfDNA in plasma [123]. In another study, a copolymer was developed and tested on animals as a new inhibitor of cfDNA in arthritis. The copolymer was composed of poly-lactic-co-glycolic acid (PLGA) and poly-2-diethylamino-ethyl methacrylate (PDMA). This copolymer in rats affected by arthritis was able to inhibit the TRL9 and scavenge cfDNA in plasma and inflamed joints. Although this copolymer's positive results have been shown, it is necessary to carry out other investigations into its toxicity and efficacy [124]. Similar results were obtained by Pan et al. [125] during their study. In fact, it was seen that the inhibition of TRL9 allowed a decrease in periodontal inflammation in rats affected by arthritis [125]. Another study investigated Hexadimethrine bromide, a cation polymer that has an affinity with mtDNA. It was seen that this cation polymer allowed a decrease of the inflammatory mediators in a rat model [126]. Narayan et al. [63] observed that the high level of TRL9 in periodontal patients influenced periodontal tissue destruction.

The coexistence of cfDNA in the inflammation mechanism of different diseases can be an alternative target for treating patients affected by periodontitis with and without other diseases.

5. Conclusions

CfDNA is a physiological biomaterial that has been observed to increase in several chronic inflammatory diseases, including periodontal disease. CfDNA actively participates in the pathology's beginning and progression in periodontitis, favoring the inflammation's continuation. The use of saliva and GCF to detect cfDNA are non-invasive methods that can be used for the future diagnosis and prognosis of periodontitis. The possibility of synthesizing nanoparticles which can remove cfDNA could be a new strategy to reduce the inflammation of periodontitis. Despite the promising results obtained about this new biomarker and new therapeutic targets in periodontitis, further studies are necessary to develop a reliable, safe and standardized protocol for the detection of cfDNA.

Author Contributions: Conceptualization, G.I.; methodology, S.S. and M.A.; validation, K.Z. and G.T.; formal analysis, P.P. and A.P.; data curation, A.P. and G.V.; writing—original draft preparation, S.S. and G.V.; writing—review and editing, G.I.; funding acquisition, G.I. All authors have read and agreed to the published version of the manuscript.

Funding: This research was funded with funds derived from the Action "Starting Grant 2020, Linea di Intervento 3, PIACERI 2020–2022" of the University of Catania, Catania, Italy Prof. G. Isola.

Institutional Review Board Statement: Not applicable.

Informed Consent Statement: Not applicable.

Data Availability Statement: Data are available from the corresponding author upon reasonable request.

Conflicts of Interest: The authors declare no conflict of interest.

References

1. Frencken, J.E.; Sharma, P.; Stenhouse, L.; Green, D.; Laverty, D.; Dietrich, T. Global epidemiology of dental caries and severe periodontitis–a comprehensive review. *J. Clin. Periodontol.* **2017**, *44*, S94–S105. [CrossRef] [PubMed]
2. Slots, J. Periodontitis: Facts, fallacies and the future. *Periodontology 2000* **2017**, *75*, 7–23. [CrossRef] [PubMed]
3. Papapanou, P.N.; Sanz, M.; Buduneli, N.; Dietrich, T.; Feres, M.; Fine, D.H.; Flemmig, T.F.; Garcia, R.; Giannobile, W.V.; Graziani, F. Periodontitis: Consensus report of workgroup 2 of the 2017 World Workshop on the Classification of Periodontal and Peri-Implant Diseases and Conditions. *J. Periodontol.* **2018**, *89*, S173–S182. [CrossRef]
4. Huang, H.; Pan, W.; Wang, Y.; Kim, H.S.; Shao, D.; Huang, B.; Ho, T.-C.; Lao, Y.-H.; Quek, C.H.; Shi, J. Nanoparticulate cell-free DNA scavenger for treating inflammatory bone loss in periodontitis. *Nat. Commun.* **2022**, *13*, 5925. [CrossRef]
5. Zhu, X.; Chu, C.-J.; Pan, W.; Li, Y.; Huang, H.; Zhao, L. The correlation between periodontal parameters and cell-free DNA in the gingival crevicular fluid, Saliva, and plasma in Chinese patients: A cross-sectional study. *J. Clin. Med.* **2022**, *11*, 6902. [CrossRef]
6. Polina, I.A.; Ilatovskaya, D.V.; DeLeon-Pennell, K.Y. Cell free DNA as a diagnostic and prognostic marker for cardiovascular diseases. *Clin. Chim. Acta* **2020**, *503*, 145–150. [CrossRef]
7. Duvvuri, B.; Lood, C. Cell-free DNA as a biomarker in autoimmune rheumatic diseases. *Front. Immunol.* **2019**, *10*, 502. [CrossRef]
8. Ullrich, E.; Heidinger, P.; Soh, J.; Villanova, L.; Grabuschnig, S.; Bachler, T.; Hirschböck, E.; Sánchez-Heredero, S.; Ford, B.; Sensen, M. Evaluation of host-based molecular markers for the early detection of human sepsis. *J. Biotechnol.* **2020**, *310*, 80–88. [CrossRef]

9. Gögenur, M.; Burcharth, J.; Gögenur, I. The role of total cell-free DNA in predicting outcomes among trauma patients in the intensive care unit: A systematic review. *Crit. Care* **2017**, *21*, 14. [CrossRef]
10. Patel, A.; Patel, S.; Patel, P.; Tanavde, V. Saliva based liquid biopsies in head and neck cancer: How far are we from the clinic? *Front. Oncol.* **2022**, *12*, 828434. [CrossRef] [PubMed]
11. Wang, Y.; Springer, S.; Mulvey, C.L.; Silliman, N.; Schaefer, J.; Sausen, M.; James, N.; Rettig, E.M.; Guo, T.; Pickering, C.R. Detection of somatic mutations and HPV in the saliva and plasma of patients with head and neck squamous cell carcinomas. *Sci. Transl. Med.* **2015**, *7*, 293ra104. [CrossRef] [PubMed]
12. Desai, A.; Kallianpur, S.; Mani, A.; Tijare, M.S.; Khan, S.; Jain, M.; Mathur, V.; Ahuja, R.; Saxena, V. Quantification of circulating plasma cell free DNA fragments in patients with oral cancer and precancer. *Gulf J. Oncol.* **2018**, *1*, 11–17.
13. Lin, L.-H.; Chang, K.-W.; Kao, S.-Y.; Cheng, H.-W.; Liu, C.-J. Increased plasma circulating cell-free DNA could be a potential marker for oral cancer. *Int. J. Mol. Sci.* **2018**, *19*, 3303. [CrossRef]
14. Ocana, A.; Díez-González, L.; García-Olmo, D.C.; Templeton, A.J.; Vera-Badillo, F.; José Escribano, M.; Serrano-Heras, G.; Corrales-Sánchez, V.; Seruga, B.; Andrés-Pretel, F. Circulating DNA and Survival in Solid TumorsCirculating DNA and Survival in Cancer. *Cancer Epidemiol. Biomark. Prev.* **2016**, *25*, 399–406. [CrossRef]
15. Cheng, J.; Tang, Q.; Cao, X.; Burwinkel, B. Cell-free circulating DNA integrity based on peripheral blood as a biomarker for diagnosis of cancer: A systematic review. *Cancer Epidemiol. Biomark. Prev.* **2017**, *26*, 1595–1602. [CrossRef]
16. Mazurek, A.M.; Rutkowski, T.; Fiszer-Kierzkowska, A.; Małusecka, E.; Składowski, K. Assessment of the total cfDNA and HPV16/18 detection in plasma samples of head and neck squamous cell carcinoma patients. *Oral Oncol.* **2016**, *54*, 36–41. [CrossRef]
17. Sayal, L.; Hamadah, O.; Almasri, A.; Idrees, M.; Thomson, P.; Kujan, O. Saliva-based cell-free DNA and cell-free mitochondrial DNA in head and neck cancers have promising screening and early detection role. *J. Oral Pathol. Med.* **2023**, *52*, 29–36. [CrossRef] [PubMed]
18. Sayal, L.; Hamadah, O.; AlMasri, A.; Idrees, M.; Kassem, I.; Habbal, W.; Alsalamah, B.; Kujan, O. Salivary-Based Cell-Free Mitochondrial DNA Level Is an Independent Prognostic Biomarker for Patients with Head and Neck Squamous Cell Carcinoma. *J. Pers. Med.* **2023**, *13*, 301. [CrossRef] [PubMed]
19. Eisenhauer, E.A.; Therasse, P.; Bogaerts, J.; Schwartz, L.H.; Sargent, D.; Ford, R.; Dancey, J.; Arbuck, S.; Gwyther, S.; Mooney, M. New response evaluation criteria in solid tumours: Revised RECIST guideline (version 1.1). *Eur. J. Cancer* **2009**, *45*, 228–247. [CrossRef]
20. Thaweboon, B.; Laohapand, P.; Amornchat, C.; Matsuyama, J.; Sato, T.; Nunez, P.; Uematsu, H.; Hoshino, E. Host β-globin gene fragments in crevicular fluid as a biomarker in periodontal health and disease. *J. Periodontal Res.* **2010**, *45*, 38–44. [CrossRef]
21. Mandel, P. Les acides nucleiques du plasma sanguin chez 1 homme. *CR Seances Soc. Biol. Fil.* **1948**, *142*, 241–243.
22. Aucamp, J.; Bronkhorst, A.J.; Badenhorst, C.P.; Pretorius, P.J. The diverse origins of circulating cell-free DNA in the human body: A critical re-evaluation of the literature. *Biol. Rev.* **2018**, *93*, 1649–1683. [CrossRef]
23. Thierry, A.R.; El Messaoudi, S.; Gahan, P.; Anker, P.; Stroun, M. Origins, structures, and functions of circulating DNA in oncology. *Cancer Metastasis Rev.* **2016**, *35*, 347–376. [CrossRef]
24. van der Vaart, M.; Pretorius, P.J. Circulating DNA. Its origin and fluctuation. *Ann. N. Y. Acad. Sci.* **2008**, *1137*, 18–26. [CrossRef]
25. Bronkhorst, A.J.; Ungerer, V.; Holdenrieder, S. The emerging role of cell-free DNA as a molecular marker for cancer management. *Biomol. Detect. Quantif.* **2019**, *17*, 100087. [CrossRef] [PubMed]
26. Lo, Y.D.; Chan, K.A.; Sun, H.; Chen, E.Z.; Jiang, P.; Lun, F.M.; Zheng, Y.W.; Leung, T.Y.; Lau, T.K.; Cantor, C.R. Maternal plasma DNA sequencing reveals the genome-wide genetic and mutational profile of the fetus. *Sci. Transl. Med.* **2010**, *2*, 61ra91. [CrossRef] [PubMed]
27. Zhang, Q.; Raoof, M.; Chen, Y.; Sumi, Y.; Sursal, T.; Junger, W.; Brohi, K.; Itagaki, K.; Hauser, C.J. Circulating mitochondrial DAMPs cause inflammatory responses to injury. *Nature* **2010**, *464*, 104–107. [CrossRef]
28. Macher, H.; Egea-Guerrero, J.J.; Revuelto-Rey, J.; Gordillo-Escobar, E.; Enamorado-Enamorado, J.; Boza, A.; Rodriguez, A.; Molinero, P.; Guerrero, J.M.; Dominguez-Roldán, J.M. Role of early cell-free DNA levels decrease as a predictive marker of fatal outcome after severe traumatic brain injury. *Clin. Chim. Acta* **2012**, *414*, 12–17. [CrossRef] [PubMed]
29. Avriel, A.; Paryente Wiessman, M.; Almog, Y.; Perl, Y.; Novack, V.; Galante, O.; Klein, M.; Pencina, M.J.; Douvdevani, A. Admission cell free DNA levels predict 28-day mortality in patients with severe sepsis in intensive care. *PLoS ONE* **2014**, *9*, e100514. [CrossRef] [PubMed]
30. Rock, K.L.; Kono, H. The inflammatory response to cell death. *Annu. Rev. Pathol.* **2008**, *3*, 99–126. [CrossRef]
31. Suzuki, N.; Kamataki, A.; Yamaki, J.; Homma, Y. Characterization of circulating DNA in healthy human plasma. *Clin. Chim. Acta* **2008**, *387*, 55–58. [CrossRef]
32. Brinkmann, V.; Reichard, U.; Goosmann, C.; Fauler, B.; Uhlemann, Y.; Weiss, D.S.; Weinrauch, Y.; Zychlinsky, A. Neutrophil extracellular traps kill bacteria. *Science* **2004**, *303*, 1532–1535. [CrossRef] [PubMed]
33. Yipp, B.G.; Petri, B.; Salina, D.; Jenne, C.N.; Scott, B.N.; Zbytnuik, L.D.; Pittman, K.; Asaduzzaman, M.; Wu, K.; Meijndert, H.C. Infection-induced NETosis is a dynamic process involving neutrophil multitasking in vivo. *Nat. Med.* **2012**, *18*, 1386–1393. [CrossRef] [PubMed]
34. Yipp, B.G.; Kubes, P. NETosis: How vital is it? *Blood J. Am. Soc. Hematol.* **2013**, *122*, 2784–2794. [CrossRef] [PubMed]

35. Papayannopoulos, V.; Metzler, K.D.; Hakkim, A.; Zychlinsky, A. Neutrophil elastase and myeloperoxidase regulate the formation of neutrophil extracellular traps. *J. Cell Biol.* **2010**, *191*, 677–691. [CrossRef] [PubMed]
36. Branzk, N.; Papayannopoulos, V. Molecular mechanisms regulating NETosis in infection and disease. *Proc. Semin. Immunopathol.* **2013**, *35*, 513–530. [CrossRef]
37. Snyder, M.W.; Kircher, M.; Hill, A.J.; Daza, R.M.; Shendure, J. Cell-free DNA comprises an in vivo nucleosome footprint that informs its tissues-of-origin. *Cell* **2016**, *164*, 57–68. [CrossRef]
38. Volik, S.; Alcaide, M.; Morin, R.D.; Collins, C. Cell-free DNA (cfDNA): Clinical significance and utility in cancer shaped by emerging technologies. *Mol. Cancer Res.* **2016**, *14*, 898–908. [CrossRef]
39. Jahr, S.; Hentze, H.; Englisch, S.; Hardt, D.; Fackelmayer, F.O.; Hesch, R.-D.; Knippers, R. DNA fragments in the blood plasma of cancer patients: Quantitations and evidence for their origin from apoptotic and necrotic cells. *Cancer Res.* **2001**, *61*, 1659–1665.
40. Breitbach, S.; Tug, S.; Simon, P. Circulating cell-free DNA: An up-coming molecular marker in exercise physiology. *Sport. Med.* **2012**, *42*, 565–586. [CrossRef]
41. Lázaro-Ibáñez, E.; Lässer, C.; Shelke, G.V.; Crescitelli, R.; Jang, S.C.; Cvjetkovic, A.; García-Rodríguez, A.; Lötvall, J. DNA analysis of low-and high-density fractions defines heterogeneous subpopulations of small extracellular vesicles based on their DNA cargo and topology. *J. Extracell. Vesicles* **2019**, *8*, 1656993. [CrossRef]
42. Torralba, D.; Baixauli, F.; Villarroya-Beltri, C.; Fernández-Delgado, I.; Latorre-Pellicer, A.; Acín-Pérez, R.; Martín-Cófreces, N.B.; Jaso-Tamame, Á.L.; Iborra, S.; Jorge, I. Priming of dendritic cells by DNA-containing extracellular vesicles from activated T cells through antigen-driven contacts. *Nat. Commun.* **2018**, *9*, 2658. [CrossRef]
43. Pös, O.; Biró, O.; Szemes, T.; Nagy, B. Circulating cell-free nucleic acids: Characteristics and applications. *Eur. J. Hum. Genet.* **2018**, *26*, 937–945. [CrossRef]
44. Kawamura, Y.; Yamamoto, Y.; Sato, T.A.; Ochiya, T. Extracellular vesicles as trans-genomic agents: Emerging roles in disease and evolution. *Cancer Sci.* **2017**, *108*, 824–830. [CrossRef]
45. Edgar, J.R. Q&A: What are exosomes, exactly? *BMC Biol.* **2016**, *14*, 46.
46. Takahashi, A.; Okada, R.; Nagao, K.; Kawamata, Y.; Hanyu, A.; Yoshimoto, S.; Takasugi, M.; Watanabe, S.; Kanemaki, M.T.; Obuse, C. Exosomes maintain cellular homeostasis by excreting harmful DNA from cells. *Nat. Commun.* **2017**, *8*, 15287. [CrossRef]
47. McGough, I.J.; Vincent, J.-P. Exosomes in developmental signalling. *Development* **2016**, *143*, 2482–2493. [CrossRef] [PubMed]
48. Warton, K.; Lin, V.; Navin, T.; Armstrong, N.J.; Kaplan, W.; Ying, K.; Gloss, B.; Mangs, H.; Nair, S.S.; Hacker, N.F. Methylation-capture and next-generation sequencing of free circulating DNA from human plasma. *BMC Genom.* **2014**, *15*, 476. [CrossRef] [PubMed]
49. Luo, H.; Wei, W.; Ye, Z.; Zheng, J.; Xu, R.-H. Liquid biopsy of methylation biomarkers in cell-free DNA. *Trends Mol. Med.* **2021**, *27*, 482–500. [CrossRef] [PubMed]
50. Di Renzo, G.C.; Bartha, J.L.; Bilardo, C.M. Expanding the indications for cell-free DNA in the maternal circulation: Clinical considerations and implications. *Am. J. Obstet. Gynecol.* **2019**, *220*, 537–542. [CrossRef] [PubMed]
51. Heitzer, E.; Auer, M.; Ulz, P.; Geigl, J.B.; Speicher, M.R. Circulating tumor cells and DNA as liquid biopsies. *Genome Med.* **2013**, *5*, 73. [CrossRef]
52. Emlen, W.; Mannik, M. Kinetics and mechanisms for removal of circulating single-stranded DNA in mice. *J. Exp. Med.* **1978**, *147*, 684–699. [CrossRef]
53. Lauková, L.; Bertolo, E.M.J.; Zelinková, M.; Borbélyová, V.; Conka, J.; Kovalcíková, A.G.; Domonkos, E.; Vlková, B.; Celec, P. Early dynamics of plasma DNA in a mouse model of sepsis. *Shock* **2019**, *52*, 257–263. [CrossRef]
54. Rathnayake, N.; Åkerman, S.; Klinge, B.; Lundegren, N.; Jansson, H.; Tryselius, Y.; Sorsa, T.; Gustafsson, A. Salivary biomarkers of oral health–a cross-sectional study. *J. Clin. Periodontol.* **2013**, *40*, 140–147. [CrossRef]
55. Chen, G.Y.; Nuñez, G. Sterile inflammation: Sensing and reacting to damage. *Nat. Rev. Immunol.* **2010**, *10*, 826–837. [CrossRef]
56. Kruger, P.; Saffarzadeh, M.; Weber, A.N.; Rieber, N.; Radsak, M.; von Bernuth, H.; Benarafa, C.; Roos, D.; Skokowa, J.; Hartl, D. Neutrophils: Between host defence, immune modulation, and tissue injury. *PLoS Pathog.* **2015**, *11*, e1004651. [CrossRef] [PubMed]
57. Yost, C.C.; Schwertz, H.; Cody, M.J.; Wallace, J.A.; Campbell, R.A.; Vieira-de-Abreu, A.; Araujo, C.V.; Schubert, S.; Harris, E.S.; Rowley, J.W. Neonatal NET-inhibitory factor and related peptides inhibit neutrophil extracellular trap formation. *J. Clin. Investig.* **2016**, *126*, 3783–3798. [CrossRef] [PubMed]
58. Lopes, D.E.; Jabr, C.L.; Dejani, N.N.; Saraiva, A.C.; de Aquino, S.G.; Medeiros, A.I.; Rossa Junior, C. Inhibition of 5-lipoxygenase attenuates inflammation and bone resorption in lipopolysaccharide-induced periodontal disease. *J. Periodontol.* **2018**, *89*, 235–245. [CrossRef] [PubMed]
59. Gong, T.; Liu, L.; Jiang, W.; Zhou, R. DAMP-sensing receptors in sterile inflammation and inflammatory diseases. *Nat. Rev. Immunol.* **2020**, *20*, 95–112. [CrossRef] [PubMed]
60. Paludan, S.R.; Bowie, A.G. Immune sensing of DNA. *Immunity* **2013**, *38*, 870–880. [CrossRef] [PubMed]
61. Kim, P.D.; Xia-Juan, X.; Crump, K.E.; Abe, T.; Hajishengallis, G.; Sahingur, S.E. Toll-like receptor 9-mediated inflammation triggers alveolar bone loss in experimental murine periodontitis. *Infect. Immun.* **2015**, *83*, 2992–3002. [CrossRef] [PubMed]
62. Crump, K.E.; Oakley, J.C.; Xia-Juan, X.; Madu, T.C.; Devaki, S.; Mooney, E.C.; Sahingur, S.E. Interplay of toll-like receptor 9, myeloid cells, and deubiquitinase A20 in periodontal inflammation. *Infect. Immun.* **2017**, *85*, e00814–e00816. [CrossRef] [PubMed]

63. Narayan, I.; Gowda, T.M.; Mehta, D.S.; Kumar, B.T. Estimation of Toll-like receptor 9 in gingival tissues of patients with chronic periodontitis with or without hyperlipidemia and its association with the presence of Porphyromonas gingivalis. *J. Indian Soc. Periodontol.* **2018**, *22*, 298. [CrossRef]
64. Chen, Y.-C.; Liu, C.-M.; Jeng, J.-H.; Ku, C.-C. Association of pocket epithelial cell proliferation in periodontitis with TLR9 expression and inflammatory response. *J. Formos. Med. Assoc.* **2014**, *113*, 549–556. [CrossRef]
65. Zhu, X.; Huang, H.; Zhao, L. PAMPs and DAMPs as the bridge between periodontitis and atherosclerosis: The potential therapeutic targets. *Front. Cell. Dev. Biol.* **2022**, *10*, 856118. [CrossRef]
66. Huang, H.; Yang, R.; Shi, B. The potential role of cfDNA-related innate immune responses in postoperative bone loss after alveolar bone grafting. *Front. Immunol.* **2022**, *13*, 1068186. [CrossRef] [PubMed]
67. Kim, Y.; Jo, A.R.; Jang, D.H.; Cho, Y.J.; Chun, J.; Min, B.M.; Choi, Y. Toll-like receptor 9 mediates oral bacteria-induced IL-8 expression in gingival epithelial cells. *Immunol. Cell Biol.* **2012**, *90*, 655–663. [CrossRef]
68. Sahingur, S.E.; Xia, X.J.; Schifferle, R.E. Oral bacterial DNA differ in their ability to induce inflammatory responses in human monocytic cell lines. *J. Periodontol.* **2012**, *83*, 1069–1077. [CrossRef] [PubMed]
69. Govindarajan, S.; Veeraraghavan, V.P.; Dillibabu, T.; Patil, S. Oral Cavity–A Resilient Source for DNA Sampling. *J. Contemp. Dent. Pract.* **2022**, *23*, 1–2.
70. Silva, L.M.; Doyle, A.D.; Greenwell-Wild, T.; Dutzan, N.; Tran, C.L.; Abusleme, L.; Juang, L.J.; Leung, J.; Chun, E.M.; Lum, A.G. Fibrin is a critical regulator of neutrophil effector function at the oral mucosal barrier. *Science* **2021**, *374*, eabl5450. [CrossRef] [PubMed]
71. Sima, C.; Glogauer, M. Neutrophil dysfunction and host susceptibility to periodontal inflammation: Current state of knowledge. *Curr. Oral Health Rep.* **2014**, *1*, 95–103. [CrossRef]
72. Bullon, P.; Newman, H.N.; Battino, M. Obesity, diabetes mellitus, atherosclerosis and chronic periodontitis: A shared pathology via oxidative stress and mitochondrial dysfunction? *Periodontology 2000* **2014**, *64*, 139–153. [CrossRef] [PubMed]
73. Wu, Z.; Oeck, S.; West, A.P.; Mangalhara, K.C.; Sainz, A.G.; Newman, L.E.; Zhang, X.-O.; Wu, L.; Yan, Q.; Bosenberg, M. Mitochondrial DNA stress signalling protects the nuclear genome. *Nat. Metab.* **2019**, *1*, 1209–1218. [CrossRef] [PubMed]
74. Liu, J.; Wang, Y.; Shi, Q.; Wang, X.; Zou, P.; Zheng, M.; Luan, Q. Mitochondrial DNA efflux maintained in gingival fibroblasts of patients with periodontitis through ROS/mPTP pathway. *Oxidative Med. Cell. Longev.* **2022**, *2022*, 1000213. [CrossRef]
75. Mikacenic, C.; Moore, R.; Dmyterko, V.; West, T.E.; Altemeier, W.A.; Liles, W.C.; Lood, C. Neutrophil extracellular traps (NETs) are increased in the alveolar spaces of patients with ventilator-associated pneumonia. *Crit. Care* **2018**, *22*, 358. [CrossRef]
76. Cedervall, J.; Hamidi, A.; Olsson, A.-K. Platelets, NETs and cancer. *Thromb. Res.* **2018**, *164*, S148–S152. [CrossRef]
77. Zheleznyak, A.; Mixdorf, M.; Marsala, L.; Prior, J.; Yang, X.; Cui, G.; Xu, B.; Fletcher, S.; Fontana, F.; Lanza, G. Orthogonal targeting of osteoclasts and myeloma cells for radionuclide stimulated dynamic therapy induces multidimensional cell death pathways. *Theranostics* **2021**, *11*, 7735. [CrossRef]
78. Kaewduangduen, W.; Visitchanakun, P.; Saisorn, W.; Phawadee, A.; Manonitnantawat, C.; Chutimaskul, C.; Susantitaphong, P.; Ritprajak, P.; Somboonna, N.; Cheibchalard, T. Blood bacteria-free DNA in septic mice enhances LPS-induced inflammation in mice through macrophage response. *Int. J. Mol. Sci.* **2022**, *23*, 1907. [CrossRef] [PubMed]
79. Konečná, B.; Gaál Kovalčíková, A.; Pančíková, A.; Novák, B.; Kovaľová, E.; Celec, P.; Tóthová, Ľ. Salivary extracellular DNA and DNase activity in periodontitis. *Appl. Sci.* **2020**, *10*, 7490. [CrossRef]
80. Palmer, L.; Chapple, I.; Wright, H.; Roberts, A.; Cooper, P. Extracellular deoxyribonuclease production by periodontal bacteria. *J. Periodontal Res.* **2012**, *47*, 439–445. [CrossRef]
81. Heitzer, E.; Haque, I.S.; Roberts, C.E.; Speicher, M.R. Current and future perspectives of liquid biopsies in genomics driven oncology. *Nat. Rev. Genet.* **2019**, *20*, 71–88. [CrossRef] [PubMed]
82. Buono, G.; Gerratana, L.; Bulfoni, M.; Provinciali, N.; Basile, D.; Giuliano, M.; Corvaja, C.; Arpino, G.; Del Mastro, L.; De Placido, S. Circulating tumor DNA analysis in breast cancer: Is it ready for prime-time? *Cancer Treat. Rev.* **2019**, *73*, 73–83. [CrossRef]
83. Chang, C.P.-Y.; Chia, R.-H.; Wu, T.-L.; Tsao, K.-C.; Sun, C.-F.; Wu, J.T. Elevated cell-free serum DNA detected in patients with myocardial infarction. *Clin. Chim. Acta* **2003**, *327*, 95–101. [CrossRef] [PubMed]
84. De Vlaminck, I.; Martin, L.; Kertesz, M.; Patel, K.; Kowarsky, M.; Strehl, C.; Cohen, G.; Luikart, H.; Neff, N.F.; Okamoto, J. Noninvasive monitoring of infection and rejection after lung transplantation. *Proc. Natl. Acad. Sci. USA* **2015**, *112*, 13336–13341. [CrossRef] [PubMed]
85. Lo, Y.D.; Tein, M.S.; Pang, C.C.; Yeung, C.K.; Tong, K.-L.; Hjelm, N.M. Presence of donor-specific DNA in plasma of kidney and liver-transplant recipients. *Lancet* **1998**, *351*, 1329–1330. [CrossRef] [PubMed]
86. Hassan, S.; Shehzad, A.; Khan, S.A.; Miran, W.; Khan, S.; Lee, Y.S. Diagnostic and Therapeutic Potential of Circulating-Free DNA and Cell-Free RNA in Cancer Management. *Biomedicines* **2022**, *10*, 2047. [CrossRef]
87. Doan, T.M.; Kriangcherdsak, Y.; Thaweboon, S.; Thaweboon, B. Evaluation of Host β-Globin Gene Fragment Lengths in Peri-implant Crevicular Fluid During the Wound Healing Process: A Pilot Study. *Int. J. Oral Maxillofac. Implant.* **2015**, *30*, 1295–1302. [CrossRef]
88. Nazar Majeed, Z.; Philip, K.; Alabsi, A.; Pushparajan, S.; Swaminathan, D. Identification of gingival crevicular fluid sampling, analytical methods, and oral biomarkers for the diagnosis and monitoring of periodontal diseases: A systematic review. *Dis. Markers* **2016**, *2016*, 1804727. [CrossRef]

89. Thaweboon, B.; Suwannagindra, S.; Kerdvongbundit, V.; Thaweboon, S. Using absorbent paper strips for the collection of cell-free DNA in patients with periodontal diseases. In Proceedings of the IOP Conference Series: Materials Science and Engineering, Harbin, China, 5–7 July 2019; p. 012010.
90. Suwannagindra, S. Correlation between cell free DNA in gingival crevicular fluid and clinical periodontal parameters by using two collection techniques. *Mahidol Dent. J.* **2020**, *40*, 165–174.
91. Song, M.; Bai, H.; Zhang, P.; Zhou, X.; Ying, B. Promising applications of human-derived saliva biomarker testing in clinical diagnostics. *Int. J. Oral Sci.* **2023**, *15*, 2. [CrossRef] [PubMed]
92. Almiñana-Pastor, P.J.; Boronat-Catalá, M.; Micó-Martinez, P.; Bellot-Arcís, C.; Lopez-Rolda, A.; Alpiste-Illueca, F.M. Epigenetics and periodontics: A systematic review. *Med. Oral Patol. Oral Cir. Bucal* **2019**, *24*, e659. [CrossRef] [PubMed]
93. Kc, S.; Wang, X.Z.; Gallagher, J.E. Diagnostic sensitivity and specificity of host-derived salivary biomarkers in periodontal disease amongst adults: Systematic review. *J. Clin. Periodontol.* **2020**, *47*, 289–308. [CrossRef] [PubMed]
94. Arias-Bujanda, N.; Regueira-Iglesias, A.; Balsa-Castro, C.; Nibali, L.; Donos, N.; Tomás, I. Accuracy of single molecular biomarkers in saliva for the diagnosis of periodontitis: A systematic review and meta-analysis. *J. Clin. Periodontol.* **2020**, *47*, 2–18. [CrossRef]
95. Toczewska, J.; Konopka, T.; Zalewska, A.; Maciejczyk, M. Nitrosative stress biomarkers in the non-stimulated and stimulated saliva, as well as gingival crevicular fluid of patients with periodontitis: Review and clinical study. *Antioxidants* **2020**, *9*, 259. [CrossRef]
96. Toczewska, J.; Maciejczyk, M.; Konopka, T.; Zalewska, A. Total oxidant and antioxidant capacity of gingival crevicular fluid and saliva in patients with periodontitis: Review and clinical study. *Antioxidants* **2020**, *9*, 450. [CrossRef]
97. Tóthová, L.u.; Celec, P. Oxidative stress and antioxidants in the diagnosis and therapy of periodontitis. *Front. Physiol.* **2017**, *8*, 1055. [CrossRef]
98. Rylander-Rudqvist, T.; Hakansson, N.; Tybring, G.; Wolk, A. Quality and quantity of saliva DNA obtained from the self-administrated oragene method—A pilot study on the cohort of Swedish men. *Cancer Epidemiol. Biomark. Prev.* **2006**, *15*, 1742–1745. [CrossRef] [PubMed]
99. Missiroli, S.; Genovese, I.; Perrone, M.; Vezzani, B.; Vitto, V.A.M.; Giorgi, C. The Role of Mitochondria in Inflammation: From Cancer to Neurodegenerative Disorders. *J. Clin. Med.* **2020**, *9*, 740. [CrossRef]
100. Kim, E.-H.; Joo, J.-Y.; Lee, Y.J.; Koh, J.-K.; Choi, J.-H.; Shin, Y.; Cho, J.; Park, E.; Kang, J.; Lee, K. Grading system for periodontitis by analyzing levels of periodontal pathogens in saliva. *PLoS ONE* **2018**, *13*, e0200900. [CrossRef]
101. Sina, A.A.I.; Carrascosa, L.G.; Liang, Z.; Grewal, Y.S.; Wardiana, A.; Shiddiky, M.J.; Gardiner, R.A.; Samaratunga, H.; Gandhi, M.K.; Scott, R.J. Epigenetically reprogrammed methylation landscape drives the DNA self-assembly and serves as a universal cancer biomarker. *Nat. Commun.* **2018**, *9*, 4915. [CrossRef]
102. Han, P.; Bartold, P.M.; Salomon, C.; Ivanovski, S. Salivary outer membrane vesicles and DNA methylation of small extracellular vesicles as biomarkers for periodontal status: A pilot study. *Int. J. Mol. Sci.* **2021**, *22*, 2423. [CrossRef]
103. Nuzzo, P.V.; Berchuck, J.E.; Korthauer, K.; Spisak, S.; Nassar, A.H.; Abou Alaiwi, S.; Chakravarthy, A.; Shen, S.Y.; Bakouny, Z.; Boccardo, F. Detection of renal cell carcinoma using plasma and urine cell-free DNA methylomes. *Nat. Med.* **2020**, *26*, 1041–1043. [CrossRef] [PubMed]
104. Ou, Z.; Li, K.; Yang, T.; Dai, Y.; Chandra, M.; Ning, J.; Wang, Y.; Xu, R.; Gao, T.; Xie, Y. Detection of bladder cancer using urinary cell-free DNA and cellular DNA. *Clin. Transl. Med.* **2020**, *9*, 4. [CrossRef]
105. Delbosc, S.; Alsac, J.-M.; Journe, C.; Louedec, L.; Castier, Y.; Bonnaure-Mallet, M.; Ruimy, R.; Rossignol, P.; Bouchard, P.; Michel, J.-B. Porphyromonas gingivalis participates in pathogenesis of human abdominal aortic aneurysm by neutrophil activation. Proof of concept in rats. *PLoS ONE* **2011**, *6*, e18679. [CrossRef]
106. Aoyama, N.; Suzuki, J.-I.; Ogawa, M.; Watanabe, R.; Kobayashi, N.; Hanatani, T.; Ashigaki, N.; Sekinishi, A.; Izumi, Y.; Isobe, M. Toll-like receptor-2 plays a fundamental role in periodontal bacteria-accelerated abdominal aortic aneurysms. *Circ. J.* **2013**, *77*, 1565–1573. [CrossRef]
107. Muller, L.; Hong, C.-S.; Stolz, D.B.; Watkins, S.C.; Whiteside, T.L. Isolation of biologically-active exosomes from human plasma. *J. Immunol. Methods* **2014**, *411*, 55–65. [CrossRef]
108. Dong, C.; Liu, Y.; Sun, C.; Liang, H.; Dai, L.; Shen, J.; Wei, S.; Guo, S.; Leong, K.W.; Chen, Y. Identification of specific joint-inflammatogenic cell-free DNA molecules from synovial fluids of patients with rheumatoid arthritis. *Front. Immunol.* **2020**, *11*, 662. [CrossRef] [PubMed]
109. Heitzer, E.; Auinger, L.; Speicher, M.R. Cell-free DNA and apoptosis: How dead cells inform about the living. *Trends Mol. Med.* **2020**, *26*, 519–528. [CrossRef]
110. Preissner, K.T.; Herwald, H. Extracellular nucleic acids in immunity and cardiovascular responses: Between alert and disease. *Thromb. Haemost.* **2017**, *117*, 1272–1282. [CrossRef] [PubMed]
111. Kaneko, C.; Kobayashi, T.; Ito, S.; Sugita, N.; Murasawa, A.; Nakazono, K.; Yoshie, H. Circulating levels of carbamylated protein and neutrophil extracellular traps are associated with periodontitis severity in patients with rheumatoid arthritis: A pilot case-control study. *PLoS ONE* **2018**, *13*, e0192365. [CrossRef] [PubMed]
112. Rao, A.; D'Souza, C.; Subramanyam, K.; Rai, P.; Thomas, B.; Gopalakrishnan, M.; Karunasagar, I.; Kumar, B.K. Molecular analysis shows the presence of periodontal bacterial DNA in atherosclerotic plaques from patients with coronary artery disease. *Indian Heart J.* **2021**, *73*, 218–220. [CrossRef]

113. Schenkein, H.A.; Papapanou, P.N.; Genco, R.; Sanz, M. Mechanisms underlying the association between periodontitis and atherosclerotic disease. *Periodontology 2000* **2020**, *83*, 90–106. [CrossRef] [PubMed]
114. Martinez-Martinez, R.E.; Abud-Mendoza, C.; Patiño-Marin, N.; Rizo-Rodríguez, J.C.; Little, J.W.; Loyola-Rodríguez, J.P. Detection of periodontal bacterial DNA in serum and synovial fluid in refractory rheumatoid arthritis patients. *J. Clin. Periodontol.* **2009**, *36*, 1004–1010. [CrossRef] [PubMed]
115. Komine-Aizawa, S.; Aizawa, S.; Hayakawa, S. Periodontal diseases and adverse pregnancy outcomes. *J. Obs. Gynaecol. Res.* **2019**, *45*, 5–12. [CrossRef] [PubMed]
116. Tang, Q.; Fu, H.; Qin, B.; Hu, Z.; Liu, Y.; Liang, Y.; Zhou, L.; Yang, Z.; Zhong, R. A Possible Link Between Rheumatoid Arthritis and Periodontitis: A Systematic Review and Meta-analysis. *Int. J. Periodontics Restor. Dent.* **2017**, *37*, 79–86. [CrossRef]
117. Oliveira, S.R.; de Arruda, J.A.A.; Schneider, A.H.; Carvalho, V.F.; Machado, C.C.; Corrêa, J.D.; Moura, M.F.; Duffles, L.F.; de Souza, F.F.L.; Ferreira, G.A. Are neutrophil extracellular traps the link for the cross-talk between periodontitis and rheumatoid arthritis physiopathology? *Rheumatology* **2022**, *61*, 174–184. [CrossRef]
118. Sanz, M.; Marco del Castillo, A.; Jepsen, S.; Gonzalez-Juanatey, J.R.; D'Aiuto, F.; Bouchard, P.; Chapple, I.; Dietrich, T.; Gotsman, I.; Graziani, F. Periodontitis and cardiovascular diseases: Consensus report. *J. Clin. Periodontol.* **2020**, *47*, 268–288. [CrossRef]
119. Zardawi, F.; Gul, S.; Abdulkareem, A.; Sha, A.; Yates, J. Association between periodontal disease and atherosclerotic cardiovascular diseases: Revisited. *Front. Cardiovasc. Med.* **2021**, *7*, 625579. [CrossRef]
120. Ziebolz, D.; Jahn, C.; Pegel, J.; Semper-Pinnecke, E.; Mausberg, R.; Waldmann-Beushausen, R.; Schöndube, F.; Danner, B. Periodontal bacteria DNA findings in human cardiac tissue—Is there a link of periodontitis to heart valve disease? *Int. J. Cardiol.* **2018**, *251*, 74–79. [CrossRef]
121. Wu, Y.; Wang, Y.; Du, L.; Wang, K.; Wang, S.; Li, G. The link between different infection forms of Porphyromonas gingivalis and acute myocardial infarction: A cross-sectional study. *BMC Oral Health* **2023**, *23*, 63. [CrossRef]
122. Carestia, A.; Frechtel, G.; Cerrone, G.; Linari, M.A.; Gonzalez, C.D.; Casais, P.; Schattner, M. NETosis before and after hyperglycemic control in type 2 diabetes mellitus patients. *PLoS ONE* **2016**, *11*, e0168647. [CrossRef] [PubMed]
123. Liu, F.; Sheng, S.; Shao, D.; Xiao, Y.; Zhong, Y.; Zhou, J.; Quek, C.H.; Wang, Y.; Hu, Z.; Liu, H. A cationic metal–organic framework to scavenge cell-free DNA for severe sepsis management. *Nano Lett.* **2021**, *21*, 2461–2469. [CrossRef] [PubMed]
124. Liang, H.; Peng, B.; Dong, C.; Liu, L.; Mao, J.; Wei, S.; Wang, X.; Xu, H.; Shen, J.; Mao, H.-Q. Cationic nanoparticle as an inhibitor of cell-free DNA-induced inflammation. *Nat. Commun.* **2018**, *9*, 4291. [CrossRef] [PubMed]
125. Pan, W.; Yin, W.; Yang, L.; Xue, L.; Ren, J.; Wei, W.; Lu, Q.; Ding, H.; Liu, Z.; Nabar, N.R. Inhibition of Ctsk alleviates periodontitis and comorbid rheumatoid arthritis via downregulation of the TLR9 signalling pathway. *J. Clin. Periodontol.* **2019**, *46*, 286–296. [CrossRef]
126. Aswani, A.; Manson, J.; Itagaki, K.; Chiazza, F.; Collino, M.; Wupeng, W.L.; Chan, T.K.; Wong, W.F.; Hauser, C.J.; Thiemermann, C. Scavenging circulating mitochondrial DNA as a potential therapeutic option for multiple organ dysfunction in trauma hemorrhage. *Front. Immunol.* **2018**, *9*, 891. [CrossRef]

International Journal of
Molecular Sciences

MDPI

Article

The Lysyl Oxidase G473A Polymorphism Exacerbates Oral Cancer Development in Humans and Mice

Yaser Peymanfar [1,†], Faranak Mahjour [2,†], Neha Shrestha [2], Ana de la Cueva [3], Ying Chen [1], Shengyuan Huang [4], Kathrin H. Kirsch [3], Xiaozhe Han [4] and Philip C. Trackman [1,2,*]

1 The Forsyth Institute, 245 First Street, Cambridge, MA 02142, USA; ypeymanfar@forsyth.org (Y.P.); ychen@forsyth.org (Y.C.)
2 Department of Translational Dental Medicine, Henry M. Goldman School of Dental Medicine, Boston University, 700 Albany Street, Boston, MA 02118, USA; faranakmahjour@gmail.com (F.M.); neha014@gmail.com (N.S.)
3 Department of Biochemistry, School of Medicine, Boston University, 72 East Concord Street, Boston, MA 02118, USA; anadelacueva.her@gmail.com (A.d.l.C.); kkirsch@mgh.harvard.edu (K.H.K.)
4 Department of Oral Science and Translational Research, College of Dental Medicine, Nova Southeastern University, Fort Lauderdale, FL 33314, USA; shuang@nova.edu (S.H.); xhan@nova.edu (X.H.)
* Correspondence: ptrackman@forsyth.org
† These authors contributed equally to this work.

Abstract: Oral cancer is primarily squamous-cell carcinoma with a 5-year survival rate of approximately 50%. Lysyl oxidase (LOX) participates in collagen and elastin maturation. The propeptide of LOX is released as an 18 kDa protein (LOX-PP) in the extracellular environment by procollagen C-proteinases and has tumor-inhibitory properties. A polymorphism in the propeptide region of *LOX* (rs1800449, G473A) results in a single amino acid substitution of Gln for Arg. Here we investigated the frequency of rs1800449 in OSCC employing TCGA database resources and determined the kinetics and severity of precancerous oral lesion development in wildtype and corresponding knockin mice after exposure to 4-nitroquinoline oxide (4 NQO) in drinking water. Data show that the OSCC is more common in humans carrying the variant compared to the wildtype. Knockin mice are more susceptible to lesion development. The immunohistochemistry of LOX in mouse tissues and in vitro studies point to a negative feedback pathway of wildtype LOX-PP on LOX expression that is deficient in knockin mice. Data further demonstrate modulations of T cell phenotype in knockin mice toward a more tumor-permissive condition. Data provide initial evidence for rs1800449 as an oral cancer susceptibility biomarker and point to opportunities to better understand the functional mechanism of LOX-PP cancer inhibitory activity.

Keywords: oral cancer; polymorphism; lysyl oxidase; human; mouse model; 4 NQO; extracellular matrix; tumor suppressor; pathogenesis

Citation: Peymanfar, Y.; Mahjour, F.; Shrestha, N.; de la Cueva, A.; Chen, Y.; Huang, S.; Kirsch, K.H.; Han, X.; Trackman, P.C. The Lysyl Oxidase G473A Polymorphism Exacerbates Oral Cancer Development in Humans and Mice. *Int. J. Mol. Sci.* **2023**, *24*, 9407. https://doi.org/10.3390/ijms24119407

Academic Editors: Marko Tarle and Ivica Lukšić

Received: 21 April 2023
Revised: 19 May 2023
Accepted: 24 May 2023
Published: 28 May 2023

1. Introduction

Lysyl oxidase (LOX) catalyzes the final enzyme reaction required for the subsequent crosslinking of elastin and collagen to promote extracellular matrix maturation [1]. LOX is synthesized and secreted as a 50 kDa proenzyme (Pro-LOX), which is cleaved extracellularly to a 30 kDa active LOX enzyme and an 18 kDa lysyl oxidase propeptide (LOX-PP) by procollagen C-proteinases [2]. Interestingly, LOX enzyme activity promotes tumor invasiveness and metastasis by modulating the extracellular matrix surrounding the tumor and actively simulating the formation of metastatic niches [3], while LOX-PP has tumor-growth inhibitory properties [4,5]. The highly disordered LOX-PP protein has multiple binding partners and several mechanisms of action [6]. LOX-PP inhibits several signaling pathways, including RAS, FGF-2, and FAK signaling. Additionally, LOX-PP targets DNA-repair pathways [4,5,7]. LOX-PP inhibits breast, pancreatic, prostate, and lung cancer, and hepatocellular carcinoma cell growth [5,8–10]. Furthermore, LOX-PP overexpression inhibits the formation of breast and prostate xenograft tumors [7,11]. By contrast, increased LOX enzyme activity derived from LOX or other *LOX* gene family members, such as LOXL2, promotes cancer and is associated with poor clinical outcomes.

A single-nucleotide polymorphism (SNP) in the *LOX* gene G473A results in an arginine (Arg) 158 substitution by glutamine (Gln) in a highly conserved region of the LOX-PP sequence. The 473A allele of the *LOX* gene in European, Asian, Sub-Saharan African, and African American populations in the HapMap database was previously found at an average frequency of 24.6%. This naturally occurring G473A polymorphism (rs1800449) appears to attenuate the ability of LOX-PP to function as a tumor suppressor [12]. The SNP was reported to associate with higher breast-cancer risk in European women [13] and African American women carrying this allele have a higher risk for triple-negative breast cancer [12]. It also correlates with breast cancer and ovarian cancer in the Chinese Han population [14,15]. In another study, the G473A polymorphism was associated with a higher risk of lung and colon cancer in cigarette smokers in a North Chinese population [16]. These data show an important role of the *LOX* G473A polymorphism in the development of solid cancers. However, the effect of this polymorphism on the occurrence of oral cancer remains unknown.

Oral squamous-cell carcinoma (OSCC) represents over 90% of oral cavity cancers [17,18]. Despite modern treatments including surgery, radiotherapy, and chemotherapy, and treatment with novel biologics, the five-year survival rate is approximately 50%. The poor prognosis of OSCC is mostly due to the late diagnosis of the disease after it reaches advanced stages [19]. In addition to gene mutations, OSCC has strong associations with environmental factors such as alcohol and tobacco abuse and human papillomavirus infections (HPV16-18) [17,18]. The genetic susceptibility of OSCC is still largely undefined because of the multifactorial nature of OSCC. The present study determined whether the G473A polymorphism results in increased oral lesion development in a chemically induced oral-cancer mouse model. In this study, we analyzed the association of the single nucleotide polymorphism at G473A (rs1800449) within the LOX propeptide in the incidence of human tongue OSCC using available TCGA data. For independent confirmation, we employed the homozygous knockin mouse that corresponds to the polymorphic human Arg/Gln polymorphism at residue 158 [20], which corresponds to residue 152 in mice. Here, we investigated the susceptibility of these mice to the DNA adduct-forming agent, 4-nitroquinoline-1 oxide (4 NQO), which is a major mutagen in tobacco smoke, according to established protocols for studying oral cancer [21]. The 4 NQO mouse protocol recapitulates human oral squamous-cell cancer development from the normal tongue epithelium and progresses through dysplastic lesions that ultimately develop into OSCC and is well suited to assess for susceptibility differences between wildtype and genetically modified mice such as our Arg to Gln LOX-PP knockin mice compared to wildtype.

Our analyses of the TCGA database indicate a significant association of OSCC with rs1800449 human polymorphism. Supporting this, we found that knockin mice are much more susceptible to oral lesion development with poor outcomes compared to wildtype mice. LOX was strongly upregulated in knockin 4 NQO-treated mouse lesions compared to wildtype, suggesting that LOX expression is downregulated by Arg LOX-PP but not Gln LOX-PP. Our in vitro studies further support that wildtype LOX-PP (Arg LOX-PP) inhibits LOX expression in an oral-tumor cell line, while mutant LOX-PP (Gln LOX-PP) has a reduced inhibitory effect. Our findings point to a novel unexpected feedback mechanism for wildtype LOX-PP suppression of LOX production that is disrupted by the variant. Since active LOX enzyme levels are strongly associated with poor clinical outcomes, our data provide at least one possible pathway for the observed poor cancer outcomes associated with rs1800449 polymorphism. Preliminary evidence for differential heightened immune suppression in knockin mice is also presented.

2. Results

2.1. Increased Human Oral-Cancer Incidence in rs1800449 Polymorphic-Variant Subjects

Analyses of the genomic-sequence data sets associated with non-specified oral sites and tongue squamous-cell neoplasms (TCGA-HNSC) retrieved from the GDC port revealed that the frequency of the LOX-PP rs1800449 polymorphism in oral-cancer patients (26.92%) is significantly higher compared to the frequency of rs1800449 in both the American population (17.57%) $p = 0.0288$ and the global (16.98%) $p = 0.0117$ population data incidence of oral cancer in patients, according to the NIH HapMap (a haplotype map) of the human genome data set (Figure 1). The data suggest that there is a strong association between LOX-PP polymorphism and the development of oral cancer.

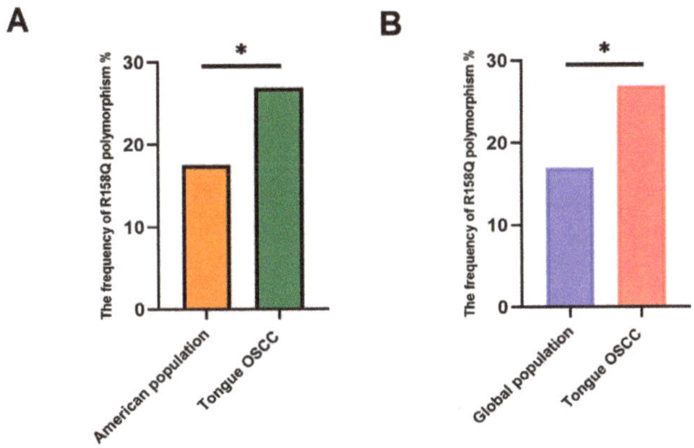

Figure 1. High frequency of rs1800449 (LOX-PP R158Q polymorphism) in OSCC. Chi-square tests: (**A**) $p = 0.0288$; $n = 156$ for cancer patients, and $n = 770$ for G > A allele frequency (NIH HapMap haplotype map) of the American population. (**B**) $p = 0.0117$; $n = 156$ for cancer patients, and $n = 1890$ for G > A allele frequency (NIH HapMap haplotype map) of the data set from the human global population. * $p < 0.05$.

2.2. Increased Lesion Occurrence in Arg to Gln LOX-PP Knockin Mice

Four-month-old LOX-PP knockin mice (Pro-LOX Gln152/Gln152), whose sequence mimics human rs1800449 G473A polymorphism, and wildtype control mice (Pro-LOX Arg152/Arg152) [20] (Figure 2) were randomly given either vehicle or 4 NQO in their drinking water for 16 weeks. All animal cages were reverted to 4 NQO-free drinking water and the mice were monitored for an additional week (Figure 3).

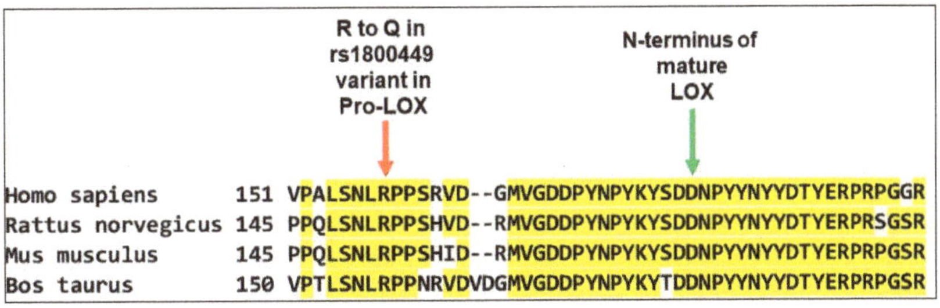

Figure 2. Conserved sequence around human residue R158 in pro-LOX, which when mutated to R158Q compromises LOX-PP tumor-suppressor function. Only the partial C-terminal end of the 14 kDa LOX-PP sequence plus the first few residues of mature LOX domains are shown. The procollagen-C proteinase processing site of pro-LOX that separates LOX-PP from active mature LOX is shown in green. Yellow highlights indicate conserved amino acid sequences.

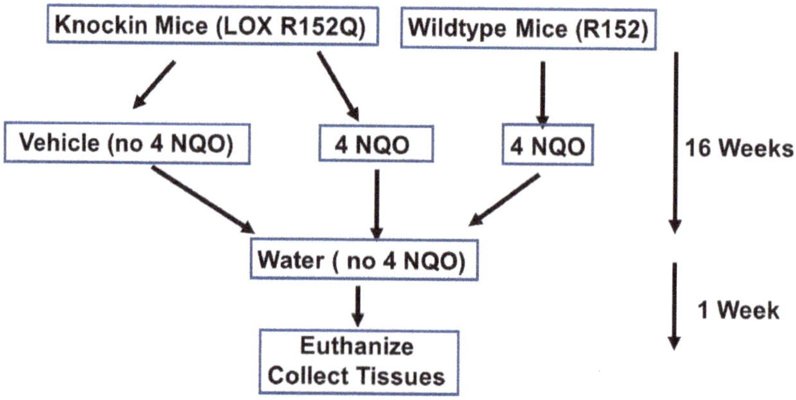

Figure 3. Experimental design.

A total of thirteen Arg to Gln LOX-PP knockin mice and seven wildtype mice were employed. Eight of the knockin mice were treated with 4 NQO and five of them were treated with vehicle. All of the wildtype mice were treated with 4 NQO. It was observed that in the Gln LOX-PP knockin group, the number of mice that developed tongue lesions was significantly higher following the 4 NQO treatment than in the wildtype group treated with 4 NQO at 17 weeks (Table 1). The mice in the LOX-PP knockin group treated with 4 NQO developed lesions with a higher incidence and faster development compared to WT mice treated with 4 NQO (Figure 4). One mouse in the LOX-PP knockin group treated with NQO developed a lesion on the floor of the mouth in the 12th week after treatment with 4 NQO and died two weeks later. Lesions developed in two LOX-PP knockin mice after the 16th week and three LOX-PP knockin mice after the 17th week of initiation of 4 NQO treatment developed cancer lesions on their tongues. Only one mouse in the wildtype group treated with 4 NQO developed tongue lesions by the 17th week. In total, six out of eight mice (75%) in the LOX-PP knockin group treated with 4 NQO developed oral cancer, while only one mouse out of seven (14%) in the 4 NQO-treated wildtype group developed tongue tumors. A chi-square test (3X2 analysis) indicated a significant number of mice with lesions in the Gln LOX-PP knockin group treated with 4 NQO compared to other experimental groups (Table 1) ($p = 0.008$). Fisher's exact test (2X2 analysis) between knockin mice treated with 4 NQO vs. wildtype (Arg LOX-PP) treated with 4 NQO indicated that the incidence of cancer in the Gln LOX-PP knockin mice treated with 4 NQO is more significant compared to the mice treated with 4 NQO ($p < 0.05$). Fisher's exact test (2X2 analysis) illustrated a remarkably high incidence of lesions in the Gln LOX-PP knockin mice treated with 4 NQO vs. Gln LOX-PP knockin mice treated with water ($p < 0.05$). At the final time point of this experiment, there was no significant statistical difference for the oral lesion incidence between knockin mice given plain water only and wildtype mice treated with 4 NQO ($p > 0.05$). In the latter group, only one mouse developed a visible tongue lesion. The mice in the knockin group exhibited a greater increase in tongue volumes compared to wildtype after 4 NQO treatment ($p < 0.05$) (Figure 4). These results suggest that LOX-PP polymorphism reduced the ability of LOX-PP to suppress tumor formation in the presence of 4 NQO.

Table 1. Tumor Incidence Among Knockin Mice and Wildtype Mice Treated with 4 NQO.

	LOX-PP Knock-in Group Treated with 4 NQO (8 Mice)	**Wild Type Group Treated with 4 NQO (7 Mice)**	**LOX-PP Knock-in Group Treated with Water (5 Mice)**
12th Week	1	0	0
16th Week	2	0	0
17th Week	3	1	0
Total	6 (75%) *	1 (14%)	0

Chi-Square test (3X2 analysis) was performed and indicated significant number of mice with oral cancer in LOX-PP knock-in group treated with 4-NQO compared to other experimental groups ($p = 0.008$). Fisher's exact test (2X2 analysis) KIPP with 4 NQO vs. WT with 4 NQO, * $p < 0.05$ indicates that LOX-PP knock-in mice treated with 4-NQO have more incidence of cancer than wild type mice treated with 4-NQO.

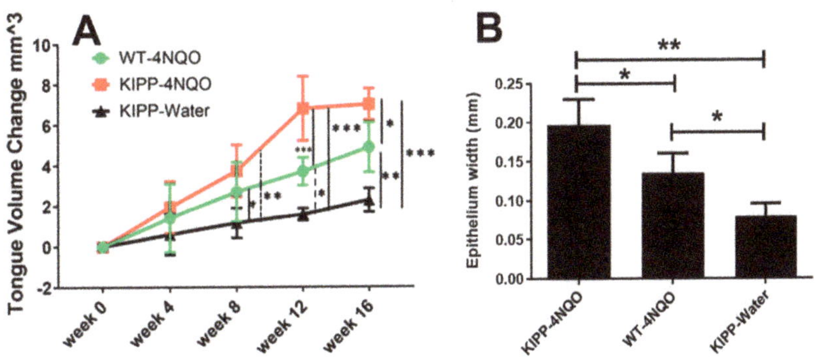

Figure 4. Tongue volume measurements in experimental mice. (**A**) tongue volumes; (**B**) epithelial thickness. Wildtype mice (WT); knockin mice (KIPP). The error bars indicate +/− SD. Two-way ANOVA, $p < 0.05$, Tukey's multiple comparison test, * $p < 0.05$, ** $p < 0.001$, *** $p < 0.0001$ indicate that the mice in the knockin group developed larger volumes of tongues compared to wildtype after 4 NQO treatment.

2.3. Histopathology of the Tongue Lesions

Histology sections stained with hematoxylin and eosin of the tongue lesions that developed in both knockin and wildtype mice treated with 4 NQO exhibited similar features of excess squamous cell accumulation, many of which exhibited a loss of close cell-to-cell contacts (red arrows in Figure 5). Specifically, atypical papillary exophytic squamous lesions were observed, some with focal dysplasia. Some cells appeared to be hyperchromatic and there was cellular discohesion with cells exhibiting increased nuclear-to-cytoplasmic ratios. Epithelial hyperplasia was also observed adjacent to the papillary outgrowths. Basal-cell hyperplasia and dysmaturation were observed. This abnormal phenotype was more apparent in the knockin mice (Figure 5). The overall finding from histopathology is that the knockin mice develop lesions characterized by an atypical pappilary exophytic squamous proliferation and general epithelial hyperplasia. Analyses of epithelial thickness showed clear generalized acanthosis in 4 NQO-treated mice with the greatest thickness observed in the 4 NQO-treated knockin mice (Figures 4B and 5). These findings are consistent with dysplastic lesions developing in 4 NQO, both wildtype and knockin mice, with knockin mice showing a stronger phenotype, while untreated knockin mice exhibited a normal morphology. Only one wildtype mouse treated with 4 NQO developed a papillary exophytic squamous proliferation, in sharp contrast to the 4 NQO-treated knockin mice (Table 1 and Figure 5).

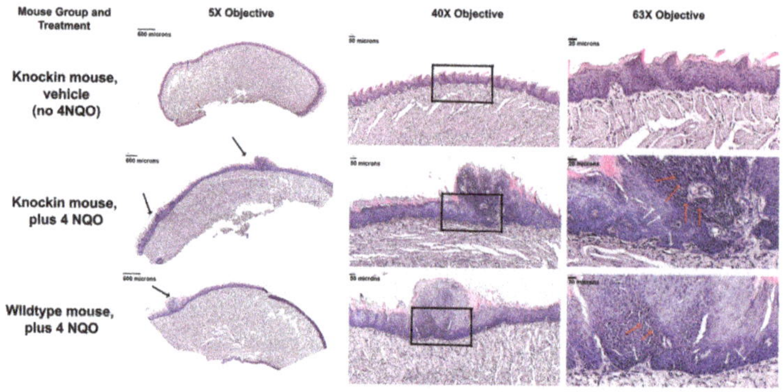

Figure 5. Hematoxylin and eosin staining of mouse tongues show dysplastic lesions generated in 4 NQO-treated especially in knockin mice with an attenuated response in the one wildtype mouse that developed a papillary lesion. Black arrows show lesion formation. Red arrows show hyperchromatic discohesive cells with increased nuclear to cytoplasmic ratios and white arrows show cohesive epithelial cells. Boxes outline areas shown at higher magnification. Images are representative of 4 mice per group subjected to histology and immunohistochemistry.

Proliferating cell nuclear antigen (PCNA) is a marker of cell proliferation. Immunohistochemistry for PCNA in vehicle-treated knockin mice exhibited normal strong nuclear expression in basal epithelial cells (Figure 6, top panels). By contrast, in 4 NQO treated knockin mice, strong nuclear staining was observed in fibroblasts in the connective tissue layer, consistent with dysplasia (Figure 6, middle panels, red arrows). Interestingly, in wildtype mice treated with 4 NQO, PCNA staining was not observed in fibroblasts, but rather in the refractile suprabasal epithelial cells in the papillary lesion, and adjacent to the papillary lesion in basal and suprabasal cells, suggesting elevated epithelial cell proliferation without as large a development of a stromal dysplastic reaction (Figure 6, bottom panels, blue arrows).

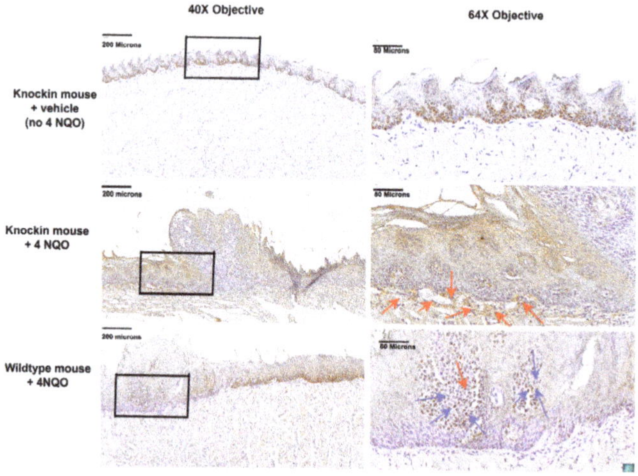

Figure 6. Differential PCNA expressions in mouse groups. Knockin mice treated with vehicle exhibit normal basal epithelial expression of PCNA (top panels), while 4 NQO treated mice exhibit lesions with connective-tissue stromal cell expression (middle panels, red arrows), while wildtype mice treated with 4 NQO exhibit suprabasal and basal epithelial staining (bottom panels, blue arrows). The boxes identify regions shown at higher magnification in the right columns. Images are representative of 4 mice per group subjected to histology and immunohistochemistry.

Lysyl oxidase is secreted as a pro-protein, and expression is typically found both inside cells and cell associated. In samples from vehicle-treated knockin mice, a typical normal staining pattern of expression associated with the basal epithelium was observed, consistent with its function in maintaining the integrity of the basal lamina (Figure 7, top panels, back arrows). Spinous epithelial staining was also observed. In 4 NQO-treated knockin mice staining for lysyl oxidase revealed a high degree of staining in fibroblasts in the stromal compartment and an apparent disorganized arrangement of cells (Figure 7, middle panels, red arrows), consistent with a strong dysplastic phenotype and profibrotic activities of LOX. In addition, a high degree of epithelial cell staining was observed primarily in suprabasal cells and spinous epithelial regions. Interestingly, in 4 NQO treated wildtype mice, epithelial cell staining was weaker and primarily associated with cells that appeared to have intact cell-cell interactions, and not the more fractile epithelial cells in the papillary lesions (Figure 7, middle panel, blue arrows). Wildtype mice treated with 4 NQO had weak staining for lysyl oxidase in and around basal epithelial cells and the connective tissue interface, unlike knockin mice (Figure 7, bottom panels, white arrows). This finding further supports the highly dysplastic nature of the knockin lesions compared to wildtype. In wildtype mice, staining was mainly observed in the suprabasal epithelial regions and little in the connective tissue. (Figure 7, bottom panels, white arrows).

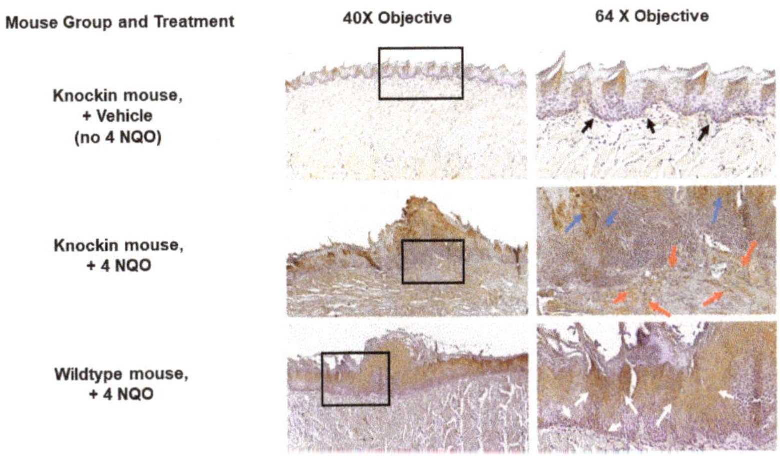

Figure 7. LOX expression is differentially regulated in knockin mice. Samples from knockin mice treated with vehicle show normal low expression of LOX in the basal epithelium (top panel, black arrows), and spinous epithelium. Knockin mice treated with 4 NQO exhibit strong staining in fibroblasts (middle panels, red arrows) and in the suprabasal epithelial cells (middle panel, blue arrows). Wildtype mice express LOX primarily in suprabasal cells (bottom panels, white arrows) with observable staining in basal epithelial cells. The boxes identify regions shown at higher magnification in the right column. Images are representative of 4 mice per group subjected to histology and immunohistochemistry.

The findings in Figure 7 suggested that wildtype Arg LOX-PP could inhibit the expression of LOX via negative feedback that is attenuated in Arg > Gln substitution in the pro-peptide domain. To investigate this possibility, we treated cultures of the mouse oral-cancer cell line LY2 with recombinant wild with vehicle type rat Arg LOX-PP or Gln LOX-PP overnight in serum-free medium followed by a Western blot of three cultures each. Data in Figure 8 shows that 50 kDa pro-LOX bands were diminished in Arg LOX-PP-treated cells, while this response was weaker in Gln LOX-PP treated cells.

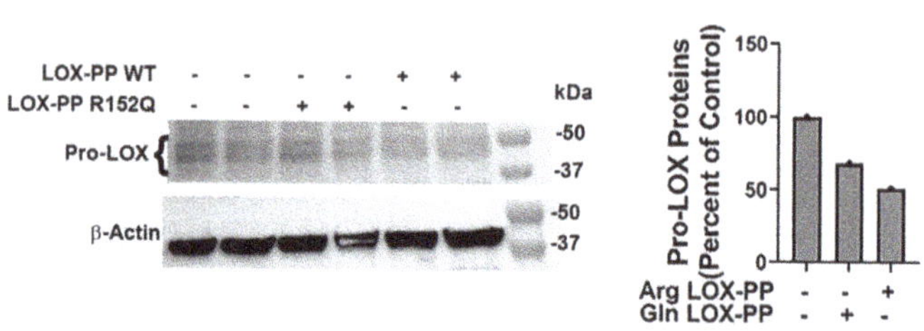

Figure 8. G152A polymorphism of LOX-PP attenuated the negative feedback inhibitory effect on LOX expression. Western blot of LY2 cell layers after treatment with 8 μg/mL rArg LOX-PP or rGln-LOXPP.

To begin to assess immune cell differences in knockin vs. wildtype mice, we assessed selected immune-marker expression patterns at the borders of lesions in histologic sections. Specifically, we compared T cell PD-L1/PD-1 expressions in cancer lesions between wildtype mice and knockin mice and $CD4^{+/-}$ and $CD8^{+/-}$ T cell expression. Immunofluorescent staining of 4 NQO tumor lesions indicated that a significant increase in PD-L1 production was observed in the lesions of knockin Gln LOX-PP mice compared to wildtype Arg LOX-PP mice, and this production was not by $CD4^+$ T cells. Cancer-cell-associated PD-1-expressing $CD4^+$ T cells were relatively high in knockin Gln LOX-PP mice, whereas PD-1-expressing $CD8^+$ T cells were decreased in knockin Gln LOX-PP mice compared to wildtype Arg LOX-PP mice. However, PD-L1-expressing $CD8^+$ T cells were relatively high in wildtype Arg LOX-PP mice (Figure 9). These results suggest that wildtype Arg LOX-PP, compared to Gln LOX-PP, could differentially modulate immune T cell PD-L1 and PD-1 expression in OSCC toward a more tumor-suppressive environment.

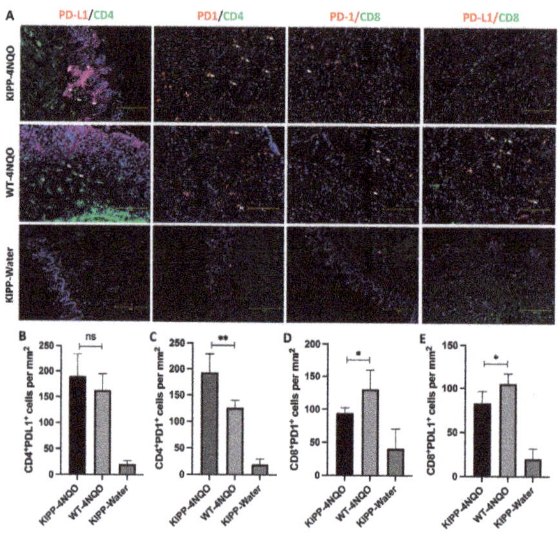

Figure 9. Differential expression of T cell immune checkpoint PD-L1 and PD-1 in tongue SCC lesions in wildtype (WT) Arg LOX-PP mice and knockin Gln LOX-PP (KIPP) mice. FFPE sections of 4 NQO-induced lesions or controls were stained with PD-L1, PD-1, CD4, and CD8 antibodies, and the images were captured by the EVOS M5000 system. (**A**) The representative images of $CD4^+PD\text{-}L1^+$, $CD4^+PD\text{-}1^+$, $CD8^+PD\text{-}1^+$, and $CD8^+PD\text{-}L1^+$ cells in each group. White arrows showed double-positive cells. (**B–E**) The numbers of double-positive cells were quantified by ImageJ and normalized in cells/mm^2. Statistical analysis was first calculated by ANOVA and then an unpaired *t*-test was used to calculate the statistical difference between the Arg LOX-PP and Gln LOX-PP groups. The significance (*p*-value) is defined as * $p < 0.05$, ** $p < 0.01$, and ns $p > 0.05$. Scale bar, 150 μm.

Taken together, the data presented here from the mouse study indicate that LOX-PP knockin mice are more susceptible to oral cancer development than wildtype mice. In vivo and in vitro data in mice and mouse cancer cells suggest a feedback pathway in which Gln LOX-PP has lost the ability to inhibit LOX expression, while wildtype Arg LOX-PP maintains a more normal LOX expression in a negative feedback pathway. Moreover, differential immune modulation by Arg LOX-PP vs. variant Gln LOX-PP is further implied by our findings. Combined with increased OSCC associated with the LOX polymorphism in humans, data point to an important role for LOX-PP in oral-tissue homeostasis with relevance to the incidence of oral cancer that must be further explored.

3. Discussion

OSCC is one of the most prevalent cancers in the world with poor clinical outcomes and a high recurrence rate [22,23]. Despite modern treatment methods such as chemotherapy, radiotherapy, surgery, and biologics, the overall 5-year survival rate is only 50%, which is mostly due to the late diagnosis of the disease [19]. Several risk factors, including tobacco and alcohol consumption, promote the development of oral cancer [24]; however, the role of genetic factors, including polymorphisms of genes important to OSCC development and progression, is unclear. The LOX family proteins are known as extracellular enzymes that are critical in the biosynthetic maturation of collagen and elastin [25]. However, LOXs were found to be highly expressed in a variety of cancers, resulting in the formation of aggressive tumors, reduced survival rate, and increased metastasis in breast, prostate, colon, and lung cancers [3,26–28]. By contrast, the propeptide domain of LOX (LOX-PP) derived from the pro-LOX has been shown to inhibit breast, pancreatic, lung, and prostate cancers [5,9,12,20]. LOX-PP polymorphism G473A (rs1800449) results in a change in amino acid residue 158 from Arg to Gln in humans and was shown to result in enhanced breast cancer development [20]. Here, we analyzed for the first time genomic oral-cancer data from the TCGA database, which mainly represents the U.S data [29,30], and found that the frequency of G > A of G473A is indeed significantly higher in OSCC patients (26.92%) compared to G > A allele frequency (17.57%) in American populations, according to the HapMap human genome project dataset ($p = 0.0288$). The frequency of rs1800449 polymorphism was even more significant ($p = 0.0117$) when genomic cancer data were compared with the global population (16.98%). These data strongly suggest that LOX-PP G473A polymorphism is associated with an increased incidence of oral cancer in patients.

To examine the role of LOX-PP polymorphism in the incidence and progress of oral cancer, Gln LOX-PP knockin mice (R152Q), which mimic human G473A and have the same Arg > Gln substitution in the propeptide domain, were employed. Oral cancer was chemically induced with 4 NQO in LOX-PP knockin and WT mice. Carcinogen 4 NQO induction of oral cancer in mice has been shown previously as a useful animal model for the study of oral cancer in both male and female mice [31]. The incidence of oral lesions in tongues was observed at a much higher rate ($p < 0.05$) in the Gln LOX-PP knockin group compared to WT mice with the same treatment. No statistically significant differences for lesion detection were observed between knockin mice treated with plain water and WT mice given 4 NQO ($p > 0.05$) under the conditions of the time of treatment in this experiment, as expected. Taken together, these results suggest an important role of the LOX-PP polymorphism in the biogenesis of oral lesions in the presence of the carcinogen 4 NQO. Consistent with our previous data, and data by others, the LOX-PP polymorphism was here demonstrated as a potential biomarker associated for OSCC.

Lesions developed under the conditions of the current study were determined by a pathologist to exhibit severe dysplasia in the 4 NQO-treated knockin mice, with milder dysplasia developing in the 4 NQO-treated wildtype mice. The 4 NQO model progresses first to hyperplasia, dysplasia, and, finally, to full-blown OSCC, and accurately mimics the development of human oral cancer [21]. For full OSCC development, wild mice must be maintained for 25 weeks [21], while our experimental design here sought to observe lesion development at an earlier time point to assess differences in the relatively early development of these oral lesions. Data suggest an accelerated developmental program that promotes early dysplasia development, and likely the early development of OSCC.

Immune modulations in the context of LOX and cancer so far have been primarily documenting elevated expression levels of increased LOX enzyme activity and its relationships to increased tissue stiffness due to increased collagen cross-linking and fibrosis [32–34]. Immune-cell phenotype has been implicated in these studies as a driving force in regulating cancer development and possibly LOX expression. We are, therefore, developing hypotheses regarding mechanisms of differential modulation of immune-cell phenotypes by wildtype and variant rLOX-PP on immune-cell phenotypes. Here, we wished to begin to assess in vivo whether such modulation could occur. We have provided initial findings that point to a link between the *LOX* polymorphic variant in the enzymatically inactive propeptide region and increased cancer susceptibility and worse outcomes. At least two mechanisms can be envisioned. One, as we have discussed above, is the loss of a feedback inhibition pathway on LOX itself. Another is that LOX-PP or secreted pro-LOX that contains the LOX-PP sequence secreted from tumor cells and associated stromal cells could have unexplored direct interactions and regulatory functions with immune cells in the microenvironment implicated by our data taken together in Figures 7–9. These possibilities are under investigation in our laboratories and are focused on the effects of LOX-PPs on cells in the microenvironment.

Previous studies revealed that LOX-PP, but not LOX, inhibits the Ras-transformed NIH3T3 fibroblast cell line [4]. It was shown that LOX-PP attenuates Her-2/neu-driven tumor development in a nude-mice breast-cancer model, via suppressing the ERK1/2, AKT, and NF-kB signaling pathways [35]. Adenoviral vector-induced LOX-PP expression reduced cell migration and suppressed angiogenic factors MMP2 and MMP9 [10]. Identification of LOX-PP polymorphism with reduced antitumor activity in several cancers may open the venue to understand the role of Arg158 in the antitumor activity of LOX-PP which is diminished in the mutant Gln158 variant. Of note, it was shown that MMP2 can cleave pro-LOX immediately adjacent to Arg158 in the most predominant form of pro-LOX, but this cleavage occurs before Gln158 in a less common form of pro-LOX [36–38]. One possibility is that Gln158 could be resistant to MMP2 proteolytic cleavage at residue 158 which then may alter the activity or substrate specificity of pro-LOX in favor of more BMP1/procollagen C-proteinase cleavage at residue 158, resulting in the formation of active LOX, which is well-known to be upregulated in a variety of cancers [39,40]. Therefore, it is possible that LOX and Arg LOX-PP play opposing effects in tumor development and metastasis by this or another still unexplored mechanism. Consistently, our data presented here indicate that overexpression of LOX occurs in connective-tissue cells adjacent to the basement membrane in Gln LOX-PP knockin mice but not in control groups (Figure 7), promoting dysplasia in the knockin mice by failing to block inhibitory pathways in fibroblasts. These findings strongly suggest that wildtype Arg LOX-PP inhibits the expression of LOX which is attenuated in the Gln LOX-PP variant. By conducting the LY2 cell-culture model of oral cancer and treating cells with Arg LOX-PP or Gln LOX-PP recombinant protein, the more pro-LOX protein was observed to be expressed following Gln LOX-PP treatment, while less was expressed after wildtype Arg LOX-PP treatment (Figure 8). This observation is fully consistent with our in vivo findings.

In summary, our in silico and in vivo data indicate that the LOX-PP polymorphism results in increased incidence and severity of oral cancer development. The mouse and cell-culture data strongly suggest a loss of naturally occurring inhibitory activity of the Gln LOX-PP variant compared to wildtype Arg LOX-PP which ultimately results in the elevation of LOX production and tumor development (Figure 10). Our findings indicate that LOX-PP G473A polymorphism could be an important biological marker with a strong association with the oral-cancer phenotype and may open new avenues for future studies and therapeutic approaches.

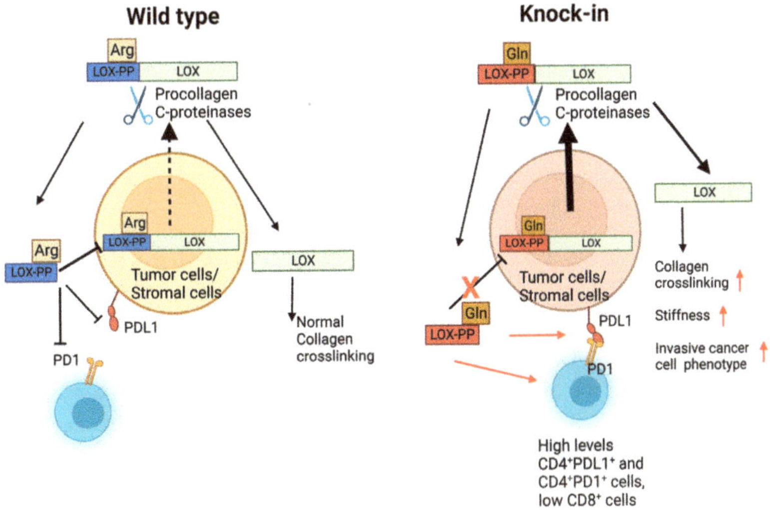

Figure 10. Summary and hypotheses regarding differences in activity between wildtype Arg LOX-PP and variant Gln LOX-PP in OSCC tissues. While Arg LOX-PP can inhibit LOX production through a negative feedback mechanism variant (left cartoon and Figure 8), Gln LOX-PP loses this inhibitory effect. This ultimately results in more secretion of LOX from oral lesions in ECM and progressing tumor formation (right cartoon). Additional differential effects of Gln LOX-PP occur on T cells in the microenvironment are suggested by high $CD4^+PD1^+$ and high $CD4^+PDL1^+$ T in the knockin mice (right cartoon and Figure 9), which could lead to enhanced immunosuppression. Created with BioRender.com.

4. Materials and Methods

4.1. LOX G473A Polymorphism in Oral-Cancer Patients

The NCI Genomic Data Commons (GDC) portal was used to access The Cancer Genome Atlas (TCGA) program. Genomic sequences from 157 male and female patients diagnosed with tongue squamous-cell neoplasms and unspecified parts of the tongue (TCGA-HNSC project) were downloaded from the TCGA database, specifically dbGap Study Accession phs000178 [29]. The genome sequences (.BAM files) were selected and sliced to include the region of interest of the lysyl oxidase gene on chromosome 5 between 122,070,800-122,078,200 bp locus, release (GRCh38.p13). To view the SNP sequences, index files (.BAI files) were constructed for all associated BAM files using an open-source software gene pattern (Broad Institute, MIT, Cambridge, MA, USA and University of California, USA). The rs1800449 (LOX-PP R158Q polymorphism) sequences [41] were analyzed for the point mutation (sequence C > T and reference sequence G > A) at 122.077.513 bp site which is located at a highly conserved region of LOX-PP (Figure 2) by employing the open-source Integrative Genomics Viewer (IGV) software, version 2.12.3 (Broad Institute, MIT, Cambridge, MA, USA and University of California, USA). TCGA datasets are primarily collected from U.S. institutions [29,30]. Analyzed data were, therefore, compared to allele frequency of rs1800449 data from the NIH HapMap (a haplotype map) of the human genome data set from the American population. TCGA is recognized as the only comprehensive cancer genomic database. Therefore, in a separate analysis, TCGA data was also compared to the global frequency of rs1800449 according to NIH HapMap [41]. Chi-square statistical analysis was performed, and the p values were determined using GraphPad Prism 9.5.1, Clarivate, Philadelphia, PA, USA.

4.2. Animals Study and 4 NQO Treatment

Animal protocols were reviewed and approved by the Boston University Medical Center Institutional Animal Care and Use Committee (IACUC). Homozygous LOX knockin mice in the C57BL/6 background were generated in the *LOX* gene (Arg152Gln change), as we described previously [20].

Thirteen knockin mice and seven wildtype mice beginning at 4 months old were used in this study. Male and female mice were analyzed together. The 4-Nitroquinoline-1-oxide (4 NQO) was obtained from Sigma-Aldrich (catalog # N8141) and was dissolved in propylene glycol (W294004, Sigma-Aldrich) at a concentration of 4 mg/mL and stored at 4 °C. Then, the solution of 4 NQO was added to red opaque sterilized water bottles for mice containing drinking water to obtain a final concentration of 100 µg/mL. This concentration of 4 NQO restricts lesion development to the tongue and oral cavity in both male and female mice that experience primary contact with the mutagen [31]. The water was changed once a week during the 16 weeks of the 4 NQO treatment. Regular chow and soft diet gel containing nutrients (Diet Gel76A, ClearH20, Westbrook, ME, USA) were provided for the mice throughout the experimental period. Mice were monitored for food consumption and weight loss.

Animals were euthanized by isoflurane inhalation, followed by cervical dislocation on the 17th week after initiation of treatment with NQO. The oral cavity, esophagus, and stomach were assessed for any pathological lesions or tumors. Tongues were fixed in 4% paraformaldehyde, embedded in paraffin, and sectioned into 5-µm sections for histology and immunohistochemistry.

4.3. Histology and Immunohistochemistry

Sections were deparaffinized, rehydrated, and stained with H&E for histopathology. Sections were stained overnight with the following primary antibodies; PCNA (dilution, 1:500, #ab92552, Abcam, Wlatham, MA, USA), and LOX antibody at 1 µg/mL [42]. The slides were incubated with a secondary biotinylated goat antirabbit immunoglobulin antibody, as recommended by the manufacturer (Vector Laboratories, Newark, CA, USA). Control slides were generated by incubating the sections with rabbit IgG (Vector Laboratories) instead of primary antibody and showed no staining at the same IgG concentrations. The slides were developed with 3, 3-diaminobenzidine (DAB Peroxidase substrate kit, Vector Laboratories, Inc.). Images were captured on a digital slide scanner and processed using CaseViewer 2.3 software (3D Histotech, Budapest, Hungary).

The epithelium thickness of the tongues was measured In 4 mice per group (10 measurements per mouse). The epithelium thickness was measured at intervals from the top to the base of the epithelium layer and from the top of the tongue towards the middle every 0.5 mm, overall, 4.5 mm in length. Data for each individual mouse were then averaged to produce the final thickness data point for each mouse.

Sections were subjected to immunofluorescence staining to detect the phenotype of T cells and the expression of PD-1 and PD-L1. FITC anti-mouse CD4 (dilution, 1:500, catalogue #100406, Biolegend, San Diego, CA, USA)), Alexa Fluor 488 antimouse CD8 (dilution, 1:500, catalogue #126628, Biolegend, San Diego, CA, USA), antimouse PD-1 (dilution, 1:500, #135202, Biolegend, San Diego, CA, USA), and antimouse PD-L1 (dilution, 1:500, #124302, Biolegend, San Diego, CA, USA) antibodies were incubated with tissue sections overnight at 4 °C, then incubated with Alexa Fluor 647 anti-rat antibody (dilution, 1:500, #407512, Biolegend, San Diego, CA, USA) for 1 h. Sections were counterstained with DAPI for cell-nucleus staining. Images were captured and recorded by EVOS M5000 Imaging System (Invitrogen, Carlsbad, CA, USA). Subsequent image analysis was performed using ImageJ software (Version, 1.53t). Briefly, the double-positive areas of Alexa Fluor 647 and FITC were selected and counted in each region of interest (ROI), which is the subepithelial connective tissue area adjacent to the squamous cancerous lesion. After measuring the area of the ROI, the number of positive cells was presented as cells/mm^2, according to the defined ROI.

4.4. Cell Culture and Western Blots

To examine the effects of mutant and wildtype LOX-PP on LOX expression, mouse oral-cancer cell line, LY2 cells [43] were cultured and, at confluency, cells were treated overnight in serum-free medium with 8 μg/mL recombinant wildtype rat Arg LOX-PP or Gln-LOX-PP. Cell layers were extracted into a 5X SDSPAGE sample buffer. Equal amounts of proteins were applied to 10% SDS PAGE gels and transferred to PVDF membranes at 66 mA overnight. Membranes were washed in TBS-T (20 mM Tris, 150 mM NaCl, and 0.01% Tween-20) and then blocked for an hour in 5% nonfat dry milk in TBS-T and incubated with primary antibody overnight at 4 °C. Antibodies employed were rabbit anti-LOX (NSJ BioReagents #32045, San Diego, CA, USA), or rabbit mAb β-actin (Cell Signaling, catalogue #4970, Danvers, MA USA). Membranes were washed in TBST 3 times for 10 min and were incubated with antirabbit IgG, HRP-linked antibody (#7074, Cell Signaling, San Diego, CA, USA) for 2 **h** at room temperature. HyGlo Quick spray (Denville Scientific, catalogue #1001354, Holliston, MA, USA) or SuperSignal™ West Femto Maximum Sensitivity Substrate (#34095, Thermo Fisher Scientific, Waltham, MA, USA) were used to visualize the signals using a chemiluminescence detector (G:BOX, Syngene, Bangalore, India). Using ImageJ software, version 1.53t, the band intensity of proteins was analyzed from three independent samples/group and normalized to their respective β-actin signals after stripping and reprobing.

4.5. Statistical Analysis

The chi-square test, Fisher's exact test, one-way ANOVA, two-way ANOVA, and post hoc tests were performed using Graphpad Prism (version 9.5.1 for windows, GraphPad Software, San Diego, CA, USA). Significance was considered when $p < 0.05$. In the graphs, asterisks on bars are representative of significant differences between the indicated columns compared to the control.

Author Contributions: Conceptualization, X.H. and P.C.T.; Methodology, Y.P.; Formal analysis, Y.P., F.M. and P.C.T.; Investigation, Y.P., F.M., N.S., A.d.l.C., Y.C. and S.H.; Resources, P.C.T.; Data curation, F.M.; Writing—original draft, F.M.; Writing—review & editing, Y.P., K.H.K. and P.C.T.; Supervision, X.H. and P.C.T.; Project administration, P.C.T.; Funding acquisition, P.C.T. All authors have read and agreed to the published version of the manuscript.

Funding: This work was supported in part by NIH grants R21 DE023973 and R21 AR077260 to P.C.T.

Institutional Review Board Statement: Human data analyzed came from NIH databases containing only de-identified DNA sequences.

Informed Consent Statement: This is not applicable. Human data analyzed came from NIH databases containing only de-identified DNA sequences.

Data Availability Statement: The data presented in this study are available on request from the corresponding author. Downloaded *LOX* sequence data are stored on the Forsyth Institute server and will be provided upon request.

Acknowledgments: We thank Vikki Noonan, Division of Oral Pathology Boston University Henry M. Goldman School of Dental Medicine for helping with the evaluation of the histopathology of the histology sections.

Conflicts of Interest: The authors declare no conflict of interest.

References

1. Kagan, H.M.; Trackman, P.C. Properties and function of lysyl oxidase. *Am. J. Respir. Cell Mol. Biol.* **1991**, *5*, 206–210. [CrossRef]
2. Trackman, P.C.; Bedell-Hogan, D.; Tang, J.; Kagan, H.M. Post-translational glycosylation and proteolytic processing of a lysyl oxidase precursor. *J. Biol. Chem.* **1992**, *267*, 8666–8671. [CrossRef]
3. Barker, H.E.; Cox, T.R.; Erler, J.T. The rationale for targeting the LOX family in cancer. *Nat. Rev. Cancer* **2012**, *12*, 540–552. [CrossRef]
4. Palamakumbura, A.H.; Jeay, S.; Guo, Y.; Pischon, N.; Sommer, P.; Sonenshein, G.E.; Trackman, P.C. The propeptide domain of lysyl oxidase induces phenotypic reversion of ras-transformed cells. *J. Biol. Chem.* **2004**, *279*, 40593–40600. [CrossRef]

5. Palamakumbura, A.H.; Vora, S.R.; Nugent, M.A.; Kirsch, K.H.; Sonenshein, G.E.; Trackman, P.C. Lysyl oxidase propeptide inhibits prostate cancer cell growth by mechanisms that target FGF-2-cell binding and signaling. *Oncogene* **2009**, *28*, 3390–3400. [CrossRef]
6. Vora, S.R.; Guo, Y.; Stephens, D.N.; Salih, E.; Vu, E.D.; Kirsch, K.H.; Sonenshein, G.E.; Trackman, P.C. Characterization of recombinant lysyl oxidase propeptide. *Biochemistry* **2010**, *49*, 2962–2972. [CrossRef]
7. Bais, M.V.; Ozdener, G.B.; Sonenshein, G.E.; Trackman, P.C. Effects of tumor-suppressor lysyl oxidase propeptide on prostate cancer xenograft growth and its direct interactions with DNA repair pathways. *Oncogene* **2015**, *34*, 1928–1937. [CrossRef]
8. Min, C.; Zhao, Y.; Romagnoli, M.; Trackman, P.C.; Sonenshein, G.E.; Kirsch, K.H. Lysyl oxidase propeptide sensitizes pancreatic and breast cancer cells to doxorubicin-induced apoptosis. *J. Cell. Biochem.* **2010**, *111*, 1160–1168. [CrossRef]
9. Wu, M.; Min, C.; Wang, X.; Yu, Z.; Kirsch, K.H.; Trackman, P.C.; Sonenshein, G.E. Repression of BCL2 by the tumor suppressor activity of the lysyl oxidase propeptide inhibits transformed phenotype of lung and pancreatic cancer cells. *Cancer es.* **2007**, *67*, 6278–6285. [CrossRef]
10. Zheng, Y.; Wang, X.; Wang, H.; Yan, W.; Zhang, Q.; Chang, X. Expression of the lysyl oxidase propeptide in hepatocellular carcinoma and its clinical relevance. *Oncol. Rep.* **2014**, *31*, 1669–1676. [CrossRef]
11. Bais, M.V.; Nugent, M.A.; Stephens, D.N.; Sume, S.S.; Kirsch, K.H.; Sonenshein, G.E.; Trackman, P.C. Recombinant lysyl oxidase propeptide protein inhibits growth and promotes apoptosis of pre-existing murine breast cancer xenografts. *PLoS ONE* **2012**, *7*, e31188. [CrossRef] [PubMed]
12. Min, C.; Yu, Z.; Kirsch, K.H.; Zhao, Y.; Vora, S.R.; Trackman, P.C.; Spicer, D.B.; Rosenberg, L.; Palmer, J.R.; Sonenshein, G.E. A loss-of-function polymorphism in the propeptide domain of the LOX gene and breast cancer. *Cancer Res.* **2009**, *69*, 6685–6693. [CrossRef] [PubMed]
13. Friesenhengst, A.; Pribitzer-Winner, T.; Schreiber, M. Association of the G473A polymorphism and expression of lysyl oxidase with breast cancer risk and survival in European women: A hospital-based case-control study. *PLoS ONE* **2014**, *9*, e105579. [CrossRef]
14. Ren, J.; Wu, X.; He, W.; Shao, J.; Cheng, B.; Huang, T. Lysyl oxidase 473 G>A polymorphism and breast cancer susceptibility in Chinese Han population. *DNA Cell Biol.* **2011**, *30*, 111–116. [CrossRef]
15. Wang, X.; Cong, J.L.; Qu, L.Y.; Jiang, L.; Wang, Y. Association between lysyl oxidase G473A polymorphism and ovarian cancer in the Han Chinese population. *J. Int. Med. Res.* **2012**, *40*, 917–923. [CrossRef]
16. Wang, G.; Shen, Y.; Cheng, G.; Bo, H.; Lin, J.; Zheng, M.; Li, J.; Zhao, Y.; Li, W. Lysyl Oxidase Gene G473A Polymorphism and Cigarette Smoking in Association with a High Risk of Lung and Colorectal Cancers in a North Chinese Population. *Int. J. Environ. Res. Public Health* **2016**, *13*, 635. [CrossRef]
17. El-Bayoumy, K.; Chen, K.M.; Zhang, S.M.; Sun, Y.W.; Amin, S.; Stoner, G.; Guttenplan, J.B. Carcinogenesis of the Oral Cavity: Environmental Causes and Potential Prevention by Black Raspberry. *Chem. Res. Toxicol.* **2017**, *30*, 126–144. [CrossRef]
18. Tanaka, T.; Ishigamori, R. Understanding carcinogenesis for fighting oral cancer. *J. Oncol.* **2011**, *2011*, 603740. [CrossRef]
19. Groome, P.A.; Rohland, S.L.; Hall, S.F.; Irish, J.; Mackillop, W.J.; O'Sullivan, B. A population-based study of factors associated with early versus late stage oral cavity cancer diagnoses. *Oral Oncol.* **2011**, *47*, 642–647. [CrossRef]
20. De la Cueva, A.; Emmerling, M.; Lim, S.L.; Yang, S.; Trackman, P.C.; Sonenshein, G.E.; Kirsch, K.H. A Polymorphism in the Lysyl Oxidase Propeptide Domain Accelerates Carcinogen-induced Cancer. *Carcinogenesis* **2018**, *39*, 921–930. [CrossRef]
21. Kanojia, D.; Vaidya, M.M. 4-nitroquinoline-1-oxide induced experimental oral carcinogenesis. *Oral Oncol.* **2006**, *42*, 655–667. [CrossRef]
22. Thomson, P.J. Perspectives on oral squamous cell carcinoma prevention-proliferation, position, progression and prediction. *J. Oral Pathol. Med. Off. Publ. Int. Assoc. Oral Pathol. Am. Acad. Oral Pathol.* **2018**, *47*, 803–807. [CrossRef]
23. Cooper, J.S.; Porter, K.; Mallin, K.; Hoffman, H.T.; Weber, R.S.; Ang, K.K.; Gay, E.G.; Langer, C.J. National Cancer Database report on cancer of the head and neck: 10-year update. *Head Neck* **2009**, *31*, 748–758. [CrossRef]
24. Ram, H.; Sarkar, J.; Kumar, H.; Konwar, R.; Bhatt, M.L.; Mohammad, S. Oral cancer: Risk factors and molecular pathogenesis. *J. Maxillofac. Oral Surg.* **2011**, *10*, 132–137. [CrossRef]
25. Trackman, P.C.; Peymanfar, Y.; Roy, S. Functions and Mechanisms of Pro-Lysyl Oxidase Processing in Cancers and Eye Pathologies with a Focus on Diabetic Retinopathy. *Int. J. Mol. Sci.* **2022**, *23*, 5088. [CrossRef]
26. Baker, A.-M.; Cox, T.R.; Bird, D.; Lang, G.; Murray, G.I.; Sun, X.-F.; Southall, S.M.; Wilson, J.R.; Erler, J.T. The role of lysyl oxidase in SRC-dependent proliferation and metastasis of colorectal cancer. *J. Natl. Cancer Inst.* **2011**, *103*, 407–424. [CrossRef]
27. Erler, J.T.; Giaccia, A.J. Lysyl oxidase mediates hypoxic control of metastasis. *Cancer Res.* **2006**, *66*, 10238–10241. [CrossRef]
28. Gao, Y.; Xiao, Q.; Ma, H.; Li, L.; Liu, J.; Feng, Y.; Fang, Z.; Wu, J.; Han, X.; Zhang, J. LKB1 inhibits lung cancer progression through lysyl oxidase and extracellular matrix remodeling. *Proc. Natl. Acad. Sci. USA* **2010**, *107*, 18892–18897. [CrossRef]
29. Tomczak, K.; Czerwińska, P.; Wiznerowicz, M. The Cancer Genome Atlas (TCGA): An immeasurable source of knowledge. *Contemp. Oncol.* **2015**, *19*, A68–A77. [CrossRef]
30. Spratt, D.E.; Chan, T.; Waldron, L.; Speers, C.; Feng, F.Y.; Ogunwobi, O.O.; Osborne, J.R. Racial/ethnic disparities in genomic sequencing. *JAMA Oncol.* **2016**, *2*, 1070–1074. [CrossRef]
31. Vitale-Cross, L.; Czerninski, R.; Amornphimoltham, P.; Patel, V.; Molinolo, A.A.; Gutkind, J.S. Chemical carcinogenesis models for evaluating molecular-targeted prevention and treatment of oral cancer. *Cancer Prev. Res.* **2009**, *2*, 419–422. [CrossRef]

32. Maller, O.; Drain, A.P.; Barrett, A.S.; Borgquist, S.; Ruffell, B.; Zakharevich, I.; Pham, T.T.; Gruosso, T.; Kuasne, H.; Lakins, J.N.; et al. Tumour-associated macrophages drive stromal cell-dependent collagen crosslinking and stiffening to promote breast cancer aggression. *Nat. Mater.* **2021**, *20*, 548–559. [CrossRef]
33. Saito, T.; Uzawa, K.; Terajima, M.; Shiiba, M.; Amelio, A.L.; Tanzawa, H.; Yamauchi, M. Aberrant Collagen Cross-linking in Human Oral Squamous Cell Carcinoma. *J. Dent. Res.* **2019**, *98*, 517–525. [CrossRef]
34. Albinger-Hegyi, A.; Stoeckli, S.J.; Schmid, S.; Storz, M.; Iotzova, G.; Probst-Hensch, N.M.; Rehrauer, H.; Tinguely, M.; Moch, H.; Hegyi, I. Lysyl oxidase expression is an independent marker of prognosis and a predictor of lymph node metastasis in oral and oropharyngeal squamous cell carcinoma (OSCC). *Int. J. Cancer J. Int. Cancer* **2010**, *126*, 2653–2662. [CrossRef]
35. Min, C.; Kirsch, K.H.; Zhao, Y.; Jeay, S.; Palamakumbura, A.H.; Trackman, P.C.; Sonenshein, G.E. The tumor suppressor activity of the lysyl oxidase propeptide reverses the invasive phenotype of Her-2/neu-driven breast cancer. *Cancer Res.* **2007**, *67*, 1105–1112. [CrossRef]
36. Nareshkumar, R.N.; Sulochana, K.N.; Coral, K. Inhibition of angiogenesis in endothelial cells by Human Lysyl oxidase propeptide. *Sci. Rep.* **2018**, *8*, 10426. [CrossRef]
37. Pichu, S.; Sathiyamoorthy, J.; Vimalraj, S.; Viswanathan, V.; Chatterjee, S. Impact of lysyl oxidase (G473A) polymorphism on diabetic foot ulcers. *Int. J. Biol. Macromol.* **2017**, *103*, 242–247. [CrossRef]
38. Griner, J.D.; Rogers, C.J.; Zhu, M.-J.; Du, M. Lysyl oxidase propeptide promotes adipogenesis through inhibition of FGF-2 signaling. *Adipocyte* **2017**, *6*, 12–19. [CrossRef]
39. Mahjour, F.; Dambal, V.; Shrestha, N.; Singh, V.; Noonan, V.; Kantarci, A.; Trackman, P.C. Mechanism for oral tumor cell lysyl oxidase like-2 in cancer development: Synergy with PDGF-AB. *Oncogenesis* **2019**, *8*, 34. [CrossRef]
40. Xiao, Q.; Ge, G. Lysyl oxidase, extracellular matrix remodeling and cancer metastasis. *Cancer Microenviron.* **2012**, *5*, 261–273. [CrossRef]
41. NIH SNP rs1800449. Available online: https://www.ncbi.nlm.nih.gov/snp/rs1800449 (accessed on 21 April 2023).
42. Hurtado, P.A.; Vora, S.; Sume, S.S.; Yang, D.; St Hilaire, C.; Guo, Y.; Palamakumbura, A.H.; Schreiber, B.M.; Ravid, K.; Trackman, P.C. Lysyl oxidase propeptide inhibits smooth muscle cell signaling and proliferation. *Biochem. Biophys. Res. Commun.* **2008**, *366*, 156–161. [CrossRef]
43. Vigneswaran, N.; Wu, J.; Song, A.; Annapragada, A.; Zacharias, W. Hypoxia-induced autophagic response is associated with aggressive phenotype and elevated incidence of metastasis in orthotopic immunocompetent murine models of head and neck squamous cell carcinomas (HNSCC). *Exp. Mol. Pathol.* **2011**, *90*, 215–225. [CrossRef]

International Journal of *Molecular Sciences*

MDPI

Article

Nutri-PEITC Jelly Significantly Improves Progression-Free Survival and Quality of Life in Patients with Advanced Oral and Oropharyngeal Cancer: A Blinded Randomized Placebo-Controlled Trial

Aroonwan Lam-Ubol [1], Jirasak Sukhaboon [2], Withee Rasio [2], Peerawitch Tupwongse [3], Thapana Tangshewinsirikul [4] and Dunyaporn Trachootham [5,*]

1 Faculty of Dentistry, Srinakharinwirot University, Bangkok 10110, Thailand; aroonwan@gmail.com
2 Lopburi Cancer Hospital, Lopburi 15000, Thailand
3 National Cancer Institute, Bangkok 10400, Thailand
4 Chonburi Cancer Hospital, Chonburi 20000, Thailand
5 Institute of Nutrition, Mahidol University, Nakhon Pathom 73170, Thailand
* Correspondence: dunyaporn.tra@mahidol.ac.th or dunyaporn.tra@mahidol.edu

Abstract: *TP53* mutation is associated with cancer progression. Novel strategies to reboot p53 are required to stabilize the disease and improve survival. This randomized placebo-controlled trial investigated safety and efficacy of Nutri-PEITC Jelly (a texture-modified nutritious diet fortified with β-phenethyl isothiocyanate (PEITC) on oral cancer. Seventy-two patients with advanced-staged oral or oropharyngeal cancer were randomly assigned to study and control groups, who consumed 200 g of Nutri-Jelly with and without 20 mg of PEITC, respectively, 5 days/week for 12 weeks. Outcomes, including adverse events, health-related quality of life (HRQOL), progression-free survival (PFS), tumor response, serum p53, and cytochrome c, were measured at 0, 1, and 3 months. Results show that the study group had a higher proportion of participants with improved HRQOL, stable disease, and increased serum p53 levels than those in the control group ($p < 0.001$). The PFS time in the study group was significantly longer than that of the control group ($p < 0.05$). Serum cytochrome c levels were non-significantly decreased in the study group. No serious intervention-related adverse events occurred in either group. In conclusion, Nutri-PEITC Jelly intake for 3 months is safe, stabilizes the disease, improves quality of life and progression-free survival, and might re-activate p53 in advanced-stage oral and oropharyngeal cancer patients.

Keywords: PEITC; Nutri-Jelly; oral cancer; tertiary chemoprevention; p53; clinical trial; survival; quality of life

Citation: Lam-Ubol, A.; Sukhaboon, J.; Rasio, W.; Tupwongse, P.; Tangshewinsirikul, T.; Trachootham, D. Nutri-PEITC Jelly Significantly Improves Progression-Free Survival and Quality of Life in Patients with Advanced Oral and Oropharyngeal Cancer: A Blinded Randomized Placebo-Controlled Trial. *Int. J. Mol. Sci.* **2023**, *24*, 7824. https://doi.org/10.3390/ijms24097824

Academic Editors: Marko Tarle and Ivica Lukšić

Received: 5 March 2023
Revised: 1 April 2023
Accepted: 4 April 2023
Published: 25 April 2023

1. Introduction

Mutations in the *TP53* gene are robust in cancer and are associated with disease progression [1–3]. Novel strategies to target p53 are required to stabilize the disease and improve the survival of advanced-stage cancer patients [4,5]. Compelling pieces of evidence from in vitro and in vivo studies suggest that β-phenethyl isothiocyanate (PEITC), a Brassica vegetable-derived compound may selectively deplete mutant p53 and reactivate p53 function. While the mechanisms were still unclear, PEITC was shown to reactivate p53 by restoring wild-type conformation and function of p53 protein and selectively depleting mutant p53 by direct binding and conformational change [6,7]. PEITC was also shown to retard the growth of several types of cancer, such as breast, oral, liver, and prostate cancer, and leukemia [8–12]. However, it is still unknown if the compound could be effective in retarding cancer progression in patients. To the best of our knowledge, there was only one published case report showing the benefit of PEITC in sensitizing B-cell prolymphocytic leukemia (B-PLL) to salvage R-CHOP (Rituximab, Cyclophosphamide, Hydroxydaunorubicin [doxorubicin hydrochloride], Oncovin [vincristine sulfate], Prednisone or Prednisolone) chemotherapy [13].

Oral and oropharyngeal cancer is the most common type of head and neck cancer, which is among the most common cancers worldwide [14]. Head and neck cancer patients suffer from the disease progression as well as the consequences of the treatments, leading to poor quality of life, diminished treatment response, and poor survival [4–16]. *TP53* mutation is associated with disease progression, unfavorable treatment response, and poor survival in head and neck cancer patients [17–19]. Malnutrition is a common problem for head and neck cancer patients due to the inability to eat and swallow properly [20,21]. To provide the nutritional support and improve the patients' quality of life, a texture-modified diet with a complete nutrient supply called Nutri-Jelly has been developed by the Dental Innovation Foundation under Royal Patronage, which is a non-profit organization. Our previous clinical trial suggested that consumption of Nutri-Jelly was proven to improve the health-related quality of life of head and neck cancer patients and reduced the necessity of tube feeding [22].

β-phenylethyl isothiocyanate (PEITC) is a phytochemical naturally present in cruciferous vegetables such as watercress, broccoli, wasabi, and cabbage [23,24]. PEITC can inhibit phase I enzymes and induce phase II detoxification enzymes, leading them to the inactivation and excretion of carcinogen metabolites [23–25]. Such mechanisms have established PEITC as a promising candidate for primary and secondary prevention of cancer [23]. Furthermore, during the past decade, numerous research studies show promising anti-cancer effects of PEITC. By conjugation with glutathione and other mechanisms, PEITC was selectively toxic to numerous types of cancer cells via reactive oxygen species, (ROS)-mediated mechanisms [26–28]. Previous studies by our group and others showed that PEITC selectively killed oral cancer cells with minimal side effects on normal cells [8,9]. Mechanistically, we showed that PEITC led to increased oxidative stress, nuclear translocation of p53 and p21, and cell cycle arrest in *TP53*-mutated oral cancer cells [9]. Consistently, our in vivo study in a *TP53*-mutated oral cancer-xenograft mouse model showed that PEITC at 5 or 10 mg per kg body weight can slow down tumor growth and prolong the survival of cancer-bearing mice along with increased p53 expression in the nucleus of tumor cells in the tissue [9]. These findings suggest that PEITC may reactivate p53 function in oral cancer cells, which could be either restoring wild-type or depleting mutant p53 as previously described in other types of cancer [6,7]. The in vitro and in vivo effects of PEITC against oral cancer cells are promising. However, the effect of PEITC as tertiary chemoprevention in oral cancer patients has never been studied.

To combine the nutritional support benefit with the potential anticancer effect of PEITC, a novel food product called Nutri-PEITC Jelly has been developed by fortification of PEITC into Nutri-Jelly. The Nutri-PEITC Jelly has been tested for its safety by acute, subacute, subchronic, and chronic toxicity tests in animals according to the OECD standardized Guidelines for the Testing of Chemicals (unpublished results). Furthermore, a pharmacokinetic and tolerable study in human volunteers showed that PEITC from Nutri-PEITC Jelly containing 40 mg of PEITC per day can be absorbed rapidly within a few hours and eliminated completely within 24 h [29]. Compared with pure PEITC, Nutri-PEITC Jelly can provide better bioavailability of PEITC evidenced by higher maximum plasma concentration (Cmax) and shorter time to reach maximum plasma level (Tmax) [29,30]. Consecutive repeated doses of Nutri-PEITC Jelly for 5 days demonstrated no accumulation of PEITC [29]. Moreover, our study in healthy volunteers showed that a 5-week continuous intake of Nutri-PEITC Jelly with 20 mg PEITC per day was safe with minimal side effects [31].

Our clinical trial showed a nutrition-improving effect of Nutri-Jelly in head and neck cancer patients. Our animal study showed a promising anti-cancer effect of PEITC against oral cancer. Our clinical trial showed the safety of Nutri-PEITC Jelly in healthy volunteers. However, the effect of Nutri-PEITC Jelly on cancer patients was still unknown. Thus, this study aimed to evaluate the clinical safety and efficacy of Nutri-PEITC Jelly in advanced-stage oral and oropharyngeal cancer patients.

2. Results

2.1. Participant Flow Chart

As shown in Figure 1, there were 72 eligible participants who were allocated randomly into the study (N = 31) and control (N = 41) groups. In the placebo control group, there were 16 participants who lost follow-up due to death and progressive disease, and 6 participants who discontinued the intervention due to adverse events and switched to herbal medicine treatment. In the Nutri-PEITC Jelly group, there were 8 participants who lost follow-up due to death and progressive disease, and 2 participants who discontinued the intervention due to adverse events or switched to herbal medicine treatment. For clinical parameters, intention-to-treat analysis was used. However, for laboratory parameters, per protocol analysis was applied due to sample unavailability.

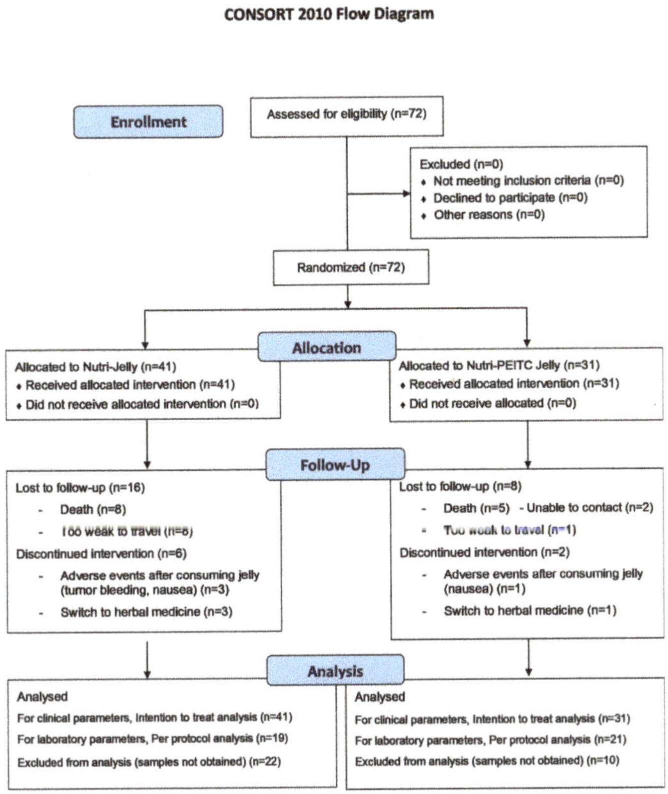

Figure 1. CONSORT participants' flow diagram. The number of recruited, randomized, and analyzed participants are shown.

2.2. Characteristics of Participants

As shown in Table 1, the baseline characteristics of participants in the placebo control group and the study group (Nutri-PEITC Jelly) were comparable. There were no statistically significant differences in gender, occupation, location of primary cancer, disease staging, BMI, age, KPS, and HRQoL scores. Table 2 shows no difference in baseline blood biochemical parameters.

Table 1. Baseline characteristics.

Characteristics	Control Group (N = 41)	Study Group (N = 31)	
	N (%)	N (%)	*p*-Value
Gender			
- Male	24 (59)	25 (81)	0.07 †
- Female	17 (41)	6 (19)	
Occupation			
- Agriculture	14 (34)	11(35)	0.99 ‡
- Employee	16 (39)	12 (39)	
- Unemployed	11 (27)	8 (26)	
Location of primary cancer			
- Oral cavity	24 (59)	18 (58)	0.83 ‡
- Tonsil and oropharynx	11 (27)	7 (23)	
- Pyriform sinus	6 (15)	6 (19)	
Staging T (tumor size)			
- T1–T2	14 (34)	9 (29)	0.79 †
- T3–T4	27 (66)	22 (71)	
Staging N (lymph node involvement)			
- N0–N1	20 (49)	16 (52)	>0.99 †
- N2–N3	21 (51)	15 (48)	
Staging M (distant metastasis)			
- M0	40 (98)	31 (100)	>0.99 †
- M1	1 (2)	0 (0)	
	mean ± SD	**mean ± SD**	***p*-value**
BMI (kg/m²)	18.3 ± 3.3	17.2 ± 3.6	0.15 §
Age (years)	63.3 ± 13.8	62.5 ± 12.1	0.67 §
KPS score (%)	69.5 ± 10.5	72.6 ± 10.3	0.22 §
HRQoL	3.7 ± 5.9	1.2 ± 4.3	0.14 §

p-values were from † Fisher's exact test, ‡ chi-squared test, and § Mann–Whitney test.

Table 2. Baseline blood biochemical parameters.

Characteristics	Control Group (N = 41)	Study Group (N = 31)	*p*-Value
Hemoglobin (gm/dL)	11 ± 1.5	10.4 ± 1.4	0.09 †
Hematocrit (%)	33.5 ± 4.3	31.8 ± 4.0	0.08 †
WBC count (cells/mm³)	8737 ± 3364	10,035 ± 5082	0.73 ‡
RBC (cells/mm³)	4114 ± 669.1	3959 ± 774.3	0.34 ‡
MCV (fL)	82.3 ± 10.7	81.1 ± 9.6	0.37 ‡
MCH (pg)	27 ± 3.7	26.7 ± 3.2	0.43 ‡
MCHC (g/dL)	32.8 ± 1.0	32.9 ± 1.0	0.63 ‡
Platelets (cells/mm³)	325,863 ± 136,124	357,355 ± 162,560	0.59 ‡
BUN (mg/dL)	12.8 ± 4.8	12.8 ± 4.9	0.94 †
Creatinine (mg/dL)	0.7 ± 0.2	0.8 ± 0.2	0.09 ‡
Cholesterol (mg/dL)	165.4 ± 42.3	174.2 ± 60.6	0.65 †
LDL (mg/dL)	100.2 ± 37	102.9 ± 49	0.87 †
HDL (mg/dL)	45.2 ± 14.4	48.4 ± 10.1	0.27 ‡
SGOT (U/L)	22.3 ± 8.8	24.7 ± 9.9	0.24 ‡
SGPT (U/L)	15.8 ± 11.4	17.6 ± 12.8	0.39 ‡
Bilirubin (mg/dL)	0.4 ± 0.2	0.4 ± 0.2	0.55 ‡

This table shows mean ± SD of each characteristic as specified. *p*-values were obtained from † unpaired *t*-test and ‡ Mann–Whitney test.

2.3. Adverse Events

As shown in Table 3, no serious intervention-related adverse events occurred in either group. Adverse events reported in both the placebo control and the study groups included nausea, vomiting, burning sensation in the mouth, constipation, dry mouth and throat, and itchy sensation. The study group that received Nutri-PEITC Jelly had a higher percentage of nausea and vomiting and a burning sensation in the mouth, but the percentage of the adverse events was still lower than 30%. Nevertheless, these adverse events may not be entirely related to the interventions as most of them were transient and disappeared without treatment. Diarrhea and tumor bleeding after food consumption was only found in one participant in the placebo control group. After having nausea and vomiting and being unable to eat anything, two participants in the control group and one participant in the study group discontinued the product. As shown in Table 4, the blood chemistry values of both groups were not different throughout the study. Overall, consuming Nutri-PEITC Jelly for 3 months is quite safe in oral and oropharyngeal cancer patients.

Table 3. Adverse events.

Adverse Events	Control Group (N = 41)	Study Group (N = 31)	Details
	N (%)	N (%)	
Nausea and vomiting	4 (9.8)	7 (22.6)	Two participants in the control group and one participant in the study group discontinued the product, the rest had transient symptoms that disappeared without treatment
Burning sensation in the mouth	4 (9.8)	5 (16.1)	Transient symptoms that disappeared without treatment
Constipation	4 (9.8)	2 (6.5)	One participant in the study group received laxatives for 3 days. The rest had transient symptoms that disappeared without treatment
Dry mouth and throat	3 (7.3)	3 (9.7)	Transient, the symptom disappeared without treatment
Itchy sensation in the mouth	1 (2.4)	1 (3.2)	Transient symptoms that disappeared without treatment
Diarrhea	1 (2.4)	0	Transient symptoms that disappeared without treatment
Tumor bleeding after food consumption	1	0	One participant in the control group discontinued the product

The table shows the number of participants with the specified adverse events. Percent of the participant from total participants was shown in parentheses.

Table 4. Changes in blood biochemical parameters.

Parameters	Baseline		1 Month Follow-Up		3 Months Follow-Up		p-Value †
	Control Group	Study Group	Control Group	Study Group	Control Group	Study Group	
Hemoglobin (gm/dL)	11 ± 1.5	10.4 ± 1.4	10.9 ± 1.5	10.4 ± 1.5	10.5 ± 1.2	9.8 ± 1.7	0.96
Hematocrit (%)	33.5 ± 4.3	31.8 ± 4.0	31.7 ± 4.7	33.3 ± 4.5	32.2 ± 3.6	29.8 ± 5.1	0.75
WBC count ($\times 10^3$ cells/mm^3)	8.7 ± 3.4	10.0 ± 5.1	9.8 ± 6.1	9.8 ± 3.6	9.8 ± 5.0	10.0 ± 4.0	0.68
RBC (10^3 cells/mm^3)	4.1 ± 0.7	3.9 ± 0.8	4.0 ± 0.7	4.0 ± 0.7	3.9 ± 0.5	3.8 ± 0.8	0.87
Platelets $\times 10^5$cells/mm^3)	3.2 ± 1.4	3.5 ± 1.6	3.5 ± 1.4	3.3 ± 1.4	3.5 ± 1.4	3.5 ± 1.7	0.88
BUN (mg/dL)	12.8 ± 4.9	12.8 ± 4.7	13.7 ± 4.5	14.9 ± 9.2	12.6 ± 6.1	13.4 ± 5.5	0.63
Creatinine (mg/dL)	0.8 ± 0.2	0.8 ± 0.2	0.7 ± 0.2	0.9 ± 0.3	0.8 ± 0.4	0.9 ± 0.2	0.36
Cholesterol (mg/dL)	165.4 ± 41.7	174.2 ± 59.1	162.4 ± 40.6	171.6 ± 41.7	165.7 ± 51.0	157.1 ± 31.2	0.09
SGOT (U/L)	22.3 ± 8.8	24.7 ± 9.8	22.25 ± 9.1	25.6 ± 9.9	23.0 ± 11.5	26.9 ± 14.8	0.96
SGPT (U/L)	15.8 ± 11.4	17.6 ± 12.7	15.7 ± 12.7	18.1 ± 8.8	18.8 ± 18.8	18.8 ± 15.1	0.98
Bilirubin (mg/dL)	0.4 ± 0.2	0.4 ± 0.2	0.5 ± 0.2	0.6 ± 0.6	0.5 ± 0.3	0.5 ± 0.3	0.82

This table shows the mean $\pm$ SD of each characteristic as specified. p-values were obtained from † Mixed-effects model (time $\times$ group).

2.4. Monitoring Plasma PEITC Levels

As shown in Figure 2, the plasma PEITC levels in the study group significantly increased up to 6 folds ($p < 0.05$) at 1 and 3 months after the intervention. The data confirm the compliance of Nutri-PEITC intake.

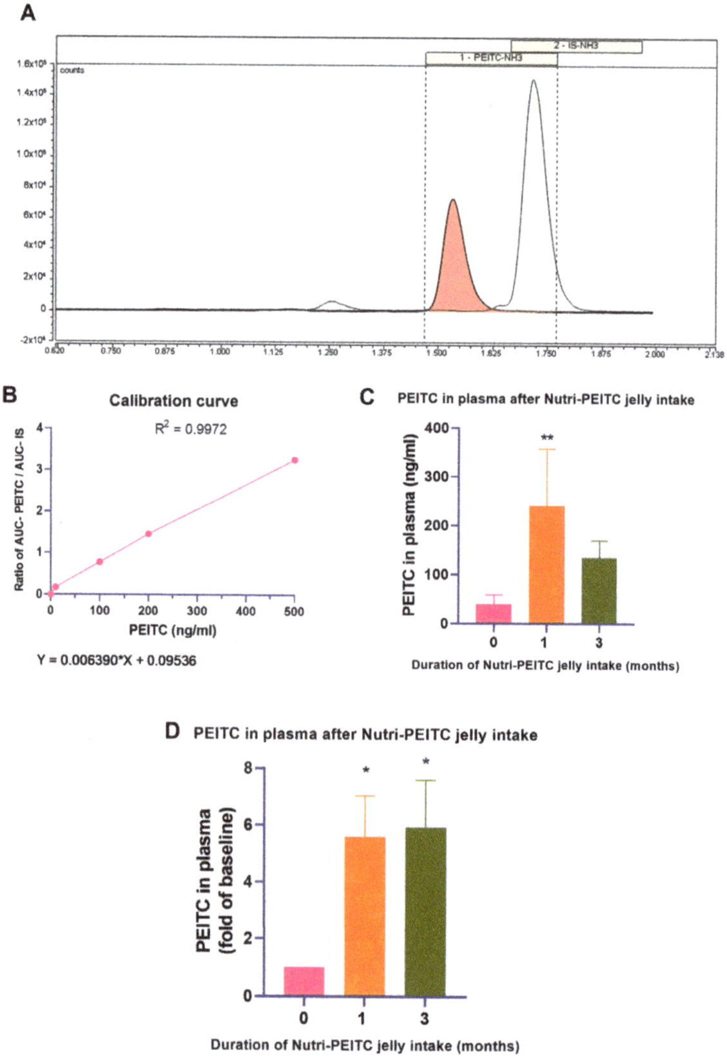

Figure 2. Changes in plasma levels of PEITC after receiving Nutri-PEITC Jelly. (**A**) Representative chromatogram of PEITC and internal standard (IS), (**B**) calibration curve for quantitation of PEITC. Line plots show the ratio between the area under the curve (AUC) of PEITC and the AUC of IS at different concentrations of PEITC (ng/mL), (**C**) comparison of PEITC levels in plasma after Nutri-PEITC Jelly for 0, 1, and 3 months. The bar graph represents mean +/− SEM. ** represents $p < 0.01$, obtained from a Friedman test and Dunn's multiple comparison test, compared with those of baseline. (**D**) Changes in plasma levels of PEITC after receiving Nutri-PEITC Jelly for 1 and 3 months. The bar graph represents mean +/− SEM of the fold number of PEITC in plasma, compared with individual baseline. * represents $p < 0.05$, a Friedman test and Dunn's multiple comparison test, compared with those of baseline.

2.5. Effects of Nutri-PEITC Jelly on Health-Related Quality of Life (HRQoL)

As shown in Figure 3A, at baseline the mean head-and-neck specific HRQoL (H&N HRQOL) score of the study group was lower than those of the control group but the difference was not statistically significant ($p = 0.1357$). As shown in Figure 3B,C, the mean H&N HRQOL of the placebo group had decreased over time, while those in the study group (Nutri-PEITC Jelly) tended to improve. As shown in Figure 3D,E, at 1 and 3 months after the intervention, the study group has a significantly higher proportion of participants with improved head-and-neck specific quality of life ($p < 0.05$ and $p < 0.0001$, respectively).

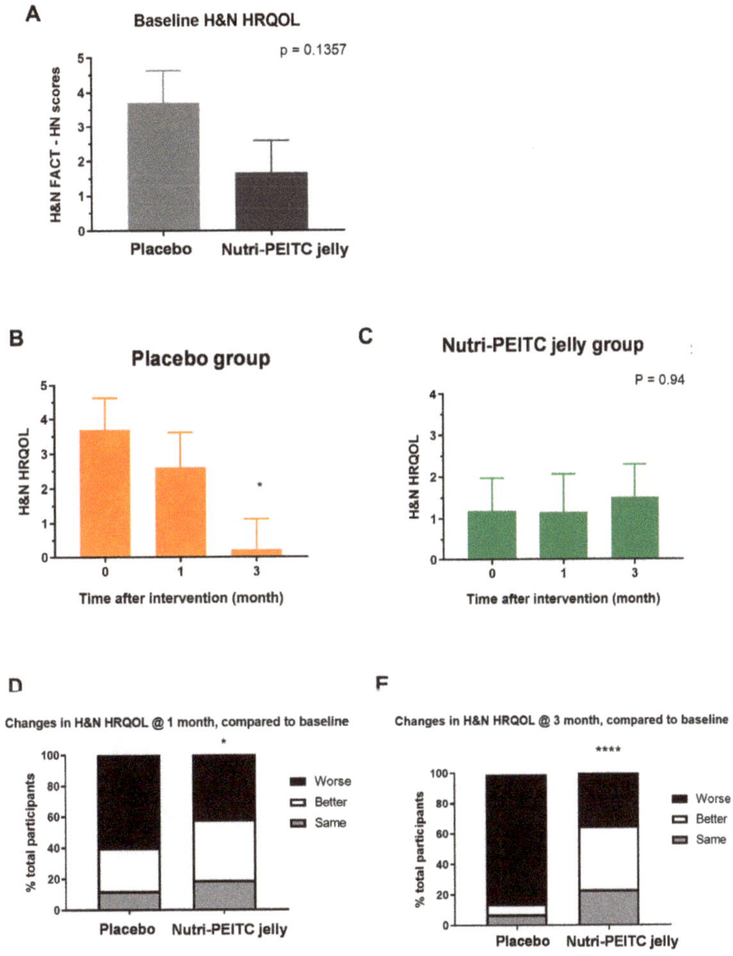

Figure 3. Changes in head and neck health-related quality of life (H&N HRQoL) scores. (**A**) Baseline H&N HRQoL in participants receiving placebo and Nutri-PEITC Jelly as labeled. Bar graph represents mean +/− SEM. p-value was from Mann–Whitney Test. (**B**,**C**) Comparison of H&N HRQoL after receiving placebo (**B**) and Nutri-PEITC Jelly (**C**) for 0, 1, and 3 months. Bar graph represents mean+/− SEM. * represents $p < 0.05$, obtained from a Friedman test and Dunn's multiple comparison test, compared with those of baseline. (**D**,**E**) Changes in H&N HRQoL after receiving placebo and Nutri-PEITC Jelly for 1 (**D**) and 3 (**E**) months. Stacked bars show percentages of participants with worse, better, and the same HRQoL scores when compared with the baseline. * and **** represent $p < 0.05$ and $p < 0.0001$, respectively, compared between groups, obtained from the chi-squared test.

2.6. Effects of Nutri-PEITC Jelly on Tumor Response and Progression-Free Survival Time

Tumor response was evaluated according to RECIST criteria and shown in Figure 4. As shown in Figure 4A, 1 month after the intervention, the study group had a significantly higher proportion of participants with stable disease (SD) or partial response (PR) than those of the placebo control group (80% vs. 40%, $p < 0.0001$). Consistently, as shown in Figure 4B, 3 months after the intervention, the Nutri-PEITC Jelly group had a significantly higher proportion of participants with SD or PR than those of the placebo control group (50% vs. 20%, $p < 0.0001$). The duration from starting the intervention to developing the progressive disease (PD) was counted as the progression-free survival time. As shown in Figure 4C, the average progression-free survival time in the Nutri-PEITC Jelly group was significantly higher than that of the control group (7.37 ± 4.45 vs. 4.93 ± 4.15 weeks, respectively; $p < 0.05$).

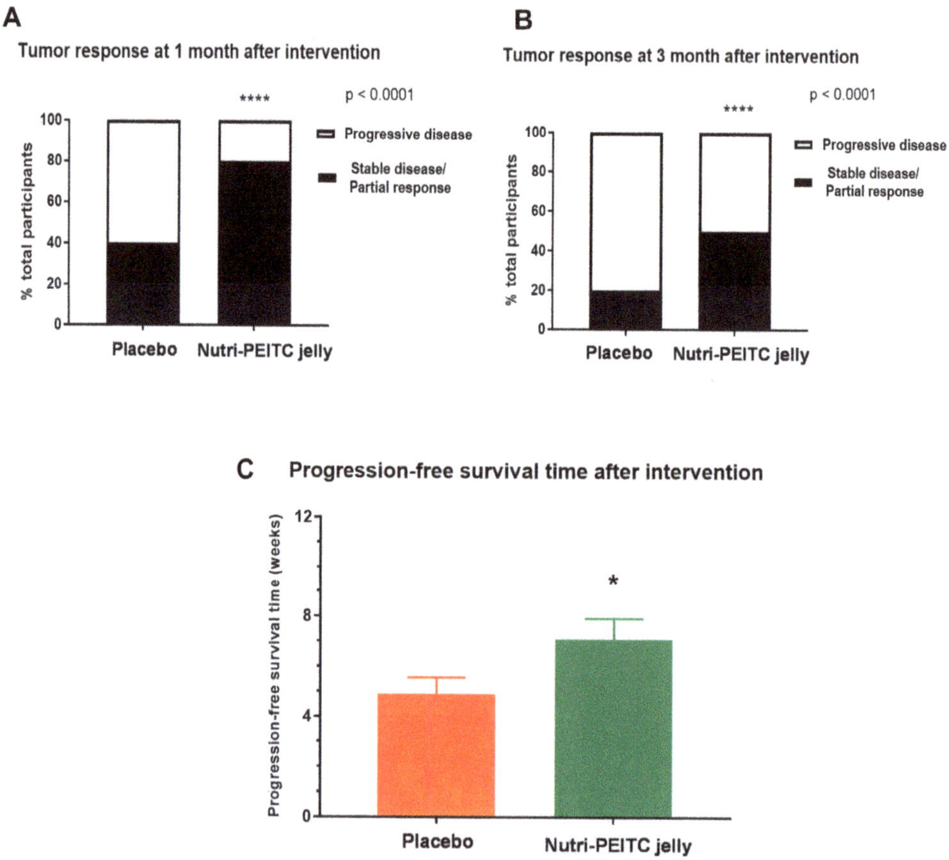

Figure 4. Tumor response and progression-free survival. (**A**,**B**) Tumor response at 1 month (**A**) and 3 months (**B**) after receiving placebo and Nutri-PEITC Jelly as labeled. Stacked bars show percentages of participants with progressive disease (white bar) and stable disease/partial response (black bar) according to RECIST criteria. * and **** represent $p < 0.05$ and $p < 0.0001$, respectively, compared between groups, obtained from the chi-squared test. (**C**) Comparison of progression-free survival between receiving placebo and Nutri-PEITC Jelly as labeled. The bar graph represents mean +/− SEM. * represents $p < 0.05$, obtained from the Mann–Whitney test.

2.7. Effects of Nutri-PEITC Jelly on Body Mass Index

As shown in Figure 5A,B, there were no significant differences in the mean body mass index after consuming placebo control or Nutri-PEITC Jelly for 1–3 months. However, as shown in Figure 5C,D, 3 months after the intervention, the Nutri-PEITC Jelly group had a significantly higher proportion of participants with improved BMI than that of the placebo control group (40% vs. 20%, $p < 0.05$), while there was no significant difference between groups at 1 month of intervention.

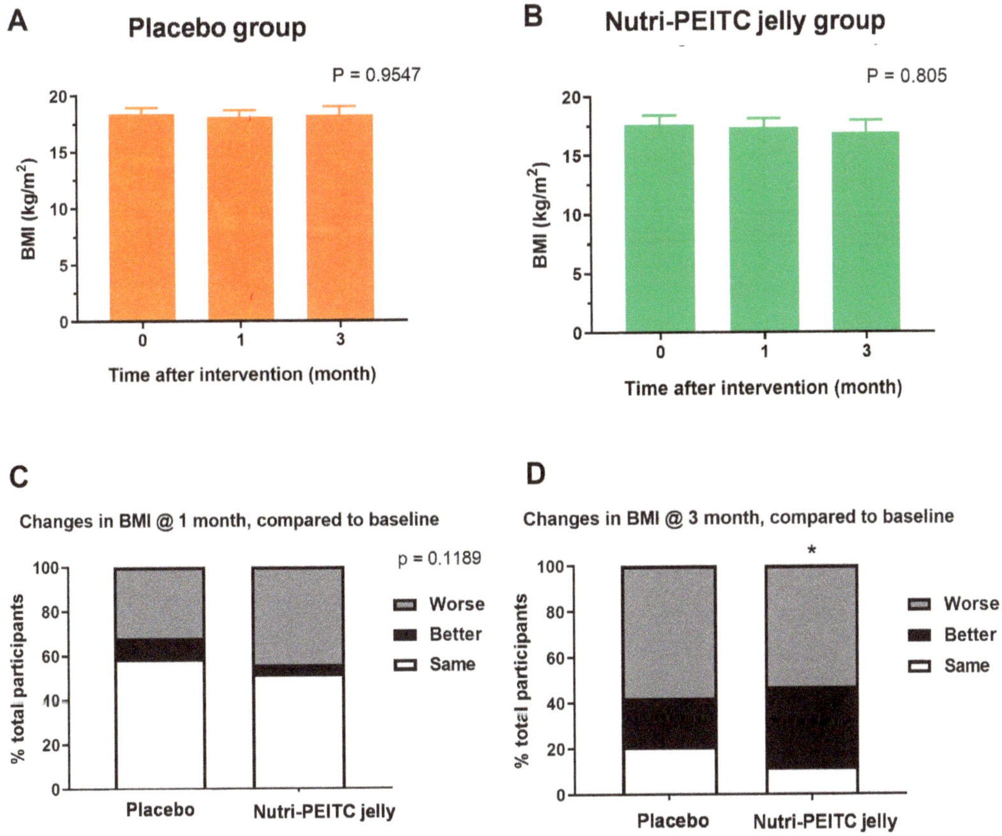

Figure 5. Changes in body mass index (BMI). (**A**,**B**) Comparison of BMI after receiving placebo (**a**) and Nutri-PEITC Jelly (**B**) for 0, 1, and 3 months. The bar graph represents mean +/− SEM. p-values were obtained from a Friedman test and compared with those of the baseline. (**C**,**D**) Changes in BMI after receiving placebo and Nutri-PEITC Jelly for 1 (**C**) and 3 (**D**) months. Stacked bars show percentages of participants with worse, better, and the same HRQoL scores when compared with the baseline. * represents $p < 0.05$, respectively, compared between groups, obtained from the chi-squared test.

2.8. Effects of Nutri-PEITC Jelly on Karnofsky Performance Status Scale (KPS)

As shown in Figure 6A–D, there were no significant differences in the KPS scores after consuming placebo control or Nutri-PEITC Jelly for 1–3 months.

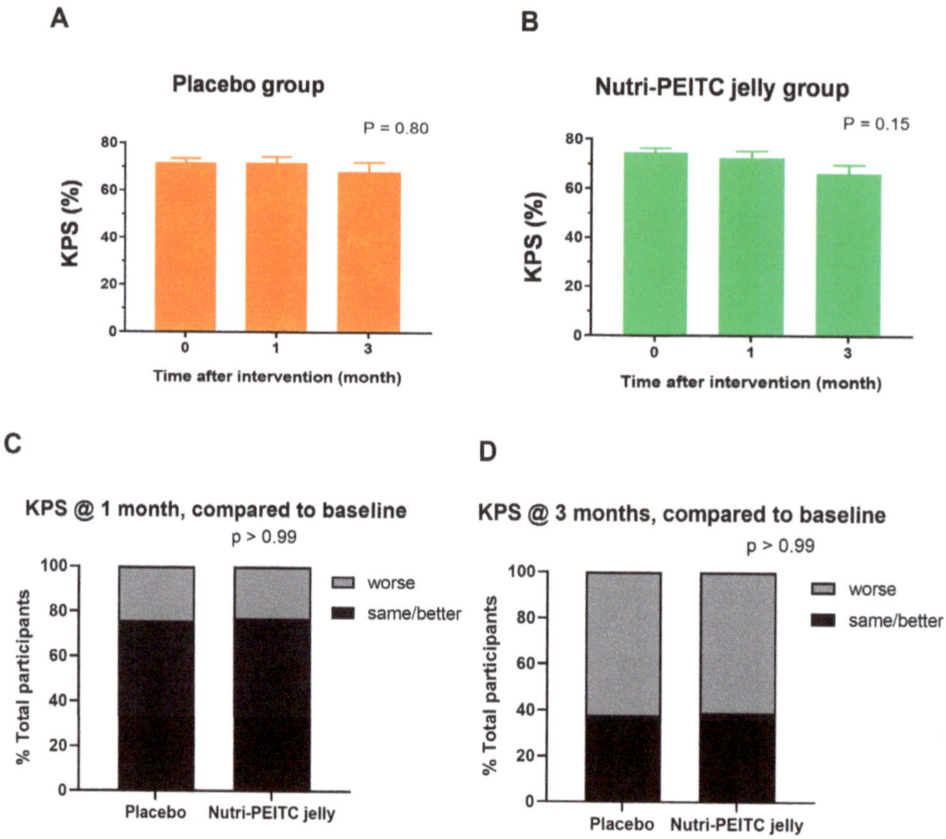

Figure 6. Changes in Karnofsky Performance Status Scale (KPS). (**A**,**B**) Comparison of KPS after receiving placebo (**A**) and Nutri-PEITC Jelly (**B**) for 0, 1, and 3 months. The bar graph represents mean +/− SEM. *p*-values were obtained from a Friedman test and compared with those of the baseline. (**C**,**D**) Changes in KPS after receiving placebo and Nutri-PEITC Jelly for 1 (**C**) and 3 (**D**) months. Stacked bars show percentages of participants with worse, and same/better KPS scores when compared with the baseline. *p*-values were obtained from Fisher's exact test.

2.9. Effects of Nutri-PEITC Jelly on Serum p53 Levels and Disease Progression

TP53 mutation is commonly found in 30–70% of oral and oropharyngeal cancer cases and is associated with poor survival [18]. Restoration of p53 function has been proposed as a new approach to stabilizing cancer progression [32,33]. In this study, we analyzed the serum level of total p53 using ELISA and pan antibodies which could react with both wild-type and mutant p53 protein (Figure 7A). As shown in Figure 7B,C, the average serum p53 levels in the study group were increased after consuming PEITC in a time-dependent manner, with statistical significance seen at 3 months. Compared to the placebo group, the Nutri-PEITC Jelly group had a significantly higher proportion of participants with increased serum p53 protein at 1 and 3 months after intervention (Figure 7D,E; $p < 0.01$ and $p < 0.001$, respectively). Since the increased level of total serum p53 protein could be either a good or bad thing, we further analyzed its association with the SD status. Interestingly, as shown in Figure 7F, at 3 months after intervention all participants with increased p53 levels had SD status, while participants with no change in p53 had either PD or SD status. The significant difference ($p < 0.0001$) suggests that the increased serum p53 level is associated with stable disease tumor status.

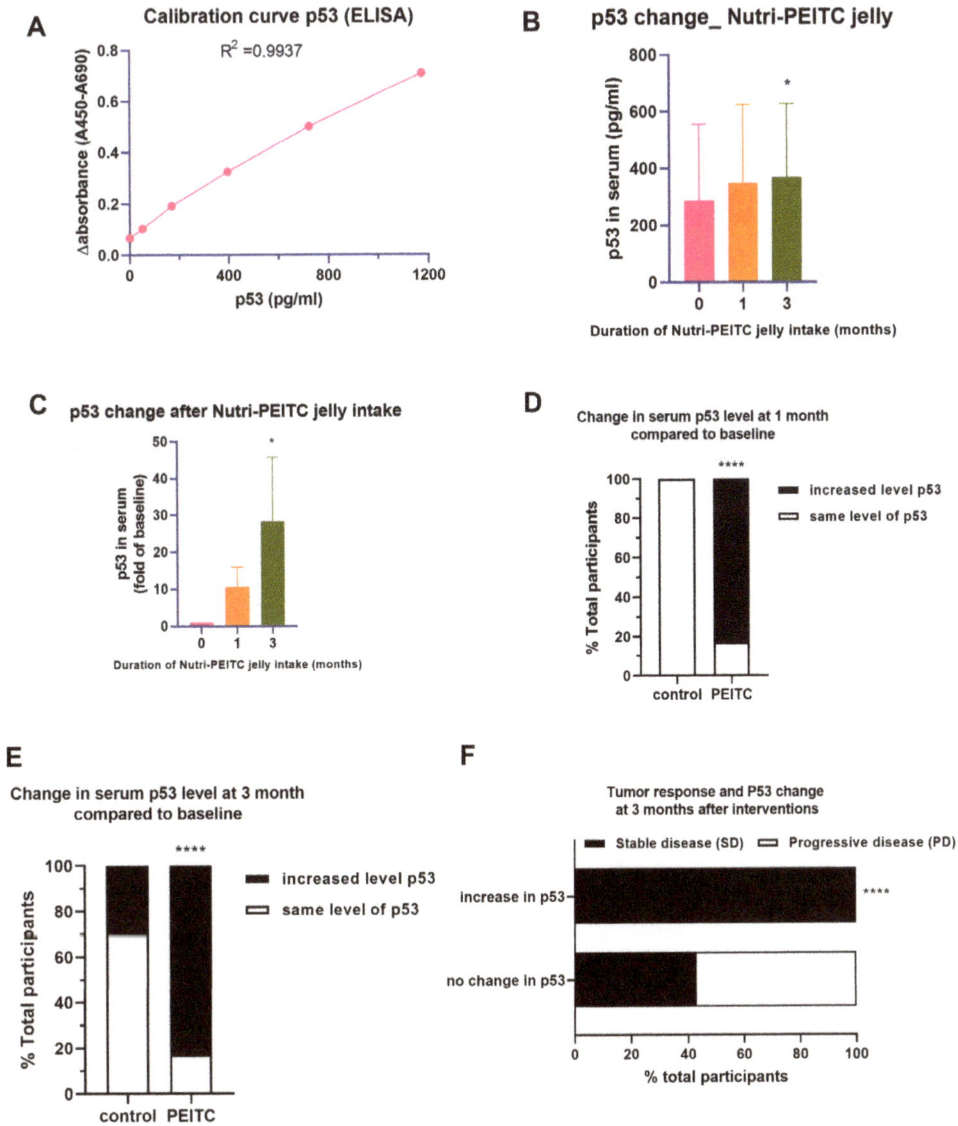

Figure 7. Changes in serum level of p53. (**A**) Calibration curve for quantitation of p53. Line plots show Δ absorbance at 450–690 nm at different concentrations of p53 (pg/mL). R^2 was obtained from linear regression. (**B**,**C**) Comparison of p53 level in serum (**B**): pg/mL, (**C**) fold number, compared with individual baseline) after receiving Nutri-PEITC Jelly for 0, 1, and 3 months. The bar graph represents mean +/− SEM. * represents $p < 0.05$, obtained from a Friedman test, compared with those of baseline. (**D**,**E**) Changes in serum level of p53 after receiving placebo and Nutri-PEITC Jelly for 1 (**D**) and 3 (**E**) months. Stacked bars show percentages of participants with increased levels of p53 when compared with the baseline. **** represents $p < 0.0001$, respectively, compared between groups, obtained from Fisher's exact test. (**F**) Tumor response in participants with an increase or no change in serum p53 level. Stacked bars show percentages of stable disease (black bar) and progressive disease (white bar) in participants with increased or no change in serum p53. **** represents $p < 0.0001$, respectively, compared between groups, obtained from Fisher's exact test.

2.10. Effects of Nutri-PEITC Jelly on Serum Cytochrome c Levels

High serum cytochrome c is associated with poor prognosis and poor survival in cancer patients [34]. In this study, we analyzed the serum level of cytochrome c using ELISA and the specific antibody (Figure 8A). Although the difference between groups was not statistically significant, Figure 8B–D showed that the serum cytochrome c level in the placebo control group tended to increase, while those of the Nutri-PEITC Jelly group tended to decrease.

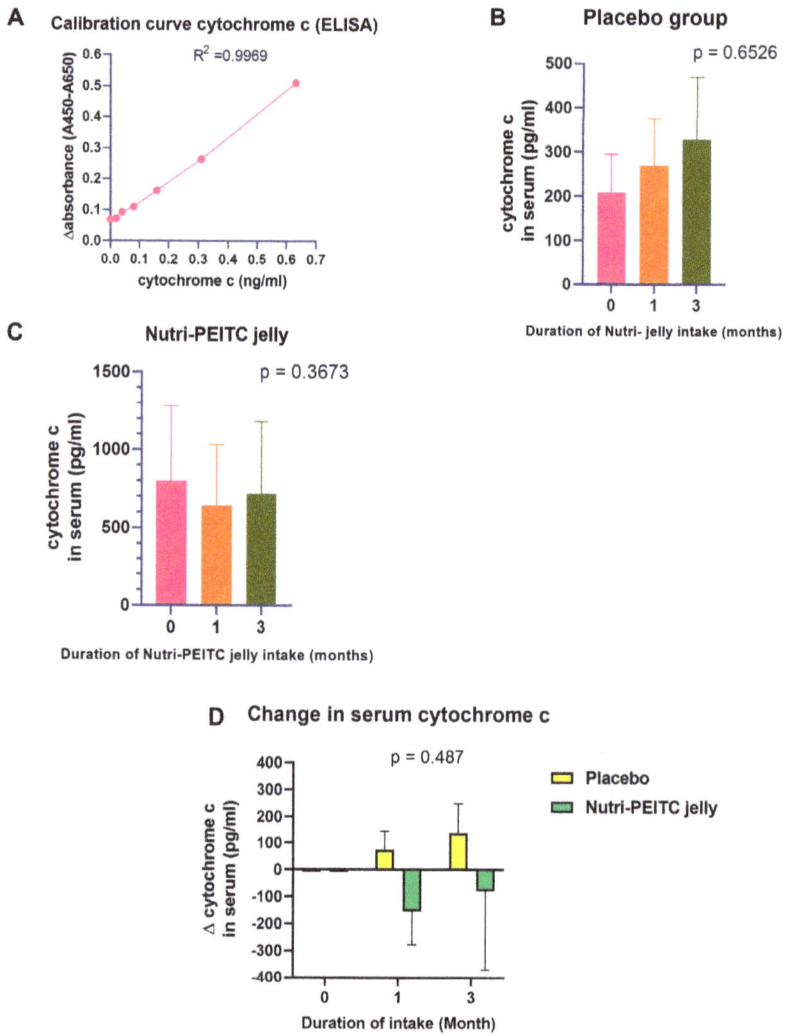

Figure 8. Changes in serum level of cytochrome c. (**A**) Calibration curve for quantitation of cytochrome c. Line plots shows Δ absorbance at 450–690 nm at different concentration of p53 (pg/mL). R^2 was obtained from linear regression. (**B**,**C**) Comparison of cytochrome c level in serum after receiving placebo (**B**) or Nutri-PEITC Jelly (**C**) for 0, 1, and 3 months. The bar graph represents mean +/− SEM. *p*-values were obtained from a Friedman test and compared with those of the baseline. (**D**) Changes in serum level of cytochrome c after receiving placebo and Nutri-PEITC Jelly for 1 and 3 months. Stacked bars show mean +/− SEM of Δ cytochrome c from individual baseline. *p*-values were obtained from two-way ANOVA.

3. Discussion

Head and neck cancer, especially oral and oropharyngeal cancers, are one of the most devastating cancers in its effect on quality of life [35,36]. Problems with chewing and swallowing, taste perception, talking, and facial appearance limit the patient's physical activities, working capability, and socialization, which eventually lead to malnutrition, low income, and psychological stress [35,36]. Treatment sequelae also severely affect the life quality of the patients [21,37,38]. Despite the advances in treatment modalities, head and neck cancer has had little improvement in survival rate during the past multiple decades [16,39,40]. Therefore, an innovation to stabilize the disease, improve the quality of life, and extend the survival of the patients is urgently needed. In this study, we reported the clinical safety and efficacy of Nutri-PEITC Jelly, an innovative texture-modified diet combining nutritional and anti-cancer properties. The findings suggest that continuous intake of Nutri-PEITC Jelly for 1 and 3 months is tolerable with minimal adverse events and can significantly improve head-and-neck specific quality of life, stable disease (SD) status, and extend the progression-free survival time. Moreover, an investigation of potential anti-cancer mechanisms revealed a significant increase in serum p53 and a non-significant decrease in serum cytochrome c levels in participants taking Nutri-PEITC Jelly.

To our knowledge, only a few human studies have investigated cancer preventive and therapeutic effects of PEITC. A clinical trial in cigarette smokers showed the benefit of PEITC to reduce metabolic activation of lung cancer-specific carcinogens [41]. Our previous clinical trial in meat-eaters showed the efficacy of PEITC-rich vegetable sauce in promoting detoxification and urinary excretion of grilled meat-derived carcinogens [25]. The previous work demonstrates the potential of PEITC in primary cancer prevention. However, the role of PEITC in tertiary prevention in cancer patients has not been reported. Thus, our present study is the first to report the efficacy of functional food containing PEITC in cancer patients. The idea of using functional food for cancer prevention is owing to the paradigm shift from aiming to cure cancer toward reducing mortality and disability by means of cost-effective approaches [42,43]. A recent in vitro study also attempted to identify tertiary chemo-preventive agents [44]. Since oral cancer survival depends on disease progression, nutritional status, and quality of life, Nutri-PEITC Jelly likely has a strong clinical implication in tertiary chemoprevention. In this study, the tumor response was graded according to the RECIST criteria as compared to baseline before the intervention. At baseline, there was no difference in TNM staging between experiment and control groups, suggesting a baseline balance of disease characteristics between the two groups. Compared to the control group, Nutri-PEITC Jelly exhibited a significantly higher percentage of SD/PR status at 1 and 3 months. Nevertheless, when comparing between 1 and 3 months the percentage of SD/PR in the study group still decreased over time. Therefore, Nutri-PEITC Jelly at the dose of 20 mg/day of PEITC did not inhibit the disease progression and the clinical application of this product is rather a functional food for tertiary chemoprevention than a therapy. Future studies with >20 mg/day of PEITC are warranted to investigates its potential therapeutic effect.

In this study, the number of interventions taken was aimed at a nutritional supplement (200 kcal per serving). Supplementation with Nutri-Jelly was previously shown to improve quality of life and reduced the requirement for an NG tube for head and neck cancer patients [22]. In the present study, fortification of PEITC into Nutri-Jelly was shown to better improve the quality of life, which is most likely related to disease stabilization as evidenced by the increased proportion of SD status. The stable disease condition and enhanced quality of life likely contributed to the extended progression-free survival time in patients receiving Nutri-PEITC Jelly. A previous systematic review suggests that cancer-related outcomes were the main factor influencing the quality of life in head and neck cancer patients [45]. Furthermore, previous studies showed that quality of life is a strong predictor of oral cancer survival [46,47].

Reactivation of p53 is a critical approach to regain apoptosis and halt cancer progression [32,33]. In vitro and in vivo studies suggested that PEITC could reactivate p53 function by at least two mechanisms. First, PEITC may selectively deplete mutant p53 by allowing wild-type p53 to regain its activity [8,48]. Second, PEITC could restore wild-type p53 conformation of the mutant p53 [7]. Both mechanisms result in resuming wild-type p53 function in tumor suppression [6–8]. Our previous animal study in the oral cancer model showed that PEITC increased total p53 protein expression and nuclear translocation of p53 [9]. This present clinical trial suggested that consuming Nutri-PEITC jelly led to a significant increase in serum p53 levels associated with stable disease status. To our knowledge, this is the first report of an increase in serum p53 associated with favorable outcomes of intervention. Previous observational studies reported elevated serum levels of mutated p53 protein as a marker of *TP53* gene mutation and advanced disease stage [48–52]. According to previous studies in other cancer models, the mechanism of p53 reactivation by PEITC could either resume wild-type p53 function or selectively deplete mutant p53 [6,7]. Unfortunately, in this study we used a p53 pan antibody to measure the total p53 protein (both wild-type and mutant in combination) in serum. Thus, our findings still cannot reveal the actual molecular mechanism. Nevertheless, the observed association between the increase in total p53 protein and stable disease response after consumption of Nutri-PEITC Jelly suggests the possibility that PEITC may favorably reactivate p53 and regain its tumor suppressive function. In fact, a previous study showed that an increase in the p53 protein level might indicate elevated transcriptional activity of *TP53* [53]. Furthermore, a secretome study showed anti-proliferative, pro-apoptotic, and chemosensitivity effects of secreted proteins in media driven by wild-type p53 [54]. Intriguingly, a recent study with a genetically knock-in mice model showed that just partial *TP53* reactivation is adequate to resume tumor suppressive function of p53 resulting in cancer regression [55]. This was quite enthusiastic for head and neck cancer since the *TP53* tumor suppressor gene was the most common somatic genomic alteration in head and neck squamous cells carcinoma (HNSCC) [18]. Although cancer *TP53* status in our participants was unknown, the significant association of increased serum p53 level and stable disease status suggested that anti-cancer effects of PEITC noted in this study likely involved p53. Numerous studies also supported PEITC as a candidate for p53 reactivation [56]. Future studies are warranted to compare responses to treatment in various p53 statuses and identify the exact molecular mechanisms of the increased serum p53 levels. Moreover, a genetic study to investigate p53 alterations in head and neck cancer patients included in the future trial will be beneficial for personalized nutrition.

The strength of this study was the triple-blinded design with matched study and control arms. In addition, we evaluated the participants in various aspects that could affect their quality of life and survival. Subject diaries to record intervention intake as well as serum PEITC levels were analyzed to ensure participants' compliance. Nevertheless, we encountered some limitations. First, dropout rates were quite high (51.22% and 32.2% in control and study groups, respectively), mostly due to death or progressive disease. Notably, the percentage of dropouts in the control group was higher than that of the study group. The difference may be a result of the intervention's efficacy in stabilizing the disease in study group [57]. Such high drop-out is commonly seen in clinical trials of late-stage cancer patients, which might affect the reliability of the result [58]. To ensure that our data were reliable, we analyzed all data obtained from the participants by using intention-to-treat analysis for clinical parameters and per protocol analysis for laboratory parameters. We also performed post-hoc power analysis which revealed adequate power based on the sample size obtained: 1.0 for changes in quality of life at 3 months (chi-squared test), 0.917 for tumor response at 1 month (Fisher's exact test), and 0.843 for progression-free survival (unpaired *t*-test). For future clinical trials in late-stage cancer patients, inclusion criteria shall be modified by recruiting only patients with life expectancy of at least 6 months. Secondly, the genetic background of participants in this study had not been characterized. Thus, the reactivation of p53 as the mechanism is speculation based on our previous in vivo studies and the result of p53 expression change in this study. Third, our study focused on serum p53 levels rather than analyzing p53 levels in tumor samples. Investigating tumor samples could provide more accurate insights into the effects of Nutri-PEITC Jelly on cancer cells and the molecular mechanisms behind its cancer-stabilizing properties. Unfortunately, these patients were biopsied earlier in their disease course in various places in the country. It would be difficult to retrieve the paraffin block of biopsied tissue, and a new tissue biopsy performed during this trial would be too invasive and unjustified. Future studies that include only patients with known genetic background information, i.e., mutated compared to wild-type *TP53* will be very useful in deciphering the p53-mediated mechanism of Nutri-PEITC Jelly. Our previous works have shown the redox-modulating effect of PEITC as a strategy to selectively kill cancer cells in vitro and in vivo [26,27,59,60]. p53 also regulates redox-modulated ferroptosis (lipid peroxidation-induced cell death) [61]. Thus, future mechanistic studies shall focus on p53 reactivation and redox-modulation pathways. Furthermore, there could be other mechanisms behind the cancer-stabilizing mechanism of PEITC, such as epigenetic modulation [62], suppression of inflammatory signaling NF-κB [59,63,64], and inhibition of epithelial-mesenchymal transition as invasion machinery [65]. Future metabolomic studies of clinical specimens from patients receiving Nutri-PEITC Jelly would be worthwhile to characterize the molecular pathways [66].

To address the above-mentioned flaws and limitations, future studies should aim to reduce dropout rates, characterize the genetic background of participants, analyze p53 levels in tumor samples, and explore additional molecular pathways that may contribute to the cancer-stabilizing effects of Nutri-PEITC Jelly.

4. Materials and Methods

4.1. Ethical Aspects and Setting

Data were collected at Chonburi Cancer Hospital, Lopburi Cancer Hospital, National Cancer Institute, and Maharat Nakhonratchasima Hospital. The study protocol was in compliance with the Declaration of Helsinki and the International Conference on Harmonization Guidelines for Good Clinical Practice (ICH-GCP), and was approved by the Ethical committees for human research of Chonburi cancer hospital (protocol No. 10/2015), Lopburi cancer hospital (Approval No. LEC5712), National cancer institute (protocol No. 302014RC_OUT360), and Maharat Nakhonratchasima hospital (Approval No. 058/2014). This trial was registered with ClinicalTrials.gov (Identifier number: NCT03034603). The protocol can be accessed at https://clinicaltrials.gov/ct2/show/NCT03034603 (accessed on 5 February 2023). All participants provided written informed consent before enrollment.

4.2. Study Design, Blinding, Random Allocation, and Concealment

A multi-center blind randomized placebo-controlled trial was conducted. Seventy-two patients with advanced-stage oral or oropharyngeal cancer were randomly assigned with minimization for age and baseline quality of life scores into the study group (n = 31) and control group (n = 41). The study and control groups received Nutri-PEITC Jelly and Nutri-Jelly without PEITC (placebo), coded as A and B to conceal their identities. Participants, data collectors, and data analyzers were blinded throughout the study. The placebo jelly and Nutri-PEITC Jelly were packed in the same container with no labels except for the capital letter stating the groups A or B, which were blinded to the investigators, all health personnel and the participants. Furthermore, the researcher who performed randomization, the researcher who provided intervention, the researcher who performed data collection and laboratory analysis, and the statistical analyzer were different people. Standard operating procedure (SOP) was developed by all investigators and used as a standard guide for data collection of all centers.

4.3. Participants

Inclusion criteria of the study population included patients with primary cancers at the lip, oral cavity, oropharynx, pyriform sinus, or hypopharynx (ICD10: C00-C14) whose treatment aimed for palliative care or who denied definitive/standard treatments. If the patients previously received radiotherapy or chemotherapy, those treatments had to be discontinued at least 1 month before enrollment. Cancer had to be diagnosed histopathologically as squamous cell carcinoma and have at least one measurable target lesion. The patients had to have a baseline Karnofsky Performance Status Scale (KPS) of at least 40% or Eastern Cooperative Oncology Group (ECOG) of 0–3, and have acceptable laboratory values (white blood cells $\geq 1.5 \times 10^9$ cells/L ($\geq$1500 cells/mm^3), platelets $\geq 100 \times 10^9$/L; Hb $\geq$ 9.0 g/dL), renal function (creatinine clearance using the CKD-EPI formula (Chronic Kidney Disease Epidemiology group) $\geq$ 50 mL/min) and hepatic function (SGOT, SGPT, serum bilirubin not more than 1.5 times of upper normal limits). Moreover, participants had to be able to consume the intervention either by mouth or tube feeding for 3 months without aspiration and able to communicate well. Exclusion criteria included patients who received N-acetylcysteine within 3 days before enrollment or continuously, ongoing dialysis, were pregnant or breastfeeding, had uncontrolled systemic diseases or infection, and had a high risk of aspiration. The participants were discontinued from the study if they demonstrated serious adverse events or stopped taking the intervention for more than 2 weeks. All participants signed written informed consent before enrollment into the study and could leave the study whenever they wished.

4.4. Sample Size

The estimated sample size was identified by a priori power analysis using G Power 3.1. The effect size was calculated from our previous study on head and neck cancer patients receiving palliative radiotherapy [22] by using quality of life as the primary outcome. Based on the calculation, at least 30 participants per group were required to achieve 90% power at $\alpha = 0.05$ significance level. Accounting for possible drop-out, no more than a total of 96 participants were expected. Data were collected for three years. Finally, completed data were from 72 patients composed of 31 patients in the study group and 41 patients in the control group. We recruited more subjects in the control than the study group to obtain enough samples for laboratory analyses on account of its higher drop-out rate. Post-hoc power analysis revealed a power of 1.0 for changes in quality of life at 3 months (chi-squared test), 0.917 for tumor response at 1 month (Fisher's exact test), and 0.843 for progression-free survival (unpaired *t*-test), which are considered adequate.

4.5. Interventions

Nutri-Jelly and Nutri-PEITC Jelly products (Figure 9) were provided by the Dental Innovation Foundation under Royal Patronage. The products were prepared according to the regulation of the Thai Food and Drug Administration (FDA) and HALAL. The products were manufactured in ultra-high temperature (UHT) processing and aseptic filling system under international standards (Good Manufacturing Practice (GMP), Hazard Analysis and Critical Control Points (HACCP), and International Organization for Standardization (ISO) 22000). The products also passed microbiological tests from outside certified laboratories according to the regulation of food in hermetically sealed containers. Nutri-Jelly Mango Flavored is a Thai FDA-registered product with No. 10-1-09760-5-0002. The product is lactose-free. Nutri-PEITC Jelly is the PEITC-fortified version of Nutri-Jelly. Nutri-Jelly and Nutri-PEITC Jelly were both made from similar ingredients (water, mango puree, milk powder, sugar, whey protein, rice bran oil, INS420(i), INS 330, INS 428, INS 406, INS 415) except food-grade PEITC (C6H5CH2CH2NCS, Sigma-Aldrich, St. Louis, MO, USA) was added in Nutri-PEITC Jelly. Each cup of 100 g Nutri-PEITC Jelly contained about 10 mg PEITC (0.01% weight/weight (*w/w*). For quality control of different batches, about 1% of the product was sampled for measurement of PEITC by LC/MS-MS [25]. The acceptable range of PEITC for each batch is 0.006–0.012% PEITC *w*/*w* with the intra-batch coefficient of variation (CV) of <15%. The products were stored at room temperature. The nutrition values of Nutri-Jelly and Nutri-PEITC Jelly were shown in Table 5. The participants in the control and study groups were asked to consume two cups of Nutri-Jelly or Nutri-PEITC Jelly, respectively. Thus, the study group received 20 mg of PEITC per day.

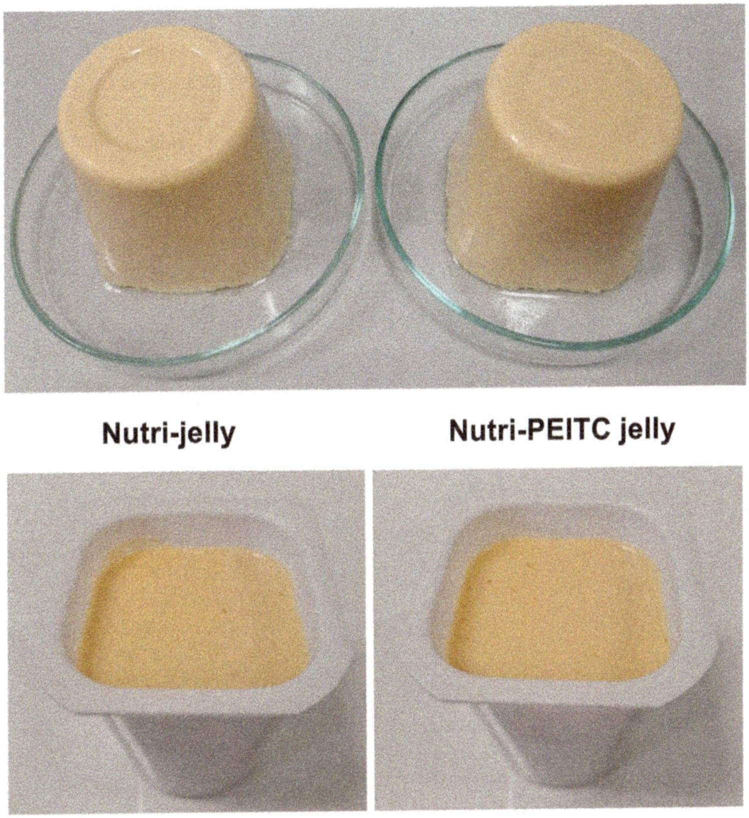

Figure 9. Nutri-Jelly and Nutri-PEITC Jelly: the similar appearance of Nutri-Jelly (left panel) and Nutri-PEITC Jelly (right panel). The bottom panel shows the 100 g cup products.

Table 5. Nutrition values of Nutri-Jelly and Nutri-PEITC Jelly per 100 g cup.

	Nutri-Jelly	**Nutri-PEITC Jelly**
Total energy (kcal)	130	110
Energy from fat (kcal)	35	30
Total fat (g)	4	3
Saturated fat (g)	2	2
Cholesterol (mg)	15	15
Protein (g)	5	5
Total carbohydrate (g)	18	16
Dietary fiber (g)	2	<1
Sugar (g)	12	9
Sodium (mg)	45	45
Vitamin A (μg RE)	64	64
Vitamin B1 (mg)	0	0
Vitamin B2 (mg)	0.17	0.34
Calcium (mg)	120	120
Iron (mg)	0.3	1.5

4.6. Study Procedure

Baseline assessment was performed before the randomization, including physical examination, cancer size, location and stage, complete blood count, and liver and kidney function tests. General information about the participants, including age, sex, height, and medical history was retrieved from patients' charts. The participants were asked to consume either 2 cups of 100 g (total of 200 g) of Nutri-Jelly or Nutri-PEITC Jelly in the morning on Monday to Friday (5 days a week) for 3 months. All participants were asked to record their use of the product daily in subject diaries to ensure adherence to the intervention protocol. The intake of paracetamol was also recorded. The outcome measures were evaluated at 0, 1, and 3 months after interventions. The primary outcome measure included adverse events, health-related quality of life (HRQoL), nutritional status, progression-free survival (PFS), and tumor response. The secondary outcome measures were functional assessment outcome (Karnofsky performance status scale: KPS) and serum p53 and cytochrome c levels.

Questionnaires, body weight measurements, blood collection, and tumor size measurement by caliper were performed at all time points. CT scan was performed at 0 and 3 months.

4.7. Outcomes

4.7.1. Adverse Events

The physicians assessed the adverse events at 1 and 3 months after the intervention by physical examination, blood hematology, and chemistry. Moreover, adverse events such as nausea, vomiting, and gastrointestinal disturbance were recorded and reported throughout the study period by the participants. The adverse events were graded by the physicians for severity, seriousness, and relatedness to the intervention.

4.7.2. Health-Related Quality of Life and Karnofsky Performance STATUS Scale

Health-related quality of life (HRQoL) was determined by using the Thai version of the FACT-HN questionnaire form after receiving approval from FACIT [67–70]. The participants were evaluated in several domains including physical, social and family, emotional and functional well-being, and head and neck-related symptoms by completing the questionnaire or interviewing. The higher scores represented better HRQoL. Karnofsky performance status scale for functional impairment was evaluated by a physician using standard criteria [68,71]. Higher scores indicated better performance.

4.7.3. Nutritional Status

Nutritional status was evaluated by body mass index and the levels of serum albumin. Body weight was measured by using a body composition monitor machine (TANITA BC-730, Tanita Corporation, Tokyo, Japan). Body mass index (kg/m^2) was calculated from body weight/height^2.

4.7.4. Tumor Responses and Progression-Free Survival Time

Progression-free survival (PFS) time was calculated from the time of the intervention until any signs or symptoms of progressive disease be recorded [69,72]. According to the National Cancer Institute, USA, tumor response is defined as a standard way to measure how well a cancer patient responds to treatment. It is based on whether tumors shrink, stay the same, or get bigger [73]. Tumor responses were investigated according to the response evaluation criteria in solid tumors (RECIST) criteria version 1.1 [73], by using a caliber or CT scan, when applicable, of the target lesion. Complete response (CR) was recorded if all target lesions disappeared after intervention. Partial response (PR) was recorded when there was a 30% decrease in the sum diameter of target lesions after intervention. Progressive disease (PD) was recorded when there was a 20%, and at least 5 mm, increase in the sum diameter of the target lesions after intervention. Stable disease (SD) was recorded when the changes were not sufficient to qualify CR, PR, or PD [73]. Therefore, the SD implies that the disease is subsided with no significant progression [74]. To measure tumor response, the baseline size of tumor mass (target lesion) was measured by using a Vernier caliper and computer tomography (CT) scan at 0 months before intervention. Then, at 1 month the tumor size was measured again using Vernier caliper. At 3 months the tumor size was re-measured by using a Vernier caliper and computer tomography (CT) scan. The tumor sizes at 1 and 3 months were compared with those of the baseline of each participant. Then, tumor response as CR, PR, SD, or PD was concluded according to the RECIST criteria.

4.7.5. Serum Levels of p53 and Cytochrome c

The serum was centrifuged at 4 °C for 10 min at 1000× *g* (3000 rpm). Then, the serum was aliquot and stored at −80 °C until ready to be tested. The p53 ELISA assay was performed by using a p53 pan ELISA kit (Catalog No. 11 828 789 001, Roche, Basel, Switzerland). The assay was designed to recognize a conserved, pantropic, denaturation-stable antigenic determinant of the p53 protein. Briefly, 100 µL of serum samples were plated in duplicate in a 96-well microtiter plate. The plate was pre-coated with biotin-labeled anti-p53 capture antibodies. Then 100 µL of anti-p53-pan-peroxidase detection antibody was added to all wells. The plate was then incubated at room temperature on a shaker for 2 h. After the washing step, tetramethylbenzidine (TMB) substrate was added, followed by a stop solution. The assay results were quantitated spectrophotometrically at 450 nm (reference wavelength 690 nm) using a microplate reader. The calibration curve was generated and used for the calculation of p53 concentration (pg/mL).

The Cytochrome c ELISA assay was performed by using a Cytochrome c Human ELISA Kit (Catalog No. ab119521, Abcam, Cambridge, UK). Briefly, 100 µL of serum samples were plated in duplicate in a 96-well microtiter plate pre-coated with anti-Cytochrome c monoclonal antibody. Then 50 µL of biotinylated detection antibody was added to each well. The plate was then incubated at room temperature for 2 h. After the washing step, 100 uL of streptavidin-horseradish peroxidase was added and incubated at room temperature for 1 h. The plate was then washed, followed by the addition of TMB substrate and stop solution. Optical density was measured by spectrophotometer at 450 nm (reference wavelength 620 nm) using a microplate reader.

4.7.6. Plasma Level of PEITC

To ensure that the participants did consume Nutri-PEITC Jelly, the plasma level of PEITC was measured by using Liquid chromatography Tandem Mass Spectrometry (LC-MS/MS), as previously described [25,75]. A standard curve was generated by using control plasma samples spiked with multiple levels of PEITC concentration (0–500 ng/mL). 3-phenyl propyl isothiocyanate (PPITC) was used as an internal standard (IS) [76]. Both PEITC and PPITC were purchased from Sigma–Aldrich. Extraction of PEITC was performed by adding 600 µL of hexane using a positive displacement pipette to 250 µL of plasma standard or sample and mixing for 30 s with a high-velocity vortex mixer. Then, the mixture was centrifuged at 1000× *g*, 25 °C for 3 min and 500 µL of the top hexane layers was collected into a 2 mL tube. The hexane extraction was performed twice and the supernatant from both times was combined. Then, 400 µL of 2 M ammonia in methanol was added to the hexane extract for ammonia derivatization. The samples were vortexed for 30 s and incubated with shaking on a microplate shaker (Fisher Scientific, Hampton, NH, USA) at room temperature for 4 h. After that, drying in a speed vacuum evaporator (CentriVap Benchtop Vacuum Concentrator, Labconco, Kansas City, MO, USA) at 55 °C for 40 min was performed to remove solvents. Then, 250 µL of acetonitrile water in a ratio of 3:2 was added to reconstitute, followed by mixing with vortex for 1 min. All samples were filtered through a 0.2 µm nylon filter and stored at −20 °C before analysis. The ammonia-derivatized PEITC and PPITC (IS) were measured by an ultra-high performance liquid chromatography-tandem mass spectrometry (LC-MS/MS) system, comprising a UHPLC model Ultimate 3000 (Thermo Scientific, Waltham, MA, USA) and a TSQ Quantis Triple Quadrupole Mass spectrometer (Thermo Scientific, Waltham, MA, USA). LC condition includes injection of

5 μL each sample and run through a Hypersil GOLD™ C18 column 100 × 2.1 mm, particle size 1.9 μm with a mobile phase of acetonitrile: 5 mM formic acid (50:50) at an isocratic flow rate of 0.3 mL/min and a run time of 3.5 min. MS condition includes positive ion electrospray ionization (+ESI) with spraying voltage at 3500 V, sheath gas of 50 arbitrary units (Arb), auxiliary gas of 10.0 Arb, ion transfer tube (ITT) of 325 °C, and vaporizing temperatures of 350 °C, respectively. The retention time of PEITC-NH3 (phenethyl thiourea) was 1.6 min with the mass-to-charge ratio (m/z) of precursor, quantified, and confirmed product ions at 181, 105.13, and 77.05, respectively. The collision energy of 18.18 and 38.82 V was used for the transition of quantified and confirmed masses, respectively. The retention time of IS-NH3 was 1.7 min with the mass-to-charge ratio (m/z) of precursor, quantified, and confirmed product ions at 195, 91, and 136, respectively. The collision energy of 26 and 14 V was used for the transition of quantified and confirmed masses, respectively. RF lenses of 129 V and 148 V were used for PEITC-NH3 and IS-NH3, respectively.

4.8. Statistical Analysis

The primary efficacy parameters were analyzed for the intention-to-treat (ITT) using the last observation carried forward (LOCF) method for the replacement of missing data points.

The normality of data distribution was verified by a D'Agostino and Pearson omnibus test. Parametric statistical tests were used only when the data passed the normality test ($p > 0.05$). Comparison of baseline characteristics in study and control groups was analyzed by independent t-test, Mann–Whitney test, chi-squared, or Fisher's exact test, as appropriate. The concentrations of plasma PEITC, serum p53, and cytochrome c were calculated by using linear regression of the calibration curve. Comparison of data among different time points was performed by using two-way ANOVA, followed by the Bonferroni test for multiple comparisons. A p-value < 0.05 was considered statistically significant. Biochemical data, which contained some missing values, were analyzed by using mixed-effects model (time × group) with the Geisser greenhouse correction. In the end, post-hoc power analysis was performed to ensure an adequate sample size to gain at least 90% power. Sample size and power were calculated by G Power 3.1. Graphing and statistical analysis were performed by GraphPad Prism 5.0.

5. Conclusions

The findings of this study suggest that intake of Nutri-PEITC Jelly with 20 mg PEITC/day for 1–3 months is safe with minimal adverse effects. The supplementation may re-activate p53, stabilize the disease, improve the quality of life and progression-free survival in patients with advanced-stage oral and oropharyngeal cancer. Further studies in a larger population and various dosages are warranted to confirm that Nutri-PEITC Jelly could be functional food for tertiary chemoprevention in oral and oropharyngeal cancer.

Author Contributions: Conceptualization, A.L.-U. and D.T.; methodology, A.L.-U. and D.T.; obtain ethical approval, A.L-U.; investigation, A.L.-U., J.S., W.R., P.T., T.T. and D.T.; data curation and formal analysis, A.L.-U. and D.T.; writing—original draft preparation, A.L.-U.; writing—review and editing, D.T.; funding acquisition, A.L.-U. and D.T. All authors have read and agreed to the published version of the manuscript.

Funding: This research was funded by Dental Innovation Foundation under Royal Patronage, Thailand. The funder has no role in design, conduct, analysis, or report. The authors have full control of all data and reports.

Institutional Review Board Statement: This study was approved by the Ethical committees for human research of Chonburi cancer hospital (protocol No. 10/2015), Lopburi cancer hospital (Approval No. LEC5712), National cancer institute (protocol No. 302014RC_OUT360), and Maharat Nakhonratchasima hospital (Approval No. 058/2014).

Informed Consent Statement: Informed consent was obtained from all subjects involved in the study.

Data Availability Statement: All data collected in this project have been described in this work. No further data are available. Since the participants only gave consent to report the summary of data, no individual data can be shared.

Acknowledgments: The authors are grateful to Kamonchanok Sakulprasert, and Ketsara Phadungrerk for their assistance in coordination with each center.

Conflicts of Interest: D.T. and A.L.-U. received a research grant and Nutri-PEITC Jelly products from a non-profit organization, Dental Innovation Foundation under Royal Patronage, Thailand. The funders had no role in the design of the study; in the collection, analyses, or interpretation of data; in the writing of the manuscript; or in the decision to publish the results. The authors have full control of all data and reports.

References

1. Zhu, G.; Pan, C.; Bei, J.X.; Li, B.; Liang, C.; Xu, Y.; Fu, X. Mutant p53 in Cancer Progression and Targeted Therapies. *Front. Oncol.* **2020**, *10*, 595187. [CrossRef] [PubMed]
2. Mantovani, F.; Collavin, L.; Del Sal, G. Mutant p53 as a guardian of the cancer cell. *Cell Death Differ.* **2019**, *26*, 199–212. [CrossRef]
3. Zhang, C.; Liu, J.; Xu, D.; Zhang, T.; Hu, W.; Feng, Z. Gain-of-function mutant p53 in cancer progression and therapy. *J. Mol. Cell Biol.* **2020**, *12*, 674–687. [CrossRef] [PubMed]
4. Athar, M.; Elmets, C.A.; Kopelovich, L. Pharmacological activation of p53 in cancer cells. *Curr. Pharm. Des.* **2011**, *17*, 631–639. [CrossRef]
5. Selivanova, G.; Wiman, K.G. Reactivation of mutant p53: Molecular mechanisms and therapeutic potential. *Oncogene* **2007**, *26*, 2243–2254. [CrossRef]
6. Wang, X.; Di Pasqua, A.J.; Govind, S.; McCracken, E.; Hong, C.; Mi, L.; Mao, Y.; Wu, J.Y.C.; Tomita, Y.; Woodrick, J.C.; et al. Selective depletion of mutant p53 by cancer chemopreventive isothiocyanates and their structure-activity relationships. *J. Med. Chem.* **2011**, *54*, 809–816. [CrossRef] [PubMed]
7. Aggarwal, M.; Saxena, R.; Sinclair, E.; Fu, Y.; Jacobs, A.; Dyba, M.; Wang, X.; Cruz, I.; Berry, D.; Kallakury, B.; et al. Reactivation of mutant p53 by a dietary-related compound phenethyl isothiocyanate inhibits tumor growth. *Cell Death Differ.* **2016**, *23*, 1615–1627. [CrossRef]
8. Yeh, Y.T.; Yeh, H.; Su, S.H.; Lin, J.S.; Lee, K.J.; Shyu, H.W.; Chen, Z.F.; Huang, S.Y.; Su, S.J. Phenethyl isothiocyanate induces DNA damage-associated G2/M arrest and subsequent apoptosis in oral cancer cells with varying p53 mutations. *Free Radic. Biol. Med.* **2014**, *74*, 1–13. [CrossRef]
9. Lam-Ubol, A.; Fitzgerald, A.L.; Ritdej, A.; Phonyiam, T.; Zhang, H.; Myers, J.N.; Huangh, P.; Trachootham, D. Sensory acceptable equivalent doses of β-phenylethyl isothiocyanate (PEITC) induce cell cycle arrest and retard the growth of p53 mutated oral cancer in vitro and in vivo. *Food Funct.* **2018**, *9*, 3640–3656. [CrossRef]
10. Wu, S.J.; Ng, L.T.; Lin, C.C. Effects of antioxidants and caspase-3 inhibitor on the phenylethyl isothiocyanate-induced apoptotic signaling pathways in human PLC/PRF/5 cells. *Eur. J. Pharmacol.* **2005**, *518*, 96–106. [CrossRef]
11. Aggarwal, M.; Saxena, R.; Asif, N.; Sinclair, E.; Tan, J.; Cruz, I.; Berry, D.; Kallakury, B.; Pham, Q.; Wang, T.T.Y.; et al. p53 mutant-type in human prostate cancer cells determines the sensitivity to phenethyl isothiocyanate induced growth inhibition. *J. Exp. Clin. Cancer Res.* **2019**, *38*, 307. [CrossRef] [PubMed]
12. Liu, J.; Chen, G.; Pelicano, H.; Liao, J.; Huang, J.; Feng, L.; Keating, M.J.; Huang, P. Targeting p53-deficient chronic lymphocytic leukemia cells in vitro and in vivo by ROS-mediated mechanism. *Oncotarget* **2016**, *7*, 71378–71389. [CrossRef]
13. Nachat, A.; Turoff-Ortmeyer, S.; Liu, C.; Mcculloch, M. PEITC in End-Stage B-Cell Prolymphocytic Leukemia: Case Report of Possible Sensitization to Salvage R-CHOP. *Perm. J.* **2016**, *20*, 74–80. [CrossRef] [PubMed]
14. Aupérin, A. Epidemiology of head and neck cancers: An update. *Curr. Opin. Oncol.* **2020**, *32*, 178–186. [CrossRef] [PubMed]
15. Yuwanati, M.; Gondivkar, S.; Sarode, S.C.; Gadbail, A.; Desai, A.; Mhaske, S.; Pathak, S.K.; Khatib, M.N. Oral health-related quality of life in oral cancer patients: Systematic review and meta-analysis. *Future Oncol.* **2021**, *17*, 979–990. [CrossRef]
16. Hoesseini, A.; Offerman, M.P.J.; van de Wall-Neecke, B.J.; Sewnaik, A.; Wieringa, M.H.; Baatenburg de Jong, R.J. Physicians' clinical prediction of survival in head and neck cancer patients in the palliative phase. *BMC Palliat. Care* **2020**, *19*, 176. [CrossRef]
17. Sasahira, T.; Kirita, T. Hallmarks of Cancer-Related Newly Prognostic Factors of Oral Squamous Cell Carcinoma. *Int. J. Mol. Sci.* **2018**, *19*, 2413. [CrossRef]
18. Zhou, G.; Liu, Z.; Myers, J.N. TP53 Mutations in Head and Neck Squamous Cell Carcinoma and Their Impact on Disease Progression and Treatment Response. *J. Cell Biochem.* **2016**, *117*, 2682–2692. [CrossRef]
19. Lindemann, A.; Takahashi, H.; Patel, A.A.; Osman, A.A.; Myers, J.N. Targeting the DNA Damage Response in OSCC with TP53 Mutations. *J. Dent. Res.* **2018**, *97*, 635–644. [CrossRef]
20. Kubrak, C.; Martin, L.; Gramlich, L.; Scrimger, R.; Jha, N.; Debenham, B.; Chua, N.; Walker, J.; Baracos, V.E. Prevalence and prognostic significance of malnutrition in patients with cancers of the head and neck. *Clin. Nutr.* **2020**, *39*, 901–909. [CrossRef]
21. Terrell, J.E.; Ronis, D.L.; Fowler, K.E.; Bradford, C.R.; Chepeha, D.B.; Prince, M.E.; Teknos, T.N.; Wolf, G.T.; Duffy, S.A. Clinical predictors of quality of life in patients with head and neck cancer. *Arch. Otolaryngol. Head Neck Surg.* **2004**, *130*, 401–408. [CrossRef] [PubMed]

22. Trachootham, D.; Songkaew, W.; Hongsachum, B.; Wattana, C.; Changkluengdee, N.; Karapoch, J.; Thirdsuttironnapumi, S.; Meennuch, E.; Klaitong, C.; Sinthusek, T.; et al. Nutri-jelly may improve quality of life and decrease tube feeding demand in head and neck cancer patients. *Support. Care Cancer* **2015**, *23*, 1421–1430. [CrossRef] [PubMed]
23. Amornsil, P.; Trachootham, D. PEITC: Functional Compound for Primary and Tertiary Chemoprevention of Cancer. *Thai J. Toxicol.* **2019**, *34*, 75–93.
24. Gupta, P.; Wright, S.E.; Kim, S.H.; Srivastava, S.K. Phenethyl isothiocyanate: A comprehensive review of anti-cancer mechanisms. *Biochim. Biophys. Acta* **2014**, *1846*, 405–424. [CrossRef] [PubMed]
25. Kaewsit, N.; Winuprasith, T.; Trachootham, D. Detoxification of Heterocyclic Aromatic Amines from Grilled Meat by PEITC-rich Vegetable Sauce: A Randomized Crossover Controlled Trial. *Food Funct.* **2021**, *12*, 10411–10422. [CrossRef] [PubMed]
26. Trachootham, D.; Alexandre, J.; Huang, P. Targeting cancer cells by ROS-mediated mechanisms: A radical therapeutic approach? *Nat. Rev. Drug Discov.* **2009**, *8*, 579–591. [CrossRef]
27. Chen, G.; Wang, F.; Trachootham, D.; Huang, P. Preferential killing of cancer cells with mitochondrial dysfunction by natural compounds. *Mitochondrion* **2010**, *10*, 614–625. [CrossRef]
28. Jutooru, I.; Guthrie, A.S.; Chadalapaka, G.; Pathi, S.; Kim, K.; Burghardt, R.; Jin, U.H.; Safe, S. Mechanism of action of phenethylisothiocyanate and other reactive oxygen species-inducing anticancer agents. *Mol. Cell Biol.* **2014**, *34*, 2382–2395. [CrossRef]
29. Sutthisawas, N.; Trachootham, D.; Wattanavijitkul, T. Pharmacokinetic, safety and tolerability studies after single and multiple oral administration of Phenethyl isothiocyanate in Nutri Jelly. *Chula. Med. J.* **2015**, *59*, 631.
30. Liebes, L.; Conaway, C.C.; Hochster, H.; Mendoza, S.; Hecht, S.S.; Crowell, J.; Chung, F.L. High-performance liquid chromatography-based determination of total isothiocyanate levels in human plasma: Application to studies with 2-phenethyl isothiocyanate. *Anal. Biochem.* **2001**, *291*, 279–289. [CrossRef]
31. Lam-ubol, A.; Wongcheunsoontorn, C.; Trachootham, D. Clinical Safety of Nutri-PEITC Jelly: A Pre-Post Study in Healthy Volunteers. *Thai J. Toxicol.* **2022**, *37*, 1–15.
32. Abdel-Magid, A.F. Reactivation of the Guardian of the Genome P53: A Promising Strategy for Treatment of Cancer. *ACS Med. Chem. Lett.* **2021**, *12*, 331–333. [CrossRef] [PubMed]
33. Duffy, M.J.; Tang, M.; Rajaram, S.; O'Grady, S.; Crown, J. Targeting Mutant p53 for Cancer Treatment: Moving Closer to Clinical Use? *Cancers* **2022**, *14*, 4499. [CrossRef] [PubMed]
34. Barczyk, K.; Kreuter, M.; Pryjma, J.; Booy, E.P.; Maddika, S.; Ghavami, S.; Berdel, W.E.; Roth, J.; Los, M. Serum cytochrome c indicates in vivo apoptosis and can serve as a prognostic marker during cancer therapy. *Int. J. Cancer* **2005**, *116*, 167–173. [CrossRef] [PubMed]
35. Murphy, B.A.; Ridner, S.; Wells, N.; Dietrich, M. Quality of life research in head and neck cancer: A review of the current state of the science. *Crit. Rev. Oncol. Hematol.* **2007**, *62*, 251–267. [CrossRef]
36. Jalili, S.; Ghasemi Shayan, R. A comprehensive evaluation of health-related life quality assessment through head and neck, Prostate, Breast, Lung, and Skin Cancer in Adults. *Front. Public Health* **2022**, *10*, 789456. [CrossRef]
37. Andreassen, R.; Jönsson, B.; Hadler-Olsen, E. Oral health-related quality of life in long-term survivors of head and neck cancer compared to a general population from the seventh Tromsø study. *BMC Oral Health* **2022**, *22*, 100. [CrossRef]
38. Martino, R.; Ringash, J. Evaluation of quality of life and organ function in head and neck squamous cell carcinoma. *Hematol. Oncol. Clin. N. Am.* **2008**, *22*, 1239–1256. [CrossRef]
39. Johnson, D.E.; Burtness, B.; Leemans, C.R.; Lui, V.W.Y.; Bauman, J.E.; Grandis, J.R. Head and neck squamous cell carcinoma. *Nat. Rev. Dis. Prim.* **2020**, *6*, 92. [CrossRef]
40. Shang, C.; Feng, L.; Gu, Y.; Hong, H.; Hong, L.; Hou, J. Impact of Multidisciplinary Team Management on the Survival Rate of Head and Neck Cancer Patients: A Cohort Study Meta-analysis. *Front. Oncol.* **2021**, *11*, 630906. [CrossRef]
41. Yuan, J.M.; Stepanov, I.; Murphy, S.E.; Wang, R.; Allen, S.; Jensen, J.; Strayer, L.; Adams-Haduch, J.; Upadhyaya, P.; Le, C.; et al. Clinical Trial of 2-Phenethyl Isothiocyanate as an Inhibitor of Metabolic Activation of a Tobacco-Specific Lung Carcinogen in Cigarette Smokers. *Cancer Prev. Res.* **2016**, *9*, 396–405. [CrossRef] [PubMed]
42. Aghajanpour, M.; Nazer, M.R.; Obeidavi, Z.; Akbari, M.; Ezati, P.; Kor, N.M. Functional foods and their role in cancer prevention and health promotion: A comprehensive review. *Am. J. Cancer Res.* **2017**, *7*, 740–769. [PubMed]
43. Trachootham, D. Chapter 7: Research and development of functional foods for specific type of cancer. In *Functional Foods and Cancer: Functional Foods in Integrative Oncology*, 1st ed.; Martirosyan, D.M., Zhou, J.R., Eds.; Functional Food Center: Dallas, TX, USA, 2017; Volume 5, pp. 135–156. ISBN 978-1976255342.
44. Mallery, S.R.; Wang, D.; Santiago, B.; Pei, P.; Bissonnette, C.; Jayawardena, J.A.; Schwendeman, S.P.; Spinney, R.; Lang, J. Fenretinide, Tocilizumab, and Reparixin Provide Multifaceted Disruption of Oral Squamous Cell Carcinoma Stem Cell Properties: Implications for Tertiary Chemoprevention. *Mol. Cancer Ther.* **2019**, *18*, 2308–2320. [CrossRef] [PubMed]
45. Parkar, S.M.; Shah, M.N. A relationship between quality-of-life and head and neck cancer: A systemic review. *South Asian J. Cancer* **2015**, *4*, 179–182. [CrossRef]
46. Tarsitano, A.; Pizzigallo, A.; Ballone, E.; Marchetti, C. Health-related quality of life as a survival predictor for patients with localized head and neck cancer treated with radiation therapy. *Oral Surg. Oral Med. Oral Pathol. Oral Radiol.* **2012**, *114*, 756–763. [CrossRef]

47. Fang, F.M.; Liu, Y.T.; Tang, Y.; Wang, C.J.; Ko, S.F. Quality of life as a survival predictor for patients with advanced head and neck carcinoma treated with radiotherapy. *Cancer* **2004**, *100*, 425–432. [CrossRef]
48. Balogh, G.A.; Mailo, D.A.; Corte, M.M.; Roncoroni, P.; Nardi, H.; Vincent, E.; Martinez, E.; Cafasso, M.E.; Frizza, A.; Ponce, G.; et al. Mutant p53 protein in serum could be used as a molecular marker in human breast cancer. *Int. J. Oncol.* **2006**, *28*, 995–1002. [CrossRef]
49. Balogh, G.A.; Mailo, D.; Nardi, H.; Corte, M.M.; Vincent, E.; Barutta, E.; GLizarraga; Lizarraga, P.; Montero, H.; Gentiliet, R. Serological levels of mutated p53 protein are highly detected at early stages in breast cancer patients. *Exp. Ther. Med.* **2010**, *1*, 357–361. [CrossRef]
50. Barbati, A.; Mariani, L.; Porpora, M.G.; Anceschi, M.; Collini, P.; Lauro, V.; EV, C. Serum evaluation of P53 protein in patients with gynaecological cancer. *Anticancer Res.* **2000**, *20*, 1033–1035.
51. Luo, J.C.; Zehab, R.; Anttila, S.; Ridanpaa, M.; Husgafvel-Pursiainen, K.; Vainio, H.; Carney, W.; DeVivo, I.; Milling, C.; Brandt-Rauf, P.W. Detection of serum p53 protein in lung cancer patients. *J. Occup. Med.* **1994**, *36*, 155–160. [CrossRef]
52. Mostaid, M.S.; Mumu, S.B.; Haque, M.A.; Sharmin, S.; Jamiruddin, M.R.; Sayedur Rahman, G.M.; Reza, H.M. Elevated serum expression of p53 and association of TP53 codon 72 polymorphisms with risk of cervical cancer in Bangladeshi women. *PLoS ONE* **2021**, *16*, e0261984. [CrossRef] [PubMed]
53. McVean, M.; Xiao, H.; Isobe, K.; Pelling, J.C. Increase in wild-type p53 stability and transactivational activity by the chemopreventive agent apigenin in keratinocytes. *Carcinogenesis* **2000**, *21*, 633–639. [CrossRef]
54. Butera, G.; Manfredi, M.; Fiore, A.; Brandi, J.; Pacchiana, R.; De Giorgis, V.; Barberis, E.; Vanella, V.; Galasso, M.; Scupoli, M.; et al. Tumor Suppressor Role of Wild-Type P53-Dependent Secretome and Its Proteomic Identification in PDAC. *Biomolecules* **2022**, *12*, 305. [CrossRef]
55. Klimovich, B.; Meyer, L.; Merle, N.; Neumann, M.; König, A.M.; Ananikidis, N.; Keber, C.U.; Elmshäuser, S.; Timofeev, O.; Stiewe, T.; et al. Partial p53 reactivation is sufficient to induce cancer regression. *J. Exp. Clin. Cancer Res.* **2022**, *41*, 80. [CrossRef] [PubMed]
56. Roszkowska, K.A.; Piecuch, A.; Sady, M.; Gajewski, Z.; Flis, S. Gain of Function (GOF) Mutant p53 in Cancer-Current Therapeutic Approaches. *Int. J. Mol. Sci.* **2022**, *23*, 13287. [CrossRef] [PubMed]
57. Mathibe, L.J. Drop-out rates of cancer patients participating in longitudinal RCTs. *Contemp. Clin. Trials* **2007**, *28*, 340–342. [CrossRef] [PubMed]
58. Bell, M.L.; Kenward, M.G.; Fairclough, D.L.; Horton, N.J. Differential dropout and bias in randomized controlled trials: When it matters and when it may not. *BMJ* **2013**, *346*, e8668. [CrossRef]
59. Trachootham, D.; Zhou, Y.; Zhang, H.; Demizu, Y.; Chen, Z.; Pelicano, H.; Chiao, P.J.; Achanta, G.; Arlinghaus, R.B.; Liu, J.; et al. Selective killing of oncogenically transformed cells through a ROS-mediated mechanism by beta-phenylethyl isothiocyanate. *Cancer Cell* **2006**, *10*, 241–252. [CrossRef]
60. Trachootham, D.; Zhang, H.; Zhang, W.; Feng, L.; Du, M.; Zhou, Y.; Chen, Z.; Pelicano, H.; Plunkett, W.; Wierda, W.G.; et al. Effective elimination of fludarabine-resistant CLL cells by PEITC through a redox-mediated mechanism. *Blood* **2008**, *112*, 1912–1922. [CrossRef]
61. Kang, R.; Kroemer, G.; Tang, D. The tumor suppressor protein p53 and the ferroptosis network. *Free Radic. Biol. Med.* **2019**, *133*, 162–168. [CrossRef]
62. Shoaib, S.; Ansari, M.A.; Ghazwani, M.; Hani, U.; Jamous, Y.F.; Alali, Z.; Wahab, S.; Ahmad, W.; Weir, S.A.; Alomary, M.N.; et al. Prospective Epigenetic Actions of Organo-Sulfur Compounds against Cancer: Perspectives and Molecular Mechanisms. *Cancers* **2023**, *15*, 697. [CrossRef] [PubMed]
63. Cykowiak, M.; Kleszcz, R.; Kucińska, M.; Paluszczak, J.; Szaefer, H.; Plewiński, A.; Piotrowska-Kempisty, H.; Murias, M.; Krajka-Kuźniak, V. Attenuation of Pancreatic Cancer In Vitro and In Vivo via Modulation of Nrf2 and NF-κB Signaling Pathways by Natural Compounds. *Cells* **2021**, *10*, 3556. [CrossRef] [PubMed]
64. Cykowiak, M.; Krajka-Kuźniak, V.; Kleszcz, R.; Kucińska, M.; Szaefer, H.; Piotrowska-Kempisty, H.; Plewiński, A.; Murias, M.; Baer-Dubowska, W. Comparison of the Impact of Xanthohumol and Phenethyl Isothiocyanate and Their Combination on Nrf2 and NF-κB Pathways in HepG2 Cells In Vitro and Tumor Burden In Vivo. *Nutrients* **2021**, *13*, 3000. [CrossRef] [PubMed]
65. Xiao, J.; Zhou, N.; Li, Y.; Xiao, Y.; Chen, W.; Ye, J.; Ma, T.; Zhang, Y. PEITC inhibits the invasion and migration of colorectal cancer cells by blocking TGF-β-induced EMT. *Biomed. Pharmacother.* **2020**, *130*, 110743. [CrossRef]
66. Brasili, E.; Filho, V.C. Metabolomics of cancer cell cultures to assess the effects of dietary phytochemicals. *Crit. Rev. Food Sci. Nutr.* **2017**, *57*, 1328–1339. [CrossRef]
67. FACIT. Functional Assessment of Cancer Therapy—Head & Neck (FACT-HN) Version 4. Available online: https://www.facit.org/measures/FACT-HN (accessed on 5 February 2023).
68. List, M.A.; D'Antonio, L.L.; Cella, D.F.; Siston, A.; Mumby, P.; Haraf, D.; Vokes, E. The Performance Status Scale for Head and Neck Cancer Patients and the Functional Assessment of Cancer Therapy-Head and Neck Scale. A study of utility and validity. *Cancer* **1996**, *77*, 2294–2301. [CrossRef]
69. Weiss, J.; Gilbert, J.; Deal, A.M.; Weissler, M.; Hilliard, C.; Chera, B.; Murphy, B.; Hackman, T.; Liao, J.J.; Olson, J.G.; et al. Induction chemotherapy with carboplatin, nab-paclitaxel, and cetuximab for at least N2b nodal status or surgically unresectable squamous cell carcinoma of the head and neck. *Oral Oncol.* **2018**, *84*, 46–51. [CrossRef]
70. Chumachote, A. Quality of life in Head and Neck Cancer Patients Received Radiotherapy. *J. Thai Assoc. Rad. Oncol.* **2016**, *22*, 24–33.

71. The National Palliative Care Research Center (NPCRC). Karnofsky Performance Status Scale Definitions Rating (%) Criteria. Available online: http://www.npcrc.org/files/news/karnofsky_performance_scale.pdf (accessed on 5 February 2023).
72. Gyawali, B.; Eisenhauer, E.; Tregear, M.; Booth, C.M. Progression-free survival: It is time for a new name. *Lancet Oncol.* **2022**, *23*, 328–330. [CrossRef]
73. National Cancer Institute, USA. Response Evaluation Criteria in Solid Tumors. Available online: https://www.cancer.gov/publications/dictionaries/cancer-terms/def/response-evaluation-criteria-in-solid-tumors (accessed on 1 April 2023).
74. Eisenhauer, E.A.; Therase, P.; Bogaerts, J.; Schwartz, L.H.; Sargent, D.; Ford, R.; Dancey, J.; Arbuck, S.; Gwyther, S.; Mooney, M.; et al. New response evaluation criteria in solid tumours: Revised RECIST guideline (version 1.1). *Eur. J. Cancer* **2009**, *45*, 228–247. [CrossRef]
75. Ji, Y.; Morris, M.E. Determination of phenethyl isothiocyanate in human plasma and urine by ammonia derivatization and liquid chromatography-tandem mass spectrometry. *Anal. Biochem.* **2003**, *323*, 39–47. [CrossRef] [PubMed]
76. Zheng, L.; Zheng, F. Development and validation of an LC-APCI-MS/MS method for the determination of phenethyl isothiocyanate in human plasma. *Biomed. Chromatogr.* **2015**, *29*, 619–625. [CrossRef] [PubMed]

MDPI
St. Alban-Anlage 66
4052 Basel
Switzerland
Tel. +41 61 683 77 34
Fax +41 61 302 89 18
www.mdpi.com

International Journal of Molecular Sciences Editorial Office
E-mail: ijms@mdpi.com
www.mdpi.com/journal/ijms

www.ingramcontent.com/pod-product-compliance
Lightning Source LLC
Chambersburg PA
CBHW040316270926
51850CB00007BC/1502
* 9 7 8 3 0 3 6 5 8 4 3 1 7 *